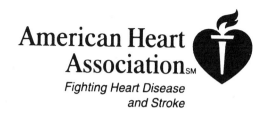

American Heart
Association℠
*Fighting Heart Disease
and Stroke*

Monograph Series

THE FETAL AND NEONATAL
PULMONARY CIRCULATIONS

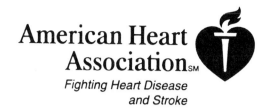

American Heart
Association℠
*Fighting Heart Disease
and Stroke*

Monograph Series

THE FETAL AND NEONATAL
PULMONARY CIRCULATIONS

Edited by

E. Kenneth Weir, MD

*Professor of Medicine
University of Minnesota
Minneapolis, Minnesota*

Stephen L. Archer, MD

*Professor of Medicine
University of Alberta
Edmonton, Alberta, Canada*

John T. Reeves, MD

*Professor Emeritus of Pediatrics and Medicine
University of Colorado
Denver, Colorado*

Futura Publishing
Company, Inc.
Armonk, NY

Library of Congress Cataloging–in–Publication Data

The fetal and neonatal pulmonary circulations / edited by E. Kenneth
Weir, Stephen L. Archer, John T. Reeves.
     p.   cm. — (American Heart Association monograph
series)
    Includes bibliographical references and index.
    ISBN 0-87993-439-5 (alk. paper)
    1. Pulmonary circulation.   2. Blood—Circulation.   3. Fetus—
Physiology.   4. Infants (Newborn)—Physiology.   I. Weir,
E. Kenneth. II. Archer, Stephen L. III. Reeves, John T.
IV. Series.
    [DNLM: 1. Pulmonary Circulation—Infant, Newborn.
2. Fetal Blood. 3. Lung—embryology.
WF 600 F419   1999]
RG618.F456   1999
612.2—dc21
DNLM/DLC
for Library of Congress   99-27196
                                                        CIP

Published by
Futura Publishing Company, Inc.
135 Bedford Road
Armonk, New York 10504

LC #99-27196
ISBN #: 0-87993-439-5

Every effort has been made to ensure that the information in this book
is as up to date and accurate as possible at the time of publication. However, due to the constant developments in medicine, neither the author,
nor the editor, nor the publisher can accept any legal or any other re-
sponsibility for any errors or omissions that may occur.

Printed in the United States of America on acid-free paper.

Preface

Birth is a cataclysmic event where the fetus must make the transition from a parasitic to an independent existence, from an aqueous to an air environment, from a zero gravitational field to the forces of earth, and from a relatively low to a high oxygen environment. The transition occurs suddenly, so that if the fetus is not well prepared for the event, it will likely perish. Further, if the transition is flawed, but the fetus survives, lifelong disability may result. Nowhere is the drama of birth played out with more intensity than in the lung circulation. Once the placental oxygen supply ceases, the fetus has only minutes to establish pulmonary oxygen transport, a transition which requires not only inflation of the lungs, but also sudden and sustained changes in the lung circulation. For fetal health, the lung arteries must be constricted to maintain low lung blood flow; but the transition to a healthy newborn requires that these arteries dilate to allow a tenfold increase in lung blood flow. Moreover, in health the arteries must remain dilated throughout life.

For the lung circulation, all of these processes—the preparation for the moment of birth, the transition at the time of birth, and the changes that must follow birth—are incompletely understood. We understand even less about how these processes are controlled. Yet, such understanding is of extreme importance, because the survival of the individual and ultimately the species depends on these processes. An understanding of these processes will be better facilitated by studying the fetus and newborn rather than the adult, because it is at this early time of life when the potential for vasoreactivity and vascular wall remodeling is greatest both in magnitude and in rate. Furthermore, pathophysiologic changes in the fetus or neonate may determine the potential for disease in adult life.

The problems for biomedical scientists are not only the rate and magnitude of the changes at birth, as great as these changes may be, but also the incorporation of the enormous growth of knowledge in this field. Only a decade or two ago, the scientific tools were largely restricted to morphology and physiology. Now the powerful techniques of cellular and molecular biology have been introduced.

These new tools have begun to elucidate the processes in the developing lung by which new blood vessels are formed; how the cells in

v

the arteries differentiate from stem cells and assume their respective functions; how diversity of cell types is sustained to accomplish the various functions; how the matrix comes to play its role and how it interacts with the cells; and how ion channels, cytokines, and humoral mediators interact with intracellular machinery to control the function of the vascular wall cells. There is enormous ferment and excitement in the field. These are the changes that will shape the future of scientific advances, as well as the clinical care of the pregnant woman, the unborn child, the newborn, and even the adult.

The present volume has brought together leading scientists to summarize where the field is and how far it has come, and to detail the advances in it. There are four main objectives, which are to examine in the developing lung circulation:

1) the cellular and molecular factors controlling vasculogenesis;
2) the genetic and molecular factors responsible for vascular cell differentiation;
3) the role of the extracellular matrix in regulating vascular cell proliferation and activity; and
4) the mechanisms controlling tone in the transition at birth.

The editors hope that the present volume will effectively serve to provide cross-fertilization of the various disciplines represented, to inform the basic scientist as well as the clinician and student, and to provide a benchmark for progress in the field as we approach the next millennium.

E. Kenneth Weir, M.D.
Stephen L. Archer, M.D.
John T. Reeves, M.D.

Contributors

Steven H. Abman, MD   The Pediatric Heart Lung Center, Section of Pulmonary Medicine, Department of Pediatrics, B-395, The University of Colorado School of Medicine and The Children's Hospital, Denver, CO

Stephen L. Archer, MD   Division of Cardiology, University of Alberta Hospital, Edmonton, Alberta, Canada

Lucas C. Armstrong, PhD   Department of Biochemistry and Medicine, University of Washington, Seattle, WA

Robert Auerbach, PhD   Laboratory of Developmental Biology, University of Wisconsin, Madison, WI

Paul Bornstein, MD   Department of Biochemistry and Medicine, University of Washington, Seattle, WA

David Bouchey, PhD   Cardiovascular Pulmonary and Developmental Biology Research Laboratories, University of Colorado Health Sciences Center, Denver, CO

Aesim Cho, PhD   Department of Pathology, University of Washington, Seattle, WA

Flavio Coceani, MD   Scuola Superiore S. Anna, Pisa, Italy

David N. Cornfield, MD   Department of Pediatrics, University of Minnesota School of Medicine, Variety Heart and Research Center, Minneapolis, MN

Mita Das, PhD   Cardiovascular Pulmonary and Developmental Biology Research Laboratories, University of Colorado Health Sciences Center, Denver, CO

Daphne E. deMello, MD   Department of Pathology, St. Louis University Health Sciences Center, Cardinal Glennon Children's Hospital, St. Louis, MO

Edward C. Dempsey, MD Cardiovascular Pulmonary and Developmental Biology Research Laboratories, University of Colorado Health Sciences Center; Denver Veterans Administration Medical Center, Denver, CO

Christopher J. Drake, PhD Department of Cell Biology and The Cardiovascular Developmental Biology Center, Medical University of South Carolina, Charleston, SC

Alexandra H. Guldemeester, MD Department of Pediatric Surgery, Sophia Children's Hospital, Rotterdam, The Netherlands

Jennifer M. W. Hausladen, MD Department of Cell Biology and Physiology, Washington University School of Medicine, St. Louis, MO

James C. Huhta, MD Clinical Professor of Pediatrics, University of South Florida School of Medicine, Tampa, FL

D. Dunbar Ivy, MD Pediatric Cardiology, The Children's Hospital and The University of Colorado Health Sciences Center, Denver, CO

John P. Kinsella, MD Section of Neonatology, Department of Pediatrics, University of Colorado School of Medicine and The Children's Hospital, Denver, CO

Kyriakos E. Kypreos, PhD Department of Biochemistry, Boston University School of Medicine, Boston, MA

Themis R. Kyriakides, PhD Department of Biochemistry and Medicine, University of Washington, Seattle, WA

B. Lowell Langille, PhD The Toronto Hospital Research Institute; Department of Laboratory Medicine and Pathobiology, and Department of Obstetrics and Gynecology, University of Toronto, Toronto, Ontario, Canada

Timothy D. Le Cras PhD Pediatric Heart Lung Center, Section of Pulmonary Medicine, Department of Pediatrics, University of Colorado School of Medicine and The Children's Hospital, Denver, CO

Charles D. Little, PhD Department of Cell Biology and The Cardiovascular Developmental Biology Center, Medical University of South Carolina, Charleston, SC

Toshiaki Mano, MD   Division of Cardiovascular Research, St. Elizabeth's Medical Center and Tufts University School of Medicine, Boston, MA

Darius J. Marhamati, MD, PhD   Department of Biochemistry, Boston University School of Medicine, Boston, MA

Robert P. Mecham, PhD   Department of Cell Biology and Physiology, Washington University School of Medicine, St. Louis, MO

Keith C. Meyer, MD   Department of Medicine, University of Wisconsin, Madison, WI

Olga Mirzoeva, PhD   Laboratory of Developmental Biology, University of Wisconsin, Madison, WI

Matthew A. Nugent, PhD   Department of Biochemistry, Boston University School of Medicine, Boston, MA

Thomas A. Parker, MD   Section of Neonatology, Department of Pediatrics, University of Colorado School of Medicine, and The Children's Hospital, Denver, CO

Marlene Rabinovitch, MD   Division of Cardiovascular Research, The Hospital for Sick Children; Department of Pediatrics, Laboratory, Medicine and Pathobiology, and Medicine, University of Toronto, Toronto, Ontario, Canada

Juha Rasanen, MD   Department of Obstetrics and Gynecology, Thomas Jefferson University, Philadelphia, PA

Helen L. Reeve, PhD   Department of Cardiology, University of Minnesota School of Medicine, Department of Research, Veterans Administration Medical Center, Minneapolis, MN

John T. Reeves, MD   Professor Emeritus, Pediatrics, Medicine, Family Medicine, University of Colorado Health Sciences Center, Denver, CO

Michael A. Reidy, PhD   Department of Pathology, University of Washington, Seattle, WA

Abraham M. Rudolph, MD   University of California, San Francisco, CA

Philip W. Shaul, MD   Department of Pediatrics, University of Texas Southwestern Medical Center, Dallas, TX

Sherif M. K. Shehata, MD, MCh   Department of Pediatric Surgery, Sophia Children's Hospital, Rotterdam, The Netherlands

Roy C. Smith, PhD   Division of Cardiovascular Research, St. Elizabeth's Medical Center and Tufts University School of Medicine, Boston, MA

Gail E. Sonenshein, PhD   Department of Biochemistry, Boston University School of Medicine, Boston, MA

Kurt R. Stenmark, MD   Cardiovascular Pulmonary and Developmental Biology Research Laboratories, University of Colorado Health Sciences Center, Denver, CO

Laurent Storme, MD   Division of Neonatology, CHRU, Lille, France

Dick Tibboel, MD, PhD   Department of Pediatric Surgery, Sophia Children's Hospital, Rotterdam, The Netherlands

Kenneth Walsh, PhD   Division of Cardiovascular Research, St. Elizabeth's Medical Center and Tufts University School of Medicine, Boston, MA

E. Kenneth Weir, MD   Department of Cardiology, Veterans Administration Medical Center, Minneapolis, MN

Mary C. M. Weiser-Evans, PhD   Developmental Lung Biology Laboratory, Department of Pediatrics, University of Colorado Health Sciences Center, Denver, CO

Contents

SECTION III
Mechanisms of Hemodynamic Control in the Neonate

Section I
Lung Growth and Development

Chapter 1

The Development of Concepts of the Ontogeny of the Pulmonary Circulation

Abraham M. Rudolph, MD

Introduction

In the middle of the 17th century, when Harvey described the course of the circulation, he recognized that the fetal circulation differed from that of the adult, but he could not explain how blood flowed in the fetal lung. Apart from occasional references to the pulmonary circulation, the fetal circulation received little consideration until the middle of the 20th century, when it was recognized that dramatic changes in blood flow through the lungs occurred after birth. Over the past 50 years, the developmental changes in the pulmonary circulation and in its responses to stresses of hypoxia, and increases in pulmonary arterial pressure and blood flow, have become subjects of increasing investigation. This chapter will provide an overview of the concepts that have been considered during this period, related to the development of the normal pulmonary circulation, with particular regard to the perinatal changes.

Early Concepts of the Pulmonary Circulation

The concept that blood is pumped from the right ventricle through the lungs, returns to the left side of the heart, and then is ejected into the systemic circulation, was first fully enunciated by Harvey in his treatise in 1628.[1] It is not generally appreciated that, in this report, Har-

From: Weir EK, Archer SL, Reeves JT (eds). *The Fetal and Neonatal Pulmonary Circulations.* Armonk, NY: Futura Publishing Company, Inc.; ©1999.

vey also presented a concept of the fetal circulation. He correctly described blood flow from the inferior vena cava through the foramen ovale, but conjectured that it then entered pulmonary veins before returning to the left atrium. It is difficult to explain this belief, but it could have been based on the fact that, because he had proposed that all blood returning in systemic veins in the adult passed through the lungs before entering the left atrium, inferior vena caval blood had to return to the left atrium via pulmonary veins in the fetus. Harvey did not recognize the purpose of blood flow through the lungs, and concluded that "hot blood is carried to and through the lungs, to be tempered by the inspired air." He also did not consider that blood passed through the lungs to the left atrium in the fetus.

The role of the pulmonary circulation in arterialization of venous blood was conceived by Lower in 1669.[2] He also believed that pulmonary blood flow was quite low during fetal life, but that it increased greatly after birth. Surprisingly, the pulmonary circulation of the fetus and newborn evoked little interest for almost 300 years following Lower's publication. In disagreement with Lower's concepts, Bichat in 1801 proposed that pulmonary blood flow progressively increased over gestation, based largely on anatomic information.[3] Kilian in 1826 suggested that pulmonary blood flow was relatively higher in the fetus than after birth.[4] Not until 1942 was pulmonary blood flow demonstrated to increase after establishment of breathing, based on angiographic studies by Barclay et al, which showed that pulmonary circulation time decreased from 2.7 seconds in the fetal lamb to 1.4 seconds within minutes after birth.[5]

Harvey, in the de motu cordis, had also proposed that, in the fetus, blood flows from the pulmonary trunk to the descending aorta through the ductus arteriosus.[1] Little consideration was given to the fact that this would require that pulmonary arterial pressure be higher than, or equal to, aortic pressure. In 1937, Hamilton et al showed, by rather crude techniques, that right and left ventricular pressures were equal in the fetus and that right ventricular pressure fell after breathing began.[6] Subsequently, in 1953, Dawes et al, by direct measurement, definitively demonstrated in fetal lambs that pulmonary blood flow increased when the lungs were ventilated with air.[7]

Pulmonary Vascular Changes at Birth

The mechanisms responsible for the increase in pulmonary blood flow and decrease in pulmonary arterial pressure after birth have evoked great interest. The concepts that have been explored to explain the decrease in pulmonary vascular resistance include:

- Expansion of the alveoli dilates pulmonary vasculature through a direct physical effect.
- Physical expansion of the lungs stimulates release of a pulmonary vasodilator agent.
- Increases in oxygen content in the lungs associated with ventilation with air result in liberation of a vasodilator agent.
- Production of a vasoconstrictor substance normally in the lungs of the fetus is inhibited by lung expansion or increased oxygenation.
- Increase in oxygen tension resulting from ventilation with air directly relaxes pulmonary arterioles.
- Increase in systemic arterial oxygen content dilates pulmonary vessels via nervous pathways.
- Exclusion of the umbilical-placental circulation by tearing or cutting the umbilical cord removes a pulmonary vasoconstrictor derived from the placenta.

Lung Expansion

The concept that gaseous expansion of the lungs was responsible for the decrease in pulmonary vascular resistance and increase in pulmonary blood flow at birth through a direct physical effect was proposed by Dawes et al in their original study.[7] They observed that ventilation not only with air, but also with nitrogen, caused a fall in pulmonary vascular resistance in fetal lambs. Also, distension of the lungs with fluid did not increase pulmonary blood flow. Subsequently, a series of studies from Dawes' laboratory demonstrated that ventilation with nitrogen or with a gas mixture of 3% oxygen and 7% CO_2 in nitrogen, which did not alter fetal blood gases, reduced pulmonary vascular resistance in fetal lambs, but that ventilation with air or oxygen, which increase fetal blood PO_2, caused a greater decrease in vascular resistance.[8]

Reynolds proposed that the decrease in pulmonary vascular resistance associated with ventilation was due to a change in architecture of the lung.[9] He suggested that the fetal lungs were collapsed and the vessels convoluted and tortuous, and expansion resulted in their straightening, thus reducing resistance to blood flow. However, the fetal lungs are normally filled with fluid, and the lung is not, as conceived by Reynolds, collapsed. Also, as mentioned, in Dawes' study pulmonary vascular resistance was not decreased by distending the lungs with fluid.

Gaseous distension or ventilation of the lungs displaces fluid from the airways and alveoli, and the establishment of a gas-fluid interface on the alveolar surface could possibly dilate pulmonary vessels by physical means. When the alveoli are filled with fluid, the forces would tend to compress adjacent vessels, but when filled with air they would tend to collapse, and a negative distending force could be applied to adjacent vessels.[10] It has been suggested by Gilbert et al that this distending force could have a greater effect on small veins, which may be acting as Starling resistors in the lung.[11] The role of direct physical forces in contributing to the reduction in pulmonary vascular resistance in association with ventilation at birth is still to be resolved.

Expansion of lungs in the fetus results in liberation of prostaglandins, which are effective pulmonary vasodilators. The decrease in pulmonary vascular resistance associated with ventilation of the lung in fetal goats was attenuated by inhibition of cyclooxygenase activity with indomethacin.[12] Leffler et al subsequently showed that ventilation induced release of prostacyclin in fetal lungs, and that this was the result of lung distension, and not an increase in oxygenation.[13,14] Prostacyclin is released from vessel walls, but how ventilation of the lungs stimulates its release has not yet been adequately explained. Prostacyclin is synthesized in increasing quantities in the lung with advancing gestation in the sheep.[15] Furthermore, its production is influenced by the state of oxygenation; at lower PO_2 levels, little prostacyclin is synthesized, but PO_2 levels above about 40 torr greatly increase its production.[16] However, despite this effect of oxygen, it does not appear that prostacyclin release by increased oxygenation is the major mechanisms by which ventilation reduces pulmonary vascular resistance because the effect of oxygen is not blocked by indomethacin.

Oxygen Effects

In the 1964 study of Cassin et al, it was clearly demonstrated that ventilation of the lamb fetus with air to increase fetal arterial PO_2 from 18 torr to 30–33 torr resulted in a marked increase in pulmonary vascular conductance and pulmonary blood flow.[8] In this study, performed in open-chest anesthetized fetuses, a cannulating flowmeter was inserted between the carotid artery and the distal end of the left pulmonary artery. Flows were quite variable, and an additional concern was that the fetuses were markedly alkalotic. To overcome many of the problems with this preparation, Teitel et al applied a cuff electromagnetic flow transducer around the left pulmonary artery and inserted a tracheal tube, which was led to the ewe's flank. Some days after surgery, the effects of ventilation with 3% O_2 and 7% CO_2 in nitrogen (which maintained fetal blood gas levels) and with 93% O_2 and 7% CO_2 were examined.[17] Pulmonary vascular resistance fell dramatically with ventilation even though fetal PO_2 did not change. However, ventilation with oxygen resulted in a further fall in pulmonary vascular resistance. The contributions of ventilation alone and of ventilation with oxygen varied greatly in different lambs. In about half of the animals, the major contribution was from physical expansion of the lungs, with only a mild further change with oxygenation, whereas in the others, the maximal effect occurred after oxygenation. The decrease in pulmonary vascular resistance associated with increased PO_2 has also been confirmed by perfusing the airways of fetal lambs with an oxygenated dextran-saline solution.[18] Also, placing the ewe in a hyperbaric oxygen chamber increased fetal arterial PO_2, and resulted in a decrease in pulmonary vascular resistance with no manipulation of the lungs.[19,20]

The initial concepts were that oxygen either had a direct relaxant effect on pulmonary vascular smooth muscle, or that the rise in fetal arterial oxygen content affected pulmonary vessels through neural pathways (vide infra). The possibility that oxygen releases a mediating substance that reduced pulmonary vascular resistance has been considered. Bradykinin, a vasoactive peptide that produced pulmonary vasodilatation in fetal lambs, has been shown to be released into fetal blood when the ewes were subjected to hyperbaric oxygenation. Furthermore, ventilation of fetal lambs with oxygen increased concentrations of bradykinin across the lungs and reduced the concentration of kininogen, a bradykinin precursor.[19] These changes did not result with nitrogen ventilation. Although bradykinin release could contribute to the reduction of pulmonary vascular resistance, it does not appear to have a continuing role, because concentration fell within an hour, even though ventilation with oxygen was maintained. Furthermore, bradykinin receptor blockade did not inhibit the rise in pulmonary blood flow induced by ventilation of fetal lambs in utero with oxygen.[21]

The discovery that the effects of some vasodilator agents, such as acetylcholine, were dependent on release of an endothelium-derived relaxing factor (EDRF), later shown to be nitric oxide (NO),[22,23] led to the exploration of its possible role in the perinatal decrease in pulmonary vascular resistance. Ventilation of fetal lambs with NO results in a considerable decrease in pulmonary vascular resistance as early as 0.75 gestation.[24] Several studies have demonstrated that administration of a blocker of NO production from arginine, N-omega-nitro-L-arginine (L-NA), markedly diminishes, or completely inhibits the pulmonary vasodilator response to oxygen. In lambs delivered by cesarean section, L-NA limited the decrease in pulmonary vascular resistance during ventilation with oxygen to about one-half of that occurring in untreated lambs.[25] Increasing fetal arterial PO_2 in lambs by exposing the ewe to hyperbaric oxygen markedly increased pulmonary blood flow, but this effect was almost completely abolished by prior administration of a blocker of NO production.[26] Ventilation with oxygen of fetal lambs in utero, in which prostaglandin production had been inhibited by administration of a synthesis inhibitor, resulted in a marked increase in pulmonary blood flow; this was almost abolished by the blocker of NO production, L-NA.[27]

The possible roles of other mediators released either by lung expansion or oxygenation, in inducing the decrease in vascular resistance at birth have been explored. Prostaglandin D_2 (PGD_2) is a pulmonary vasodilator in the lamb in the fetal and early neonatal periods, but by 7–10 days postnatally it has a vasoconstrictor effect.[28] It has been postulated that release of PGD_2 from mast cells may be stimulated at birth either by lung expansion or oxygenation. However, inhibition of prostaglandin synthesis in fetal lambs with indomethacin did not affect the decrease of fetal pulmonary vascular resistance resulting from hyperbaric oxygenation of the ewe.[29]

Calcitonin gene-related peptide and adrenomedullin have both recently been shown to produce a prolonged reduction of pulmonary vascular resistance in fetal lambs, and it has been suggested that they may have a role at the time of birth,[30,31] but this has not as yet been explored further.

Based on the previously described studies, the current concept regarding the increase in pulmonary blood flow after birth is that two main mechanisms are responsible, both of which involve liberation of mediating substances. Gaseous expansion of the lungs appears to exert its effect predominantly by liberation of prostaglandins, particularly prostacyclin. The increase in oxygen concentration in alveoli, and in blood, associated with ventilation with air, seems to be the more important factor. Oxygen acts predominantly by releasing EDRF-NO from endothelial cells, and this dilates the pulmonary vessels. Although it is currently assumed that oxygen acts directly on endothelial cells to increase NO production, it is possible that it stimulates release of another agent, such as bradykinin, calcitonin gene-related peptide, or adrenomedullin, which in turn stimulates NO production. It is known that the vasodilation resulting from these agents is largely abolished by NO blockers.

Prostacyclin and NO release are not the only factors involved in the postnatal decrease in pulmonary vascular resistance, because administration of both a prostaglandin synthesis inhibitor and an NO blocker to fetal lambs does not completely inhibit an increase in pulmonary blood flow when ventilated with air.[27] If NO release is a crucial factor in the increase in pulmonary blood flow after birth, one might anticipate that animals would not survive after birth if NO were not produced. Yet in the model of mice homozygous for a defective gene for endothelial nitric oxide synthase (eNOS), the animals survived, and appeared healthy.[31,32] They did, however, have resting arterial hypertension,[32] but no information was obtained regarding pulmonary arterial pressure. These knockout mice demonstrate, however, that other mechanisms for pulmonary vasodilation can be invoked to compensate for lack of endothelial NO synthesis.

Pulmonary Vasoconstrictors

It has been postulated that the high pulmonary vascular resistance in the fetus is maintained by the production of vasoconstrictors in the lung. Leukotrienes (LTs), derived from arachidonic acid through the lipoxygenase pathway, include some potent pulmonary constrictors. Both LTC_4 and LTD_4 increase pulmonary vascular resistance in fetal lambs,[33] and leukotriene end-organ blockers have been shown to increase pulmonary blood flow. Evidence opposing this concept is the observation that LTC_4 synthesis is actually higher in isolated newborn, as compared with fetal, pulmonary vessels, and it is greater in pulmonary veins than arteries.[34] Endothelin is a potent vasoconstrictor in the adult. In fetal lambs, endothelin-1 (ET-1) causes transient pulmonary vasodilation, but continued infusion results in an increase in pulmonary vascular resistance.[35] Blood ET-1 concentration is relatively high in the fetus, and the possibility that it contributes to the high pulmonary vascular resistance was examined by administering ET_A and ET_B receptor antagonists to fetal lambs.[36] Pulmonary vascular resistance did decrease, indicating that ET-1 did have some influence on resting tone, but the magnitude of change was not significant enough to support the removal of ET-1 influence at birth, as the only mechanism for the marked postnatal increase of pulmonary blood flow.

Direct Effect of Oxygen on Vessels

Oxygen has been shown to induce eNOS in the lungs of fetal lambs and in isolated endothelial cells,[37] and this could be the manner in which NO is produced. Recently, however, there has been a resurgence in interest in the concept that the vasodilator action of oxygen could be due to a direct local effect on vascular smooth muscle. The possible role of oxygen-sensitive potassium channels in the effects of oxygen are being explored. Type I glomus cells in the mammalian carotid body, which are the chemoreceptor sensors, demonstrate inhibition of potassium channel activity when PO_2 is reduced.[38] A similar potassium channel, which is inhibited by hypoxia, has been described in central neurons.[39] Vascular smooth muscle cells derived from pulmonary arteries also showed evidence of a potassium channel, which was inhibited by hypoxia with resultant membrane depolarization; this was not evident in mesenteric artery smooth muscle cells.[40] A similar role of potassium channels in hypoxia in pulmonary vessels was reported by Post et al.[41]

The vasoconstrictor effects of hypoxia on the pulmonary circulation could be explained by these oxygen-sensitive potassium channels, but opening of these channels could also account for the drop in pulmonary vascular resistance associated with oxygen content increase at the time of birth.

Role of the Autonomic Nervous System

The possibility has been considered that nervous stimulation resulting from lung expansion and increased arterial oxygenation, associated with ventilation, may contribute to pulmonary vasodilation. In the fetal lamb, there is evidence that sympathetic nervous stimulation causes some increase in pulmonary vascular resistance in late gestation. Also, vagal stimulation causes vasodilatation. However, these effects are not striking, and it is unlikely that the autonomic neurons have a significant role because α- or β-adrenergic receptor blockade, or parasympathetic blockade, has not had a significant effect on pulmonary vascular responses to hypoxia or increased oxygenation. The influence of the autonomic nervous system has been reviewed previously.[42]

Role of Elimination of Umbilical-Placental Circulation

The placental metabolism is extremely active and releases many substances into the fetal circulation, including several hormones and prostaglandins. The possibility has been considered of production by the placenta of a substance that maintains the high pulmonary vascular resistance in the fetus. There is little evidence to support this concept, but in studies in which fetal lambs were ventilated in utero, injection of blood collected from the umbilical vein, into the fetal pulmonary artery, induced a rise in pulmonary vascular resistance during its administration (personal observation).

In summary, numerous mechanisms have been proposed to explain the decrease in pulmonary vascular resistance associated with ventilation. The change is dramatic, resulting in an 8- to 10-fold increase in pulmonary blood flow. The relative roles of rhythmic lung expansion and increased oxygenation have varied in individual lamb fetuses, and this variability has not been explained. Although the role of NO in inducing the response to oxygenation appears to be a major factor in pulmonary vasodilation, homozygous eNOS knockout mice do survive after birth. Further studies are therefore indicated to determine whether physical expansion and oxygenation are complementary or whether either alone can produce an increase in pulmonary blood flow necessary for postnatal survival.

Maintenance of Pulmonary Blood Flow After Birth

Although the mechanisms responsible for the immediate changes in the pulmonary circulation after birth have been explored, little attention has been directed toward understanding how the high pulmonary blood flow is maintained after the initial increase. It has generally been assumed that the continuation of rhythmic expansion and of the high levels of oxygenation are the factors involved. However, administration of prostaglandin synthesis inhibitors or NO blockers in the early neonatal period do not reduce pulmonary blood flow to fetal levels. Also, eNOS activity, which is prominent in fetal lungs, is greatly decreased within a few days after birth.[43]

As discussed below, there is a rapid change in the precapillary pulmonary arteries after birth, with a decrease in their medial thickness due to thinning of the smooth muscle layer. The pulmonary vascular response to hypoxia is reduced as compared with the fetus because there is a lesser amount of muscle. However, there is not only a reduced response of the circulation, but frequently also a change in the direction of response. Thus, several agents that cause pulmonary vasodilation in the fetus, such as acetylcholine, histamine, and PGD_2, result in vasoconstriction within a few days postnatally. This has usually been explained as a difference in response based on resting vasomotor tone, because if the pulmonary vascular resistance is increased by hypoxia or vasoconstrictor drugs, a mild vasodilation occurs with acetylcholine.

Inadequate consideration has been given to possible changes in the pulmonary vascular smooth muscle cells from perinatal factors other than those occurring locally in the lungs. Thus, in the myocardium, changes in expression of myosin heavy chain from β-MHC to α-MHC, increase in β-adrenoreceptors, and in Na^+K^+ ATPase all occur after birth. Several hormonal changes, such as the postnatal increase in plasma triiodothyronine concentration could be responsible. Recently, the potential importance of cortisol has been examined. In the myocardium, glucocorticoids induce the change of MHC to the alpha type.[44] We have shown that glucocorticoids inhibit myocyte hyperplasia when administered to fetal lambs in utero (Rudolph AM et al, personal observations). A similar inhibitory effect of glucocorticoid on smooth muscle hyperplasia has been described in airway smooth muscle[45] and in aortic smooth muscle cells.[46] Fetal plasma cortisol concentrations increase markedly in the few days prior to delivery of the lamb, and this could markedly influence both growth characteristics and physiological responses of pulmonary vessels after birth.

Vascular Development in the Lung

The lung develops from the embryonic foregut, and in the human, the bronchial tree is fully developed by the 16th week of gestation. Subsequent growth is by formation of new acini, or respiratory units. The lung vessels arise as a plexus within the lung, which later becomes connected with the main circulation through the sixth branchial arches. In the fetus, the walls of the larger vessels are largely of elastic composition, but smooth muscle is evident in the acinar and preacinar arteries, with diameters of 30–200 μm. Smaller precapillary vessels have an incomplete muscular coat, and at the capillary level, no muscle is evident. The development of the intra-acinar circulation closely follows that of the alveolar units, and this process continues until about 10 years after birth.[47]

The muscularized arteries at the fifth to sixth generation, 30–50 μm in diameter, appear to be the main resistance vessels in the fetal lung. Although earlier studies suggested there is a progressive increase in the amount of smooth muscle in these vessels over the last trimester of gestation in the human,[48] subsequent studies, both in the human[49] and the lamb,[50] indicate there is no change in the morphology of these small arteries. The differences in these observations can probably be explained by the fact that the amount of muscle was based on the ratio of media to vessel diameter. If vessels were collapsed, the ratio would be greater, but if distended to the pressure present during life, the ratio would decrease. The total number of fifth- and sixth-generation vessels increases with lung growth; in the fetal lamb right lung, the total number increased from 0.1×10^6 at 85 days gestation to 4.1×10^6 at 140 days. Furthermore, the number of arteries per unit lung volume increased about 10-fold.

The smooth muscle in media of the small arteries regresses after birth. In the resistance vessels, the quantity of muscle approximates adult vessel values by 6–8 weeks after birth, but in larger arteries, of greater than 200 μm diameter, the regression is somewhat slower; adult levels are reached in 2–3 years. This regression is also accompanied by extension of smooth muscle more peripherally, so that by 10 years of age, the intra-acinar portion of the arteries is fully muscularized.[47]

During fetal life, the lung does not serve the function of gas exchange, and a large blood flow through the lung would considerably increase work-load on the heart. The thick medial muscle layer in fetal pulmonary arteries allows a high pulmonary vascular resistance to be maintained. Blood is largely directed away from the lung through the ductus arteriosus, and the high pulmonary arterial pressure is not transmitted to the capillary circulation. The regression of smooth muscle after birth results in a decrease of pulmonary arterial pressure. However, the rationale for the peripheral extension of smooth muscle in adult vessels has yet to be explained.

The normal pattern of growth of the pulmonary vessels changes dramatically during development. During fetal life, smooth muscle cells replicate rapidly, and an increase in smooth muscle mass is almost exclusively by hyperplasia. However, within 2–3 months after birth, smooth muscle cell division is almost completely inhibited.[51] The fetal smooth muscle cells are smaller than adult cells. Adult cells show a high incidence of polyploidy, whereas fetal cells are mononucleate. In vitro, neonatal bovine smooth muscle cells show greater growth potential than adult cells, and show a greater response to insulin-like growth factor (IGF_1).[52] The mechanisms responsible for these differences pre- and postnatally have not yet been delineated.

Developmental Changes in Pulmonary Circulation

In the adult, the total cardiac output passes through the lungs, but in the fetus, only a small proportion of the combined ventricular output (CVO) is distributed to the pulmonary circulation. Pulmonary blood flow has been measured in fetal lambs at various gestational ages.[53] At 60 days (0.4) gestation, pulmonary blood flow is about 3.5% of CVO; this proportion does not change significantly until 0.7–0.8 gestation (115–120 days), when it increases gradually to reach about 8% of CVO at term. The actual pulmonary blood flow increases from about 3–5 mL/min to about 140 mL/min. In relation to fetal body weight, at term pulmonary flow is 35–40 mL/kg/min. After birth, flow rises about 8- to 10-fold to about 350 mL/kg/min. Few measurements of pulmonary blood flow in human fetuses have been reported; measurements by Doppler ultrasound techniques have indicated that pulmonary blood flow represents about 25% of combined ventricular output.[54] No significant differences in this proportion appeared evident between 20–26 weeks and 31–36 weeks gestation. It is not unexpected that pulmonary blood flow should represent a higher proportion of CVO in the human than in the sheep fetus, because of relative brain size. The blood ejected from the left ventricle is distributed to the brain and upper body; in the sheep, the brain is only 3% of body weight, whereas in the human it is approximately 12–13% of fetal body weight. It is, however, interesting to speculate about what factors determine the magnitude of the proportion of the cardiac output distributed to the pulmonary circulation. Thus, the greater output of the left ventricle to provide the brain blood flow could be achieved by a larger flow through the foramen ovale.

Pulmonary vascular resistance is very high in the lamb fetus at 0.4 gestation—6 mm Hg/mL/min. It decreases progressively through gestational development to reach a level of 0.30–0.35 mm Hg/mL/min near term.[53] Calculated pulmonary vascular resistance represents the total cross-sectional area of the pulmonary vascular bed. The decrease in resistance during fetal development could be explained by the increase in the number of vessels per unit of lung volume, as well as the increase in lung size.

Although pulmonary vascular resistance decreases with fetal development, there is some evidence that the resistance pulmonary arteries develop increased basal tone. Late-gestation pulmonary resistance arteries show greater responses to a number of influences than in more immature fetuses. Thus, hypoxemia, which induces fetal pulmonary vasoconstriction, causes a progressively greater decrease in pulmonary blood flow and increase in pulmonary vascular resistance in fetal lambs from 0.75 gestation to term.[55] Similarly, increasing oxygen tension in the fetus by placing the ewe in a hyperbaric oxygen chamber resulted in a 10-fold increase in pulmonary blood flow in lambs of 145–148 days gestation, as compared with only a 0.2-fold increase in lambs at 93–95 days gestation.[56] Another manifestation of the changes in pulmonary vascular response during fetal development is the relatively much greater rise in pulmonary blood flow in response to acetylcholine in late-gestation lambs as compared with lambs at about 0.7 gestation.[55] A difference in response of the pulmonary circulation to oxygen has also been reported in the human fetuses. Administration of 60% oxygen to mothers did not significantly change pulmonary blood flow in fetuses at 20–26 weeks gestation, but increased flow at 31–36 weeks gestation.[54]

The mechanisms responsible for the change in response of the pulmonary vasculature with advancing gestational age have not been determined. Possible explanations include immaturity of production of vasoactive substances, poorly developed receptors on smooth muscle cells, and poor contractile ability of smooth muscle cells. Studies on endothelium-derived NO in fetal lambs have shown that as early as 115 days gestation, pulmonary vasodilation occurs with inhaled NO, and although NO synthase activity is demonstrable, it has been suggested that the endothelium lacks the ability to maintain NO production.[24] Little information is available regarding possible changes in contractility of smooth muscle.

Patterns of Blood Flow

In the fetus, the phasic flow contour in the left and right pulmonary arteries is different from that in the main pulmonary trunk, as shown by both electromagnetic and ultrasonic flowmeters in fetal lambs. In the pulmonary trunk, forward flow occurs throughout systole; a small amount of backflow is detectable at the end of systole. In the pulmonary arteries, there is a short period of forward flow in early systole, extending through one-third to one-half of systole, followed by reverse flow through the remainder of systole and early diastole, and no flow in either direction during the remainder of diastole.[55] This pattern of flow in the branch pulmonary arteries is probably related to the low compliance of the pulmonary circulation. During the high velocity of early systole, blood enters the pulmonary vasculature and distends the large arteries. Flow into the small arteries is restricted by the high resistance in the peripheral circulation. Blood flows preferentially across the ductus and because, as pressure falls in late systole, the recoil of the arteries forces it to flow toward the ductus, backflow is recorded in the left and right pulmonary arteries. If pulmonary vascular resistance is decreased, as during administration of acetylcholine, the duration of forward flow in systole is increased, no backflow occurs, and the flow contour assumes the characteristics of that in the pulmonary trunk. Postnatally, the patterns of flow in the main and branch pulmonary arteries are similar, showing only forward flow during systole. If pulmonary vascular resistance is increased by hypoxia in the fetus, the duration and magnitude of systolic forward flow are reduced, and greater backflow occurs. These changes in the blood flow contours in the left and right pulmonary arteries could be useful in estimating pulmonary vascular resistance levels in the fetus.

References

1. Harvey W. *Exercitatio anatomica de motu cordis et sanguinis in animalibus.* London: 1628. Translated by Barnes WR. Surrey, England: 1847.
2. Lower R. Tractatus de Corde. In: Gunther RT, ed: *Early Science in Oxford.* Oxford: Clarendon Press; 1932.
3. Bichat X. *Anatomie générale, appliqueé à la physiologie et à la médecine.* Paris: Brosson, Gabon; 1801.
4. Kilian HF. *Ueber den Kreislauf des Blutes im Kinde, welches noch nicht geathmet hat.* Karlsruhe: Muller; 1826.
5. Barclay AE, Barcroft J, Barron DH, et al. A radiographic demonstration of the circulation through the heart in the adult and in the foetus, and the identification of the ductus arteriosus. *Br J Radiol* 1939;12:505.
6. Hamilton WF, Woodbury RA, Woods EB. The relation between systemic and pulmonary blood pressures in the fetus. *Am J Physiol* 1937;119:206.
7. Dawes GS, Mott JC, Widdicombe JG, et al. Changes in the lungs of the newborn lamb. *J Physiol (Lond)* 1953;121:141.
8. Cassin S, Dawes GS, Mott JC, et al. The vascular resistance of the foetal and newly ventilated lung of the lamb. *J Physiol* 1964;171:61–79.
9. Reynolds SRM. The fetal and neonatal pulmonary vasculature in the

guinea pig in relation to hemodynamic changes at birth. *Am J Anat* 1956;98:97.

10. Enhorning G, Adams FH, Norman A. Effect of lung expansion on the fetal lamb circulation. *Acta Paediatr Scand* 1966;55:441–451.

11. Gilbert RD, Hessler JR, Eitzman DV, et al. Site of pulmonary vascular resistance in fetal goats. *J Appl Physiol* 1972;32:47–53.

12. Leffler CW, Tyler TL, Cassin S. Effect of indomethacin on pulmonary vascular response to ventilation of fetal goats. *Am J Physiol* 1978;234:H346-H351.

13. Leffler CW, Hessler JR, Terragno NA. Ventilation-induced release of prostaglandin-like material from fetal lungs. *Am J Physiol* 1980;238:H282-H286.

14. Leffler CW, Hessler JR, Green RS. Mechanism of stimulation of pulmonary prostaglandin synthesis at birth. *Prostaglandins* 1984;28:877–887.

15. Brannon TS, North AJ, Wells LB, et al. Prostacyclin synthesis in ovine pulmonary artery is developmentally regulated by changes in cyclooxygenase-1 gene expression. *J Clin Invest* 1994;93:2230–2235.

16. Shaul PW, Campbell WB, Farrar MA, et al. Oxygen modulates prostacyclin synthesis in ovine fetal pulmonary arteries by an effect on cyclooxygenase. *J Clin Invest* 1992;90:2147–2155.

17. Teitel DF, Iwamoto HS, Rudolph AM. Changes in the pulmonary circulation during birth-related events. *Pediatr Res* 1990;27:372–378.

18. Lauer RM, Evans JA, Aoki K, et al. Factors controlling pulmonary vascular resistance in fetal lamb. *J Pediatr* 1965;67:568–577.

19. Heymann M, Rudolph A, Nies A, et al. Bradykinin production association with oxygenation of the fetal lamb. *Circ Res* 1969;25:521–534.

20. Assali NS, Kirschbaum TH, Dilts PV Jr. Effects of hyperbaric oxygen on uteroplacental and fetal circulation. *Circ Res* 1968;22:573–588.

21. Banerjee A, Roman C, Heymann MA. Bradykinin receptor blockade does not affect oxygen-mediated pulmonary vasodilation in fetal lambs. *Pediatr Res* 1994;36:474–480.

22. Furchgott RF, Zawadzki JV. The obligatory role of endothelial cells in the relaxation of arterial smooth muscle by acetylcholine. *Nature* 1980;288:373–376.

23. Ignarro LJ, Buga GM, Wood KS, et al. Endothelium-derived relaxing factor produced and released from artery and vein is nitric oxide. *Proc Natl Acad Sci USA* 1987;84:9265–9269.

24. Kinsella JP, Ivy DD, Abman SH. Ontogeny of NO activity and response to inhaled NO in the developing ovine pulmonary circulation. *Am J Physiol* 1994;267:H1955-H1961.

25. Abman SH, Chatfield BA, Hall SL, et al. Role of endothelium-derived relaxing factor during transition of pulmonary circulation at birth. *Am J Physiol* 1990;259:H1921-H1927.

26. Tiktinsky MH, Morin FC III. Increasing oxygen tension dilates fetal pulmonary circulation via endothelium-derived relaxing factor. *Am J Physiol* 1993;265:H376-H380.

27. Moore P, Velvis H, Fineman JR, et al. EDRF inhibition attenuates the increase in pulmonary blood flow due to oxygen ventilation in fetal lambs. *J Appl Physiol* 1992;73:2151–2157.

28. Soifer SJ, Morin FC III, Kaslow DC, et al. The developmental effects of prostaglandin D_2 on the pulmonary and systemic circulations in the newborn lamb. *J Dev Physiol* 1983;5:237–250.

29. Morin FC III, Egan EA, Norfleet WT. Indomethacin does not diminish the pulmonary vascular response of the fetus to increased oxygen tension. *Pediatr Res* 1988;24:696–700.
30. de Vroomen M, Takahashi Y, Roman C, et al. Calcitonin gene-related peptide increases pulmonary blood flow in fetal sheep. *Am J Physiol* 1998;274: H277-H282.
31. Godecke A, Decking U, Ding Z, et al. Coronary hemodynamics in endothelial NO synthase knockout mice. *Circ Res* 1998;82:186–194.
32. Shesely EG, Maeda N, Kim HS, et al. Elevated blood pressures in mice lacking endothelial nitric oxide synthase. *Proc Natl Acad Sci USA* 1996;93: 13176-13181.
33. Soifer SJ, Loitz RD, Roman C, et al. Leukotriene end organ antagonists increase pulmonary blood flow in fetal lambs. *Am J Physiol* 1985;249:H570-H576.
34. Ibe BO, Anderson JM, Raj JU. Leukotriene synthesis by isolated perinatal ovine intrapulmonary vessels correlates with age-related changes in 5-lipoxygenase protein. *Biochem Mol Med* 1997;61:63–71.
35. Chatfield BA, McMurtry IF, Hall SL, et al. Hemodynamic effects of endothelin-1 on ovine fetal pulmonary circulation. *Am J Physiol* 1991;261: R182-R187.
36. Ivy DD, Kinsella JP, Abman SH. Physiologic characterization of endothelin A and B receptor activity in the ovine fetal pulmonary circulation. *J Clin Invest* 1994;93:2141–2148.
37. Black SM, Johengen MJ, Ma ZD, et al. Ventilation and oxygenation induce endothelial nitric oxide synthase gene expression in the lungs of fetal lambs. *J Clin Invest* 1997;100:1448–1458.
38. López-López J, Gonzalez C, Ureña J, et al. Low PO_2 selectively inhibits K channel activity in chemoreceptor cells of the mammalian carotid body. *J Gen Physiol* 1989;93:1001–1015.
39. Jiang C, Haddad GG. A direct mechanism for sensing low oxygen levels by central neurons. *Proc Natl Acad Sci USA* 1994;91:7198–7201.
40. Yuan X-J, Goldman WF, Tod ML, et al. Hypoxia reduces potassium currents in cultured rat pulmonary but not mesenteric arterial myocytes. *Am J Physiol* 1993;264:L116-L123.
41. Post JM, Hume JR, Archer SL, et al. Direct role for potassium channel inhibition in hypoxic pulmonary vasoconstriction. *Am J Physiol* 1992;262: C882-C890.
42. Rudolph AM, Heymann MA, Lewis AB. Physiology and pharmacology of the pulmonary circulation in the fetus and newborn. In: Hodson WA, ed: *Lung Biology in Health and Disease: The Development of the Lung*. New York: Marcel Dekker; 1977:487–523.
43. Halbower AC, Tuder RM, Franklin WA, et al. Maturation-related changes in endothelial nitric oxide synthase immunolocalization in developing ovine lung. *Am J Physiol* 1994;267:L585-L591.
44. Bian X, Briggs MM, Schachat FH, et al. Glucocorticoids accelerate the ontogenetic transition of cardiac ventricular myosin heavy-chain isoform expression in the rat: Promotion by prenatal exposure to a low dose of dexamethasone. *J Dev Physiol* 1992;18:35–42.
45. Young PG, Skinner SJ, Black PN. Effects of glucocorticoids and beta-adrenoceptor agonists on the proliferation of airway smooth muscle. *Eur J Pharmacol* 1995;273:137–143.
46. Longenecker JP, Kilty LA, Johnson LK. Glucocorticoid inhibition of vas-

cular smooth muscle cell proliferation: Influence of homologous extracellular matrix and serum mitogens. *J Cell Biol* 1984;98:534–540.

47. Hislop A, Reid LM. Pulmonary arterial development during childhood: Branching pattern and structure. *Thorax* 1973;28:129–135.

48. Naeye RL. Arterial changes during the perinatal period. *Arch Pathol* 1961; 71:121–128.

49. Hislop A, Reid L. Intrapulmonary arterial development during fetal life—branching pattern and structure. *J Anat* 1972;113:35–48.

50. Levin DL, Rudolph AM, Heymann MA, et al. Morphological development of the pulmonary vascular bed in fetal lambs. *Circulation* 1976;53: 144–151.

51. Stenmark KR, Weiser MC. Vascular development and function. In: Gluckman PD, Heymann MA, eds: *Pediatrics and Perinatology: The Scientific Basis*. London: Arnold; 1996:683–693.

52. Dempsey EC, Badesch DB, Dobyns EL, et al. Enhanced growth capacity of neonatal pulmonary artery smooth muscle cells in vitro: Dependence on cell size, time from birth, insulin-like growth factor I, and auto-activation of protein kinase C. *J Cell Physiol* 1994;160:469–481.

53. Rudolph AM, Heymann MA. Circulatory changes during growth in the fetal lamb. *Circ Res* 1970;26:289–299.

54. Rasanen J, Wood DC, Debbs RH, et al. Reactivity of the human fetal pulmonary circulation to maternal hyperoxygenation increases during the second half of pregnancy. *Circulation* 1998;97:257–262.

55. Lewis AB, Heymann MA, Rudolph AM. Gestational changes in pulmonary vascular responses in fetal lambs in utero. *Circ Res* 1976;39:536–541.

56. Morin FC III, Egan EA. Pulmonary hemodynamics in fetal lambs during development at normal and increased oxygen tension. *J Appl Physiol* 1992;73:213–218.

Chapter 2

The De Novo Formation of Blood Vessels in the Early Embryo and in the Developing Lung

Christopher J. Drake, PhD, and
Charles D. Little, PhD

Introduction

This chapter is a combination of a brief overview of our recent work on early vascular morphogenesis, and a speculation regarding two questions facing vascular developmental biologists:

1. Is the fate of vascular cells determined locally, or is it established at gastrulation?
2. Are all endothelial and vascular smooth muscle progenitors derived from an epithelial-to-mesenchymal transformation?

Where possible we will relate our work on de novo blood vessel formation, at very early stages, to similar processes during lung development.

Background

During the past 10 years we have studied the de novo formation of blood vessels in avian embryos. The quail embryo has several technical

This work was supported by National Institutes of Health Grants RO1 HL57375 and American Heart Association S98651S to C.J. Drake and NIH RO1 HL 57645 and March of Dimes Birth Defects Foundation 95–0453 to C.D. Little.

From: Weir EK, Archer SL, Reeves JT (eds). *The Fetal and Neonatal Pulmonary Circulations.* Armonk, NY: Futura Publishing Company, Inc.; ©1999.

advantages which make it suitable for experimental manipulation and optical analysis. First, it is easy to obtain at the requisite stages. Second, an extremely useful antibody is available, QH1, which marks endothelial cells. Third, because of its planar nature, it is possible to observe vascular morphogenesis through the entire thickness of an entire embryo. Finally, because the early vasculature develops in a head-to-tail progression, it is possible to observe the entire vasculogenic process in a single embryo.

Morphogenesis of the embryonic vascular system can be thought of as having two phases: (1) establishment of an interconnected network of endothelial tubes; and (2) assembly of a vessel wall. The two stages are separated in time and space. In the first case, a continuous network of small caliber endothelial tubes must form *before* blood flow can begin. In avians this process occurs during the 2nd day of development. The first smooth muscle progenitors are not seen for almost 24 hours after circulation is established. Eventually, vascular endothelial cells and smooth muscle cells tailor individual vessel segments to meet local physiological requirements. Our studies focus on mechanisms regulating the formation of the first blood vessels and their organization into networks. Additionally, our research addresses the recruitment and behavior of smooth muscle progenitors and their extracellular matrix expression pattern.

In the early embryo, initial vasculogenic activity establishes a network of endothelial tubes arranged in a precise spatial pattern. This process may be divided into several steps including: (1) commitment of mesodermal cells to an endothelial lineage; (2) ventral repositioning of endothelial precursor cells (angioblasts) into an extracellular matrix compartment; (3) formation of primitive endothelial cords; (4) the formation of the vessel lumen; and (5) morphogenesis of large caliber vessels.

Recently, we showed that the transcription factor TAL1/SCL is a marker of angioblasts,[1] a discovery that permitted studies on the behavior of vascular precursor cells as they begin to acquire endothelial characteristics. Using TAL1 antibodies, we showed that in the early embryo, endothelial progenitors, or angioblasts, are born in the splanchnic mesoderm proper. Next, these cells reposition themselves so as to lie in a ventral extracellular matrix compartment (the splanchnopleural ECM). We believe that endothelial precursor cells respond to this new extracellular matrix environment by initiating protrusive/extension behavior that results in the formation of vascular cords and subsequently vessels. That this process requires integrin-mediated adhesions was shown using our in vivo microinjection assay. In this system, vasculogenic stage quail embryos are injected with a reagent and then cultured for varying periods of time. When embryos were injected with inhibitory antibodies to β_1 integrin (CSAT) or $\alpha_v\beta_3$ integrin (LM 609),[2,3] vasculogenesis was severely compromised. The neutralization of both categories of integrins resulted in a failure of primordial endothelial cells to change shape and form the characteristic polygonal pattern of early vascular networks. Also, the ability of the cells to form lumens was impaired. Therefore, a wide spectrum of integrins is actively employed by primordial endothelial cells during the process of vessel formation.

We next turned our attention to vascular endothelial growth factor (VEGF) as a possible regulator of vessel morphogenesis. VEGF is a well-known endothelial mitogen; however, we were interested in the possibility that VEGF might also function as a vascular morphogen. When recombinant VEGF$_{165}$ was injected into embryos, dramatic vascular malformations were observed, including a complete disruption of normal vessel patterning.[4] The predominant anomalies were the inappropriate formation of vascular sinuses (vascular hyperfusion) with an accompanying loss of the normal spatial pattern. Our in vivo studies on intact embryos suggest a model whereby VEGF plays two roles in vasculogenesis: one as a mitogen, and an equally important second role as a vascular morphogen (for instance, as a regulator of endothelial cell protrusive activity). We hypothesize that local fine-tuning of VEGF bioavailability regulates whether a particular region forms a large caliber vessel such as the sinus venosus or endocardium, or the fine caliber vessels in a polygonal network.[1,5]

Unlike vasculogenesis, morphogenesis of the vessel wall does not begin until well after circulation is established. Avian embryos begin the task of assembling a vessel wall during the 3rd day of gestation. The first evidence of a vessel wall is the presence of mesenchymal cells near the aortic tube. The molecules that induce mesenchymal cells to associate with endothelial tubes are being investigated by others.[6,7]

Our work has entailed the identification of a marker for smooth muscle progenitor cells. This reagent is a monoclonal antibody, 1E12, which recognizes an isoform of smooth muscle α-actinin.[8,9] Approximately 8 hours after the first mesenchymal cells associate with the aortic tube, the 1E12 isoform of α-actinin is expressed in a radial fashion beginning with the cells closest to the basal surface of the endothelium. We contend that these cells represent the progenitors of vascular smooth muscle and that such cells are recruited locally from splanchnic mesoderm. We believe that 1E12 is a unique marker of cells committed to a smooth muscle fate, while the expression of smooth muscle α-actin is not evidence of such a commitment. This speculation is based mainly on the fact that multiple embryonic cell types express smooth muscle α-actin that are not progenitors of smooth muscle (ie, cardiac myoblasts, skeletal myoblasts, endocardial cushion cells, neural crest cells, and fibroblasts).

While we believe that, at the developmental stages we study, the progenitors of vascular smooth muscle cells (VSMCs) arise directly from the mesoderm, we are intrigued by recent work suggesting that endothelial cells may also be capable of contributing to this lineage.[10–12] In the study of de Ruiter and colleagues,[10] colloidial gold was injected to label the luminal surface of endothelial cells. When the fate of labeled cells was examined, gold-lectin was observed in a restricted population of subendothelial mesenchymal cells. Additionally, a transitional population of cells was also noted that were labeled with both gold-lectin and a marker of endothelial cells. The work of Williams and colleagues[11,12] also supports the hypothesis that vascular smooth muscle can be derived from endothelial cells. As part of bioengineering studies to prepare prosthetic vessels, these workers isolated and then transplanted an autologously derived pure population of endothelial cells onto the luminal surface of synthetic vascular grafts. When examined later, the prosthesis had acquired a coherent endothelial layer as expected and, in addition, multiple layers of vascular smooth muscle. While still open to debate, given the plasticity of primordial cells, it is not totally surprising that embryonic endothelial cells can give rise to smooth muscle precursor cells. However the possibility that adult endothelial cells have this capacity is remarkable.

Additional efforts on our part to understand the assembly of the vessel wall have been directed at identifying extracellular matrix glycoproteins associated with forming vessels. Our immunolabeling studies show that mesenchymal or fibroblastic cells surrounding the vessel produce an extracellular matrix that is distinct between vessel types. This diversity in extracellular matrix glycoproteins surrounding nascent vessels is detectable at morphogenetic stages well before VSMCs could be identified. For example, at a stage when cells thought to be progenitors of aortic smooth muscle are secreting the molecule fibulin-1, vascular smooth muscle progenitors associated with smaller vessels of the body wall are expressing fibrillin-2; the reverse, however, is not true.

Based on the above, it appears that an early event in the assembly of the vessel wall is the production by smooth muscle progenitors of an extracellular matrix tailored to a specific vessel fate. We therefore postulate that presumptive smooth muscle cells are fibroblasts—in the classic sense of that term. Further, we envision that the term vascular smooth muscle describes a diverse repertoire of cells that exist along a continuum, between mainly matrix-producing cells and cells in which contractility is the predominant cellular feature. The spectrum of VSMC types varies from inner to outer layers, as well as along the length of the circulatory route. In our view, there is no single cell type that in itself represents vascular smooth muscle in embryos or in adult organisms. Moreover, we contend that smooth muscle cell diversity is best exemplified by the extracellular matrix expression program.[13]

Lung Vasculogenesis and Vessel Wall Assembly

Neovascular processes include both angiogenesis and vasculogenesis. Until recently, vasculogenesis was widely thought to be restricted to very early embryonic stages. There is now compelling evidence that vasculogenesis, the de novo formation of blood vessels from nonendothelial precursors, occurs repeatedly in embryos, fetuses, and possibly adults. In contrast to this process of blood vessel formation, neovascularization occurring via angiogenesis is defined as the formation of new vessels from preexisting vessels.

In the remainder of this chapter, we will use the term primary vasculogenesis to refer to events that occur during, or shortly after, gastrulation. In contrast, we will refer to vasculogenesis that occurs at any later stage(s) as secondary vasculogenesis. We have no reason to think that the mechanisms regulating primary and secondary vasculogenesis differ in any manner.

While our work has focused entirely on primary vasculogenesis, the work of others provides compelling data that secondary vasculogenesis occurs throughout embryonic development, for example during lung development and during formation of coronary vessels.[14,15] A review of all of the literature pertinent to lung neovascularization is beyond the scope of this chapter; instead we will focus on a few lung-related articles that highlight concepts we hope to convey. We will also attempt to apply our understanding of primary vasculogenesis to lung vasculogenesis.

The studies of Pardanaud and colleagues have addressed lung vasculogenesis in a manner that is closely related to our work on primary vasculogenesis.[14] Their experimental data strongly support the contention that the first blood vessels that form in the lung primordia do so by vasculogenesis. This study used chimeric grafting techniques to evaluate the vasculogenic potential of lung primordia. Cross-transplantation of lung primordia between chicken and quail embryos demonstrated that the vessels of the lung were derived from the rudiment and not the host.

Beginning with the assumption that the principles of primary vasculogenesis relate directly to "secondary" sites of vasculogenesis, it would follow that there are similarities between the two events. Secondary vasculogenesis in the lung compares favorably to primary vasculogenesis. In both events vasculogenesis is driven by an interaction between splanchnic mesoderm and endoderm, with angioblasts being derived from the mesoderm and the endoderm being a source of VEGF.

While we postulate that the mechanisms regulating the de novo assembly of vessels are identical in primary and secondary vasculogenesis, there is potentially a distinct difference between the two—the source of angioblasts. This possibility was recently brought to light in studies showing that cells selected from peripheral blood, using antibodies closely associated with the endothelial lineage, were able to differentiate into endothelial cells, both in vitro and in vivo.[16,17] If similar cells are present in embryonic circulation, it is possible that lung vasculogenesis begins with two sources of angioblasts—those derived from lung splanchnic mesoderm, and those derived from the circulation.

Direct evidence that mechanisms regulating primary and secondary vasculogenesis are similar is found in the work of Zeng and colleagues.[18] These workers overexpressed VEGF under the control of the promotor for human surfactant protein C (SP-C). Experimental mice carrying this transgene exhibited vascular anomalies which are compatible with our model of vascular fusion. As mentioned above, our studies showed that injection of human recombinant $VEGF_{165}$ into avian embryos resulted in the formation of oversized blood vessels. Similar oversized vessels were observed in the SP-C mice. In our studies, we attribute this endpoint to a mechanism whereby multiple small vessels fuse to form larger caliber vessels. This proposed mechanism of vascular development is distinct from other vascular processes (ie, "interstitial growth" and dilation) which can also increase the diameter of vessels. Zeng and colleagues appear to favor interstitial growth or dilation as the cause of the increase in vessel diameter that they observed in the lung. In contrast, we feel it is equally likely that the increase is due to vascular fusion. While the exact mechanism may be debatable, it is clear that elevated levels of VEGF in both a primary and secondary vasculogenesis lead to similar morphogenetic anomalies.

An interesting, and perhaps unexpected, result of overexpression of VEGF in the lung was the disruption of the morphogenesis of the airway primordium. It has long been recognized that epithelomesenchymal interactions establish the branching pattern of parenchymal organs.[19,20] This concept of reciprocal induction between epithelial and mesenchyme has also been demonstrated in the establishment of the branching pattern of the lung.[21] That such reciprocal interactions extended to vascular development has also been suggested.[22]

Consistent with these older studies is the observation by Zeng and colleagues that the airway epithelium can ultimately be influenced by a vascular morphogen. Of course, the effect is not direct, as presumptive lung endoderm does not express VEGF receptors (VEGF-R1/flt-1 and VEGF-R2/flk-1); indeed, such receptors are confined to mesodermal cells of the endothelial lineage.

A simple explanation for the observed results is that excessive amounts of VEGF change the balance or composition of the mesoderm. For example, VEGF may influence the fate of mesodermal cells, causing the recruitment of an abnormally large proportion of the mesodermal cells to an endothelial lineage. This would result in a deficiency of nonvascular mesoderm, which in turn would impede the normal induction of the airway epithelium to branch its characteristic pattern. Alternatively, the excess VEGF may influence the production of extracellular matrix by endothelial cells, which in turn may influence airway morphogenesis.

Initial vasculogenic activity in the embryo establishes an extensive network of nascent endothelial tubes embedded in an extracellular matrix scaffold. This phase of vessel development is followed immediately by two important events, the initiation of blood flow and the recruitment of VSMC progenitors. At the present time, there is no reason to believe that recruitment of vascular smooth muscle from primary splanchnic mesoderm differs from recruitment of smooth muscle from lung splanchnic mesoderm.

By analogy with the formation of the aortic wall, as described above, it is reasonable to assume that lung splanchnic mesoderm contains uncommitted cells that are capable of responding to inducing signals. Such signals would presumably be produced by the nascent lung vasculature, and may include proteins such as platelet-derived growth factor (PDGF) family members.[23] Recent studies examining the role of the receptor tyrosine kinase tie-2, and its ligands, the angiopoietins, in vascular morphogenesis indicate that the signaling system for the recruitment of VSMCs may be complex.[24-26] These studies suggest that while signaling is ultimately derived from endothelial cells, the generation of the signal requires a dynamic interaction between the mesoderm, a source of ligand, and endothelial cells expressing the receptor. To date neither the existence of, nor the nature of, such an endothelial-derived signaling molecule has been demonstrated. In regard to the recruitment of VSMC progenitors, it is important to note that as discussed above, endothelial cells (a mesodermal epithelium) may also be a source of VSMCs.

Efforts to dissect the signaling molecules involved in the recruitment of VSMCs from mesoderm should benefit from a newly described in vitro assay.[6] This system uses 10T1/2 fibroblasts and endothelial cells seeded in adjacent culture wells, separated by agarose. In this assay, fibroblasts spontaneously migrate toward the endothelial cells, and a subpopulation of these cells begins to express smooth muscle markers. Using this assay, these workers have shown that both PDGF-β and TGF-β are factors that influence 10T1/2 fibroblasts toward a smooth muscle response.

A mechanism common to early and late embryos is epithelial-to-mesenchymal transformations. This important morphogenetic process is a recurring event throughout embryogenesis. This morphogenic process is often associated with the mesoderm, though not solely confined to this germ layer (ie, gastrulation and neural crest). In early development, prominent transitions involving the mesoderm include somitogenesis, endocardial cushion formation, and epicardial development. In a recent review Muñoz-Chápuli and colleagues suggested that epithelial-to-mesenchymal transformation may be relevant to vasculogenesis.[27] This hypothesis suggests that angioblasts are derived from mesodermal epithelia (mesothelia). If we accept the view of early workers that the splanchnic mesoderm is itself a loose columnar epithelium,[28] then primary and lung vasculogenesis would fulfill this criteria. Several other vasculogenic events meet this criteria as well, for example, the generation of angioblast from somites and the epicardium.[15,29,30]

The questions posed at the beginning of this chapter could each be the basis of an entire book. In the following sections, we will arbitrarily offer a few studies and observations that have influenced our thinking regarding these important questions. Clearly, valid arguments and differing interpretations of data could lead to a view that would be significantly different from the one we present below.

Is the fate of vascular cells determined locally, or is it established at gastrulation?

We believe that the determination of an angioblast fate versus a vascular smooth muscle fate is locally controlled. We postulate that mesodermal cells giving rise to these lineages are not determined at gastrulation; rather we contend that stochastic processes control fate. One factor that appears to play a fundamental role in the establishment of the endothelial lineage is basic fibroblast growth factor (bFGF).[31,32] Flamme and Riseau[31] showed that while both bFGF-treated and untreated blastodiscs form mesoderm in culture, induction of the endothelial lineage was only observed in treated blascodiscs. The events initiated in response to bFGF have yet to be elucidated. It is likely that there will be a number of competing extracellular/cell surface signaling molecules that act on mesodermal cells. Depending on the balance of signals received by a given cell, its fate is determined. For the angioblast, expression of factors such as the transcription factor TAL1/SCL[1,33] or the VEGF receptor flk-1/VEGF-R2[34] are among the earliest indicators of a decision toward the angioblastic fate. Work, primarily in zebra fish, has advanced our understanding of the relationship between these molecules. Two sets of experiments suggest that factors regulating TAL1 expression may be central to the endothelial lineage. First, it has been demonstrated that vascular development in the *cloche* mutant, an embryo deficient in flk-1 expression,[35] could be rescued by the forced expression of TAL1.[36] Second, overexpression of TAL1 changed the fate of mesoderm toward the hematopoietic/endothelial lineage at the apparent expense of other mesodermal population.[33]

Considering our view that the microenvironment determines both the endothelial and vascular smooth muscle lineage, it is of interest that the first smooth muscle cells do not appear in the embryo for almost 36 hours after the first angioblasts. This separation of the two lineages in time was also observed in the blastodisc culture system described above. We believe that the early splanchnic mesoderm is competent to form VSMC, and attribute the lack of such cells to the lack of and/or the proper balance of signaling molecules such as angiopoietins and PDGF.

Are all endothelial and vascular smooth muscle progenitors derived from an epithelial-to-mesenchymal transformation event?

The idea that an epithelial-to-mesenchymal transition is fundamental to vasculogenesis is supported by both morphological and experimental data. The transformation of angioblasts from somites is the best evidence for this concept.[29,30,37] Briefly, these workers noted that transplanted somites give rise to an extensive population of angioblasts, thus establishing the angiogenic potential of somites. It is virtually certain that had the somites in question been left in their original location, far fewer angioblastic cells would have been induced. There is also evidence for epithelial-to-mesenchymal transformation during coronary vessel formation. Recently, Pérez-Pomares and coworkers demonstrated evidence consistent with the possibility that angioblasts are derived from the epicardium. Their data show VEGF-R2/flk-1 in the subepicardial mesenchyme of hampster embryos.[15] Confirmation of the source of epicardial angioblasts will require cell lineage tracing. Regardless of the exact source tissue, it is virtually certain that coronary angioblasts descend from some component of the splanchic mesoderm.

The argument for epithelial-to-mesenchymal transformations in vasculogenesis can also be extended to include secondary vasculogenesis in the lung, particularly if we consider the primitive lung mesotheliem as a possible source of angioblasts. Assuming that this speculation is correct, then the angiogenic mechanisms described above also induce the primitive lung mesothelium to undergo an epithelial-to-mesenchymal transformation whereby TAL1- and VEGF-R2/flk-positive epithelial (mesothelial) cells give rise to vascular precursors in the primitive lung.

The general proposition that epithelial-to-mesenchymal transformations are an essential part of vasculogenesis was recently advanced by Muñoz-Chápuli and colleagues. Their model is based on morphological, evolutionary, and experimental grounds, and is consistent with the known features of primary vasculogenesis.[27] For example, our work using early avian embryos demonstrated that primary vasculogenesis has a dorsal-to-ventral component whereby angioblasts, within the epithelial-like splanchnic mesoderm, become elongated and move ventrally to occupy a space filled with the splanchnopleural ECM.[1] This ventral repositioning is tantamount to an epithelial-to-mesenchymal transformation. Further, initial vessel assembly proceeds once the presumptive endothelial cells are within this cell-free environment. We propose that the ventral repositioning of angioblasts from primary splanchnic mesoderm (stages 7–10) represents a mesenchymal transformation event as envisioned by Muñoz-Chápuli and Pérez-Pomares.

As discussed above, if the splanchnic mesoderm is considered to be an epithelium, then both angioblast and VSMC progenitors are derived as part of an epithelial-to-mesenchymal transformation. The argument that epithelial-to-mesenchymal transformations play a role in the formation of vascular smooth muscle cells is supported by the data presented above suggesting that endothelial cells (a mesodermal epithelium) are capable of giving rise to vascular smooth muscle.[10–12]

Acknowledgments   We would like to thank Dr. Jose Pérez-Pomares for his critical comments and input toward this review.

References

1. Drake CJ, Brandt SJ, Trusk TC, et al. TAL1/SCL is expressed in endothelial progenitor cells/angioblasts and defines a dorsal-to-ventral gradient of vasculogenesis. *Dev Biol* 1997;191:1–14.
2. Drake CJ, Davis LA, Little CD. Antibodies to beta 1 integrins cause alterations of aortic vasculogenesis, in vivo. *Dev Dyn* 1992;193:83–91.
3. Drake CJ, Cheresh DA, Little CD. An antagonist of integrin αvβ3 prevents maturation of blood vessels during embryonic neovascularization. *J Cell Sci* 1995;108:2655–2661.
4. Drake CJ, Little CD. Exogenous vascular endothelial growth factor induces malformed and hyperfused vessels during embryonic neovascularization. *Proc Natl Acad Sci USA* 1995;92:7657–7661.
5. Drake CJ, Little CD. The morphogenesis of primordial vascular networks. In: Little CD, Mironov V, Sage EH, eds: *Vascular Morphogenesis, In Vivo, In Vitro, In Mente.* Boston: Birkhauser; 1998:3–21.
6. Hirschi KK, Robovsky SA, D'Amore PA. PDGF, TGF-β, and heterotypic cell-cell interactions mediate endothelial cell-induced recruitment of 10T1/2 cells and their differentiation to a smooth muscle fate. *J Cell Biol* 1998;14:804–814.
7. Little CD, Mironov V, Sage H, eds. *Vascular Morphogenesis: In Vivo, In Vitro, In Mente.* Boston: Birkhauser; 1998.
8. Hungerford JE. Development of the vessel wall. University of Virginia. 1995.
9. Hungerford JE, Owens GK, Argraves WS, Little CD. Development of the aortic vessel wall as defined by vascular smooth muscle and extracellular matrix markers. *Dev Biol* 1996:375–392.
10. de Ruiter MC, Poelmann RE, Van Munsteren JC, et al. Embryonic endothe-

lial cells transdifferentiate into mesenchymal cells expressing smooth muscle actins in vivo and in vitro. *Circ Res* 1997;80(4):444–451.

11. Williams SK, Rose DG, Jarrell BE. Microvascular endothelial cell seeding of ePTFE vascular grafts: Improved patency and stability of the cellular lining. *J Biomed Mater Res* 1994;28:203–212.

12. Williams SK, Jarrell BE, Kleinert LB. Endothelial cell transplantation onto polymeric arteriovenous grafts evaluated using a canine model. *J Invest Surg* 1994;7:503–517.

13. Drake CJ, Hungerford JE, Little CD. Morphogenesis of the first blood vessels. In: Fleischmajer R, Timpi R, Werb Z, eds: *Annals of the New York Academy of Science. Morphogenesis: Cellular Interactions*. New York: New York Academy of Science; 1998:155–180.

14. Pardanaud L, Yassine F, Dietrelen-Lievre F. Relationship between vasculogenesis, angiogenesis and haemopoiesis during avian otogeny. *Development* 1989;105:473–485.

15. Pérez-Pomares JM, Macías D, García-Garrido L, et al. Immunolocalization of the vascular endothelial growth factor receptor-2 in the subepicaradial mesenchyme of hamster embryos: Identification of the coronary vessel precursors. *Histochem J* 1998;30:1–8.

16. Asahara LT, Murohara T, Sullivan A, et al. Isolation of putative progenitor endothelial cells for angiogenesis. *Science* 1997;275:964–967.

17. Rivard A, Isner JM. Angiogenesis and vasculogenesis in treatment of cardiovascular disease. *Mol Med* 1998;4:429–440.

18. Zeng X, Wert SE, Federici R, et al. VEGF enhances pulmonary vasculogenesis and disrupts lung morphogenesis in vivo. *Dev Dyn* 1998;211:215–227.

19. Grobstein C. Induction interaction in the development of the mouse metanephros. *J Exp Zool* 1995;130:319–340.

20. Grobstein C, Cohen J. Collagenase: Effect on the morphogenesis of embryonic salivary epithelium in vitro. *Science* 1965;150:626–628.

21. Wessells NK. Mammalian lung development: Interactions in formulation and morphogenesis of tracheal buds. *J Exp Zool* 1970;175:455–466.

22. Stenmark KR, Mecham RP. Cellular and molecular mechanisms of pulmonary vascular remodeling. *Ann Rev Physiol* 1997;59:89–144.

23. Beck L Jr, D'Amore PA. Vascular development: Cellular and molecular regulation. *FASEB J* 1997;11:365–373.

24. Sato TN, Tozawa Y, Deutsch U, et al. Distinct roles of the receptor tyrosine kinases Tie-1 and Tie-2 in blood vessel formation. *Nature* 1995;376:70–74.

25. Suri C, Jones PF, Patan S, et al. Requisite role of angiopoietin-1, a ligand for the Tie2 receptor, during embryonic angiogenesis. *Cell* 1996;87:1172–1190.

26. Maisonpierre PC, Suri C, Jones PF, et al. Angiopoietin-2, a natural antagonist for Tie2 that disrupts in vivo angiogenesis. *Science* 1997;277:55–60.

27. Muñoz-Chápuli R, Pérez-Pomares JM, Macías D, et al. Differentation of hemangioblast from embryonic mesothelial cells? A model on the origin of the vertebrate cardiovascular system. In press.

28. Trelstad RL, Revel JP, Hay ED. Tight junctions between cells in the early chick embryo as visualized with the electron microscopy. *J Cell Biol* 1996; 31(1):6–10.

29. Eichmann A, Marcelle C, Breant C, et al. Two molecules related to the VEGF receptor are expressed in early endothelial cells during avial embryonic development. *Mech Dev* 1993;42:33–48.

30. Wilting J, Brand-Saberi B, Huang R, et al. Angiogenic potential of the avian somite. *Dev Dyn* 1995;202:165–171.

31. Flamme I, Risau W. Induction of vasculogenesis and hematopoiesis in vitro. *Development* 1992;116:435–439.
32. Krah K, Mironov V, Risau W, et al. Induction of vasculogenesis in quail blastodisc-derived embryoid bodies. *Dev Biol* 1994;164:123–132.
33. Gering M, Rodaway ARF, Gottgens B, et al. The SCL gene specificies haemangioblast development from early mesoderm. *EMBO J* 1998;17:4029–4045.
34. Shalaby F, Rossant J, Yamaguchi TP, et al. Failure of blood-island and vasculogenesis in Flk-1-deficient mice. *Nature* 1995;376:62–66.
35. Liao W, Bisgrove BW, Sawyer H, et al. The zebrafish gene cloche acts upstream of a flk-1 homologue to regulate endothelial cell differentiation. *Development* 1997;124:381–389.
36. Liao EC, Paw BH, Oates AC, et al. SCL/Tal-1 transcription factor acts downstream of cloche to specify hematopoietic and vascular progenitors in zebrafish. *Genes Dev* 1998;12:621–626.
37. Poole TJ, Coffin JD. Vasculogenesis and angiogenesis: Two distinct morphogenetic mechanisms establish embryonic vascular pattern. *J Exp Zool* 1989;251:224–231.

Chapter 3

Early Development of the Vascular System of the Mouse Lung:
Ontogeny of Endothelial Cell Heterogeneity

Robert Auerbach, PhD, Olga Mirzoeva, PhD, and Keith C. Meyer, MD

Blood vessel development during mouse embryonic development can first be observed in the yolk sac of embryonic day 9 (E9) mice.[1] This stage corresponds to the 3rd week of human development.[2,3] The first clear indication of lung development occurs 2 days later, when, at E11 (equivalent to human week 16), lung rudiments can be identified, dissected, and grown in vitro in organ culture.[4,5]

How blood vessels develop in the lung has not been firmly established. There is general consensus that there are two different modes of blood vessel development: vasculogenesis and angiogenesis.[5-8] Vasculogenesis is defined as the formation of blood vessels by proliferation and organization of endothelial cell precursors, or angioblasts. Angiogenesis is defined as the formation of blood vessels by sprouting and distal extension of previously established vessels. The two processes are not mutually exclusive and recent evidence indicates that both processes occur during the formation of many, if not all, organs.[9] Angioblasts have been shown to migrate to distant sites, settling in various organ rudiments.[10-12] There they can divide, aggregate, and differentiate to produce new capillaries (vasculogenesis) which then join up with larger vessels that arrive in these rudiments by extension from the major large arteries or veins (angiogenesis). In addition, angioblasts either resident in the developing rudiments or available through the circulation, may participate in the formation of angiogenic vessels.[13]

Whereas the endothelium was once thought to be a relatively inert, homogeneous tissue, it is now clear that the endothelium is, on the

Supported in part by Grants HL52148 and EY3243 from the National Institutes of Health.

From: Weir EK, Archer SL, Reeves JT (eds). *The Fetal and Neonatal Pulmonary Circulations.*
Armonk, NY: Futura Publishing Company, Inc.; ©1999.

contrary, highly reactive and heterogeneous with respect to transport properties, secretion of cytokines, synthesis of specific enzymes, affinities for blood and tumor cells, and the presence of receptors for various factors regulating endothelial cell growth and differentiation.[14-16] In this respect, the lung vasculature is one of the most complex of all vasculatures. Not only are endothelial cells within this vasculature different from endothelial cells found in other organs, but there are also major differences even among the endothelial cells found within the lung. It can readily be accepted that all large vessels differ from the microvascular small capillaries in structure and function, and that the pulmonary vein is different from the pulmonary artery. Not as well recognized is the fact that endothelial cells within the bronchial circulation respond to angiogenic stimuli, whereas endothelial cells comprising the alveolar circulation are refractory to these stimuli.[17]

This chapter will not address the many aspects of heterogeneity that are observed during postnatal lung development, nor will it discuss the many research studies that document changes and responses of endothelial cells to physiological stimuli. Rather, it will focus on the acquisition of organ specificity of lung blood vessels during embryogenesis, a phenomenon that of necessity precedes pulmonary function.

New blood vessel development is regulated by many factors. The earliest of these are basic fibroblast growth factor (bFGF; FGF-2), vascular endothelial cell growth factor (VEGF; also known as vascular permeability factor [VPF] and vasculotropin), and beta transforming growth factor (TGF-β). Receptors for these factors (FGF-R1, FGF-R2, VEGF-R1 [flk-2/flt-1], VEGF-R2 [flk-1]) and endoglin (CD105) are found in early embryonic angioblast populations as well as in some hematopoietic stem cells.[7,9] The factor most specific for angioblast differentiation and growth of endothelial cells is VEGF. Indeed, VEGF is of such importance that mice lacking even one allele for the VEGF gene or its receptor do not develop beyond E9 or E10, and die of vascular defects.[18-21] A second specific set of endothelial growth factors is the angiopoietins (ang-1 and ang-2), and their receptors (tie-1 [presumed] and tie-2/tek), which can be identified in the yolk sac by day E10 and shortly thereafter in newly forming embryonic vessels.[22,23] The angiopoietin system appears to be involved in the three-dimensional restructuring of endothelial cells to form patent tubes. None of these factors, however, leads us to an understanding of endothelial cell heterogeneity. This heterogeneity, which can begin to be recognized during organogenesis, appears to be regulated by microenvironmental influences specific to each developing organ rudiment.

There are many organ-selective properties that define lung endothelial cells. For example, angiotensin-converting enzyme (ACE), synthesized by many endothelial cells, is up to 10 times more abundantly produced by lung endothelial cells, and ACE present on the cell membrane serves as a useful marker of early lung endothelial cell differentiation.[24] Elastin is another protein present in lung endothelium, where it acts as a selective adhesion molecule for circulating tumor cells.[25] Lung endothelial cells secrete up to 100-fold more plasminogen activator-1 (PAI-1) than other endothelial cells or fibroblasts, 1.5–15 times more urokinase-type plasminogen activator (uPA), and lesser amounts of tissue plasminogen activator (tPA) when compared to other endothelial cells.[26]

Cell adhesion molecules differ among endothelial cells from different organs. For example, lung endothelial cells express a lung-specific adhesion molecule (LuECAM) serving to anchor circulating leukocytes.[27] Antibodies to LuECAM as well as to other cell surface antigens such as endothelium-specific molecule-1 (ESM-1) selectively identify lung endothelial cells.[27,28] Surface-associated glycoconjugates present a unique pattern on lung endothelial cells, as exemplified by the unusual number of binding sites for peanut agglutinin.[14,29] Preproendothelin-1, present as early as E9.5 in the yolk sac, is high in lung endothelial cells and increases during subsequent embryonic development so that within a few days it is higher in lung endothelial cells than any other cell type.[30] Transcription factors involved in endothelial cell signaling are also selective. For example, HLF, a helix-loop-helix hypoxia-inducible factor that binds to a specific hypoxia response element, is most abundantly expressed in the lung where it appears to regulate VEGF production important for lung blood vessel development.[31,32] Among the negative markers of lung endothelium is the mannose receptor, which is found on most murine endothelial cells but is absent from lung endothelium.[33]

In our laboratory we have now established many endothelial cell lines, including those from the mouse lung and embryonic yolk sac.[34-37] The yolk sac cell lines, derived from E8–E12 embryos, are composed of primitive cells which can be induced to differentiate under the influence of appropriate organ microenvironments. We have recently shown, for example, that day 9 yolk sac endothelial cells can, when cocultured with brain rudiments from day 12 embryos, develop brain-specific properties.[37] This was illustrated by the expression and function of the brain-specific transporter gene *glut-1* and by the brain-specific activation of the multidrug resistance *(mdr-1)* gene responsible for drug resistance and the production of P-glycoprotein. Identification of the yolk sac-derived cells was achieved by transfecting the endothelial cells with a lac-Z reporter gene.

Experiments are now in progress to determine the effect of the lung rudiment environment in coculture on the differentiation of these yolk sac endothelial cells. To this end we have now labeled yolk sac endothelial cells with green fluorescence protein (GFP) as well as lac-Z, enabling us to follow the lung-specific differentiation of yolk sac-derived cells after coculture. We have obtained antibodies from Dr. Philippe Lasalle (ESM-1) and Dr. Benedict Pauli (LuECAM) that could serve as markers of lung-specific differentiation. The pattern of lectin binding to PNA and the downregulation of the mannose receptor will provide additional evidence of lung-specific differentiation. Following differentiation in coculture, cell sorting using GFP fluorescence will permit us to further characterize the endothelial cells generated in coculture.

The long-term goal of our research is, of course, to go beyond the establishment of markers and to determine the molecular basis for differentiation. By isolating endothelial cells before their exposure to the lung microenvironment and by procuring cells at various time points following coculture, we may be in a position to determine, by differential display and subtractive cloning, what genetic programs are activated and what specific genes are newly expressed or newly downregulated during the acquisition of organ specificity. Subsequently, these studies combined with the new information now being generated by the use of transgenic technologies in mice and the analysis of analogous genes in the Drosophila tracheal system, may place us in a better position to determine the basis of normal pulmonary functions as well as various pulmonary pathologies.

Acknowledgment   We thank Wanda Auerbach for editorial and bibliographic assistance.

References

1. Wagner RC. Endothelial cell embryology and growth. *Adv Microcirc* 1980; 9:45–75.
2. Reid L. The embryology of the lung. In: DeReuck AVS, Porter R, eds: *Development of the Lung*. CIBA Foundation Symposium. Boston: Little Brown & Co; 1967:109–124.
3. Demello DE, Sawyer D, Galvin N, et al. Early fetal development of lung vasculature. *Am J Respir Cell Mol Biol* 1997;16:568–581.
4. Taderera JV. Control of lung differentiation in vitro. *Dev Biol* 1967;16:489–512.
5. Gilbert SF. *Developmental Biology. 5th ed.* Sunderland, MA: Sinauer Associates; 1997.
6. Risau W, Flamme I. Vasculogenesis. *Annu Rev Cell Dev Biol* 1995;11:73–91.
7. Risau W. Mechanisms of angiogenesis. *Nature* 1997;386:671–674.
8. Auerbach W, Auerbach R. Angiogenesis inhibition: A review. *Pharmacol Ther* 1994;63:265–311.
9. Auerbach R, Auerbach W. Profound effects on vascular development caused by perturbations during organogenesis. *Am J Pathol* 1997;151: 1183–1186.
10. Noden DM. Origins and assembly of avian embryonic blood vessels. *Ann NY Acad Sci* 1990;588:236–249.

11. Noden DM. Embryonic origins and assembly of blood vessels. *Am J Resp Dis* 1989;140:1097–1103.
12. Poole TJ, Coffin JD. Vasculogenesis and angiogenesis: Two distinct morphogenetic mechanisms establish embryonic vascular pattern. *J Exp Zool* 1989;251:224–231.
13. Asahara T, Murohara T, Sullivan A, et al. Isolation of putative progenitor endothelial cells for angiogenesis. *Science* 1997;275:964–967.
14. Auerbach R. Vascular endothelial cell differentiation: Organ-specificity and selective affinities as the basis for developing anti-cancer strategies. *Int J Radiat Biol* 1991;60:1–10.
15. Auerbach R. Endothelial cell heterogeneity: Its role as a determinant of selective metastasis. In: Simionescu N, Simionescu O, eds: *Endothelial Cell Dysfunction*. New York: Plenum Press; 1992:427–437.
16. Ryan U, ed. *Endothelial Cells. Vol. 1–3*. Boca Raton, FL: CRC Press; 1989.
17. Charan NB, Baile EM, Pare PD. Bronchial vascular congestion and angiogenesis. *Eur Respir J* 1997;10:1173–1180.
18. Carmeliet P, Ferreira V, Breier G, et al. Abnormal blood vessel development and lethality in embryos lacking a single VEGF allele. *Nature* 1996; 380:435–439.
19. Ferrara N, Carver-Moore K, Chen H, et al. Heterozygous embryonic lethality induced by targeted inactivation of the VEGF gene. *Nature* 1996; 380:439–442.
20. Shalaby F, Rossant J, Yamaguchi TP, et al. Failure of blood-island formation and vasculogenesis in Flk-1-deficient mice. *Nature* 1995;376:62–66.
21. Fong G-H, Rossant J, Gertsenstein M, et al. Role of Flt-1 receptor tyrosine kinase in regulating the assembly of vascular endothelium. *Nature* 1995; 376:66–70.
22. Hanahan D. Signaling vascular morphogenesis and maintenance. *Science* 1997;277:48–50.
23. Maisonpierre PC, Suri C, Jones PF, et al. Angiopoietin-2, a natural antagonist for tie2 that disrupts in vivo angiogenesis. *Science* 1997;277:55–60.
24. Auerbach R, Alby L, Grieves J, et al. A monoclonal antibody against angiotensin-converting enzyme: Its use as a marker for murine, bovine, and human endothelial cells. *Proc Natl Acad Sci USA* 1982;279:7891–7895.
25. Zetter BR. Tumor cell interactions with elastin: Implications for pulmonary metastasis. *Am Rev Resp Dis* 1989;140:1456–1462.
26. Takahashi K, Uwabe Y, Sawasaki Y, et al. Increased secretion of urokinase-type plasminogen activator by human lung microvascular endothelial cells. *Am J Physiol* 1998;275:L47-L54.
27. Elble RC, Widom J, Gruber AD, et al. Cloning and characterization of lung-endothelial cell adhesion molecule-1 suggest it is an endothelial chloride channel. *J Biol Chem* 1997;272:27853-27861.
28. Lassalle P, Molet S, Janin A, et al. ESM-1 is a novel human endothelial cell-specific molecule expressed in the lung and regulated by cytokines. *J Biol Chem* 1996;271:20458-20464.
29. Belloni PN, Nicolson GL. Differential expression of cell surface glycoproteins on various organ-derived microvascular endothelia and endothelial cell cultures. *J Cell Physiol* 1988;136:398–410.
30. Chan TS, Lin CX, Chan WY, et al. Mouse preproendothelin-1 gene cDNA cloning, sequence analysis and determination of sites of expression during embryonic development. *Eur J Biochem* 1995;234:819–826.
31. Ladoux A, Frelin C. Cardiac expressions of HIF-1 alpha and HLF/EPAS,

two basic loop helix/PAS domain transcription factors involved in adaptative responses to hypoxic stresses. *Biochem Biophys Res Commun* 1997; 240:552–556.

32. Ema M, Taya S, Yokotani N, et al. A novel bHLH-PAS factor with close sequence similarity to hypoxia-inducible factor 1α regulates the VEGF expression and is potentially involved in lung and vascular development. *Proc Natl Acad Sci USA* 1997;94:4273–4278.

33. Takahashi K, Donovan MJ, Rogers RA, et al. Distribution of murine mannose receptor expression from early embryogenesis through to adulthood. *Cell Tissue Res* 1998;29:2311–2323.

34. Gumkowski F, Kaminska G, Kaminski M, et al. Heterogeneity of mouse vascular endothelium: In vitro studies of lymphatic, large blood vessel and microvascular endothelial cells. *Blood Vessels* 1987;24:11–23.

35. Auerbach R, Lu WC, Pardon E, et al. Specificity of adhesion between tumor cells and capillary endothelium: An in vitro correlate of preferential metastasis in vivo. *Cancer Res* 1987;47:1492–1496.

36. Wang SJ, Greer P, Auerbach R. Isolation and propagation of yolk sac-derived endothelial cells from a hypervascular transgenic mouse expressing a gain-of-function *fps/fes* proto-oncogene. *In Vitro Cell Dev Biol* 1996;32:292–299.

37. Yu D, Auerbach R. Induced brain-specific differentiation of mouse yolk sac endothelial cells. (Submitted for publication.)

Chapter 4

Structural Elements of Human Fetal and Neonatal Lung Vascular Development

Daphne E. deMello, MD

Introduction

A discussion of lung vascular structure requires consideration of the overall architectural arrangement of its tubes and of the cellular and matrix components that are its building blocks. The lung has a double arterial supply from the pulmonary and bronchial arteries and a double venous drainage through the pulmonary and bronchial veins.[1] It has an arterial and venous connection to each side of the heart.

The pulmonary artery supplies the respiratory units and pleura. It has two types of branches: (1) the conventional arteries that arise at an acute angle from the axial vessel and run a long course to the respiratory units at the distal end of the axis; and (2) the supernumerary arteries that arise as a side branch, at right angles to the main trunk and run a short course to supply respiratory units adjacent to the main axis. The supernumerary arteries are more numerous than the conventional—the ratio between the two is from 3:1 to 4:1 (Figure 1). The luminal cross-sectional area of the supernumerary arteries at their origin is a significant portion of all side branches. At different levels in the arterial tree it varies, but ranges from 25% to 45%.[2] This suggests a significant capacity and a role for the supernumeraries in recruitment of the pulmonary circulation as on exercise. The bronchial arteries supply

Supported in part by the National Institutes of Health Grant HL56000.

From: Weir EK, Archer SL, Reeves JT (eds). *The Fetal and Neonatal Pulmonary Circulations.*
Armonk, NY: Futura Publishing Company, Inc.; ©1999.

19 Week Fetus

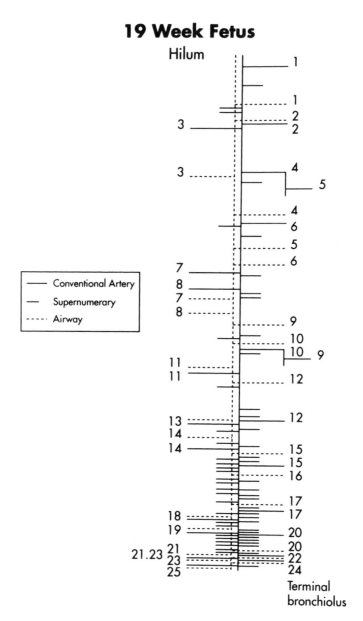

Figure 1. Reconstruction of the posterior basal artery and airway of the left lower lobe in a 19-week fetus. The airway branches and their accompanying conventional arteries are numbered, and the 58 supernumerary arteries are also shown. Actual length is 16 mm. (Reproduced with permission from Reference 2.)

the airway walls, ie, bronchi, bronchioli, and the large hilar structures.[3] The drainage pattern of the pulmonary veins is similar to the branching pattern of the pulmonary arteries in that there are conventional and supernumerary venous tributaries.[4] Of clinical significance is the fact that all intrapulmonary venous tributaries, whether from the airway walls or alveolar region, drain to the main pulmonary vein and to the *left* atrium, except for a small region around the hilum that drains to the systemic (azygos) system. Along the length of any vessel, the cellular/structural composition of each vessel, ie, elastic tissue and smooth muscle components, changes dramatically so that each segment of the lung's vascular tree is unique in its pattern of development, and in its normal mature structure as well as in its physiological response. Here, the pulmonary artery to pulmonary vein loop, of major importance in pulmonary hemodynamics, will be discussed.

Early Fetal Vascular Development

In the Mouse

Noden[5] described two processes involved in the assembly of blood vessels in the embryo, with particular reference to the yolk sac: angiogenesis, the branching of new vessels from preexisting ones, and vasculogenesis, the development of blood lakes that transform to vessels. However, little was known about development of the vasculature within an organ, and virtually nothing was known about the earliest events in the development of the lung's vasculature. Our study of the mouse lung[6] was undertaken to determine whether the processes that contribute to blood vessel assembly could be detected in early lung vascular development. Mouse embryos from 9 to 20 days in age were studied using a combination of techniques—light and transmission electron microscopy (TEM), Mercox vascular casts, and scanning electron microscopy (SEM)—which permitted interpretation of developmental processes during early gestation. The production of vascular casts at progressive gestational ages provides a means for obtaining a series of "stills" with which to unfold the evolving process of vascular development. The techniques used demonstrate that both arterial and venous systems develop concurrently (see following section, "In the Human"). Between 9 and 10 days, primitive angioblast precursors within the mesenchyme surrounding the lung bud form vascular lakes around hematopoietic cells (Figure 2). The earliest vascular cast obtained at 12 days (Figure 3) shows about four generations of central branches with no connection to the peripheral lung mesenchyme where, at this time, a dense collection of "lakes" containing

9 Days   10 Days

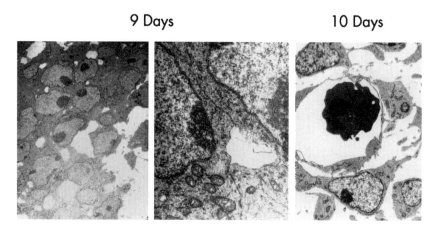

Figure 2. Transmission electron micrographs of fetal thorax. At 9 days, inter-
cellular spaces begin to appear within the densely packed mesenchyme
around the developing lung bud. Membrane bound vesicles and membranous
fragments within the spaces suggest that they result from discharge of intra-
cytoplasmic vesicles. (Reproduced with permission from Reference 6.) At 10
days, mesenchymal cells around the spaces have thinned to assume an en-
dothelial-like morphology. A hematopoietic precursor is seen within the space.

hematopoietic cells has developed independently. By 14 days, five to
seven generations of central branches, supernumerary, and conventional arteries can be recognized (Figures 3 and 4). The smallest central
vessels (~25μm in diameter) have established a connection with the
peripheral system so that now, casts of these peripheral vessels can
also be obtained. Between 15 days and term, the increasing complexity of the peripheral casts reflects an increase in connections between
the central and peripheral systems (Figures 3 and 5). At this time, the
decreased tortuosity and smoother profiles of the peripheral vessels
suggest a structural remodeling probably as a consequence of the increased blood flow that is now possible (Figure 6). Thus, in the mouse
lung, the two processes of vascular development, angiogenesis and
vasculogenesis, occur separately though concurrently. We emphasize
the significance of a third process, fusion, or communication between
the two separate systems, which is necessary to establish the completed circulation.

In the Human

The mouse experiments described above would be difficult to repeat
in the human in an effort to determine whether these three processes also

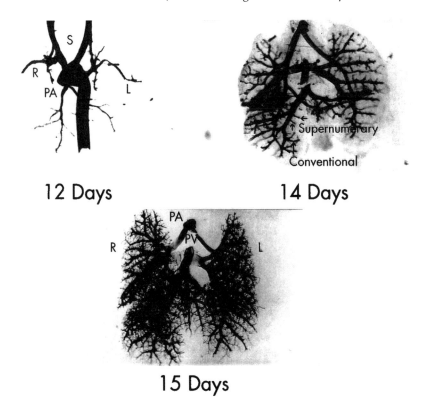

12 Days

14 Days

15 Days

Figure 3. Photomicrographs of pulmonary Mercox casts. At 12 days, only up to four generations of central branches are present, with no connection to the periphery. At 14 days, peripheral connections have been established so that casts of these vessels appear. The arterial (upper) and venous (lower) systems are both seen. At 15 days, increased connections with the peripheral system result in an increased complexity of the cast. S = systemic; R = right; L = left; PA = pulmonary artery; PV= pulmonary vein. (Reproduced with permission from Reference 6.)

contribute to development of the human lung vasculature. Consequently, for this study,[7] we utilized the unique resource of the Carnegie Collection of human embryos from the Carnegie Institution of Washington. The Collection is presently housed in the Museum of Human Development in the Armed Forces Institute of Pathology in Washington, D.C. We are grateful for the philanthropy of the industrialist Andrew Carnegie (Figure 7), who founded the Carnegie Institution, the foresight

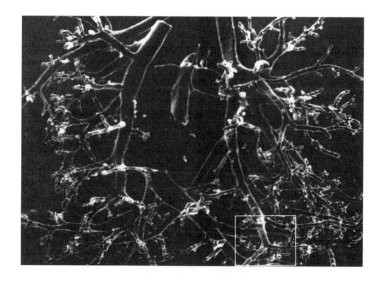

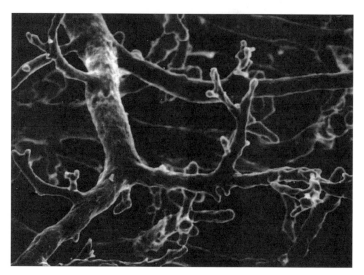

14 days

Figure 4. Scanning electron micrographs of lung vascular casts. Filling of some terminal buds suggests that fusion between the central and peripheral systems has occurred. The bottom panel is a magnified view of the boxed area in upper panel. (Reproduced with permission from Reference 6.)

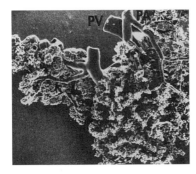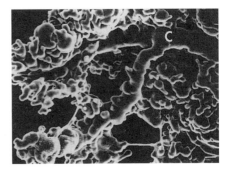

15 Days

Figure 5. Scanning electron micrographs of lung vascular casts. A complex peripheral network reflects extensive connections between the central and peripheral systems. The blind ending precapillary branches approach the future capillary bed at right angles. The arrow points to the most likely junction between the peripheral and central (C) systems. Note that the central vessels have a smooth profile whereas the peripheral vessels are irregular, perhaps reflecting their derivation by angiogenesis or vasculogenesis. (Reproduced with permission from Reference 6.)

and diligence of the anatomist Wilhelm His, the embryologist Franklin Mall who bequeathed this invaluable resource, and to George Streeter whose standardized stages of embryonic development facilitated this study.

Age Range of Embryos

Embryos from stages 10 to 23 were studied in addition to fetuses from 12 to 23 weeks. The availability of complete serial sections of entire embryos permitted determination of the sites of origin, pathway, and ending of a structure. Lakes are the first to form, being present within the primitive mesenchyme around the lung bud in the neck between stages 14 and 18 (32–44 days) (Figures 8 and 9). At stage 20 (50 1/2 days) (Figure 10), when five to six airway branches have formed, lakes are present in abundance in the subpleural mesenchyme. The pulmonary artery accompanies the bronchi only as far as the third or fourth generation. No continuity between the peripheral and central systems is detected as yet. This is first seen at stage

14 days

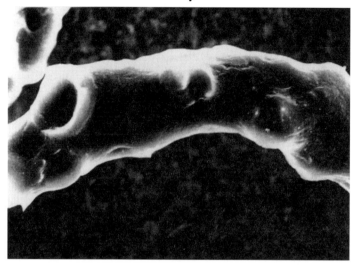

15 days

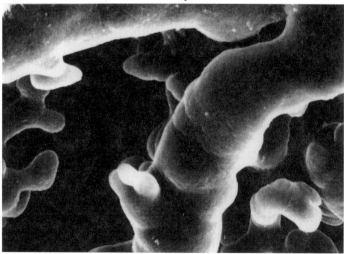

Figure 6. Scanning electron micrographs of lung vascular casts reveal surface pits at 14 days, probably indicating sites at which filamentous connections have broken. At 15 days, the surface is smoother and several filamentous structures are seen, probably identifying sites of future vascular connections. (Reproduced with permission from Reference 6.)

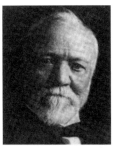 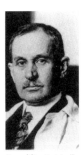 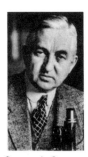 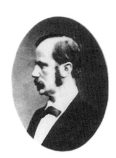

| Andrew Carnegie | Franklin P. Mall | George L. Streeter | Wilhelm His |
| (1835-1919) | (1862-1917) | (1873-1948) | (1831-1904) |

Figure 7. Important contributors to the invaluable Carnegie Collection of human embryos which are presently housed in the Human Developmental Anatomy Center at the Armed Forces Institute of Pathology in Washington, D.C.

32 days

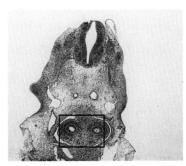 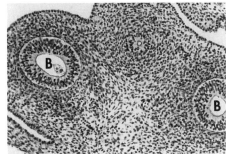

Stage 14

Figure 8. Low **(left)** and high **(right)** magnification views of a transverse section of a human embryo reveal dense mesenchyme enveloping right and left bronchi at the level of bifurcation. The thick-walled structure with a small lumen at rear is the esophagus. Blood lakes containing hematopoietic precursors **(box)** are already present in the mesenchyme; no pulmonary artery accompanies the bronchus as yet.

44 days

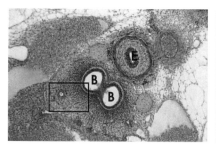

Stage 18

Figure 9. Low (left) and high (right) magnification views of a transverse section of a human embryo shows the bronchi (B) surrounded by mesenchyme, sectioned transversely at the bifurcation. The esophagus (E) is seen at the rear. Blood lakes (L) are now more numerous within the mesenchyme (box).

50 ½ days

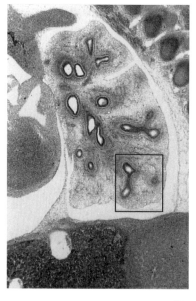

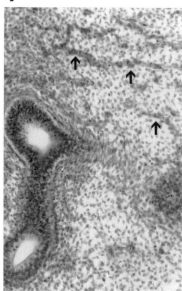

Stage 20

Figure 10. Low (left) and high (right) magnification views of a sagittally sectioned human embryo. At low power, the heart is seen at left and the bronchial generations at right. The bronchial artery accompanies only the first few generations of bronchi, while in the peripheral subpleural region (box), an extensive network of sinusoids resulting from coalescence of blood lakes has formed. No connection is seen between the central and peripheral systems.

54 days

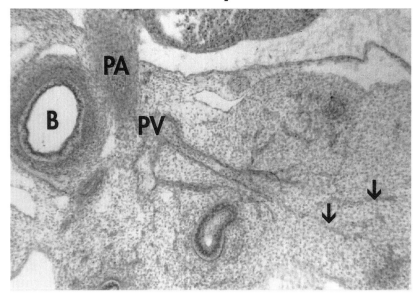

Stage 22

Figure 11. High power photomicrograph of the human embryonic lung shows a vascular channel extending from the peripheral network into the pulmonary vein (PV) at the hilum. The lobar pulmonary artery (PA) accompanies the bronchus (B) at the hilum.

22 (54 days), when a connection between peripheral lakes and a central thin walled structure, a hilar vein, is present, indicating that venous drainage is established first (Figure 11). Between stages 22 and 23, pulmonary arterial branches appear alongside airways but lag behind the airway by two to three generations (Figures 12 and 13). The artery is thick walled and the blind end is a solid cord of cells. Between 12 and 16 weeks, an extensive capillary network is developed in the mesenchyme surrounding the most distal airway buds that are beneath the pleura (Figure 14). The network is still separated from the airway buds by mesenchyme, and the distal tip of the pulmonary artery is still two to three generations behind the end of the airway. By 22 to 23 weeks, the capillary network is intimately associated with airway epithelium and bulges into the airspace, ie, the air-blood barrier has formed (Figure 15). By this time, the pulmonary artery accompanies the most distal airway branch just beneath the pleura. Thus, it appears that the three processes of vascular development occur in the human as well, but that the venous circulation is the first to be completed.

54 days

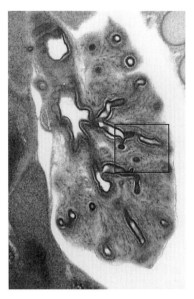
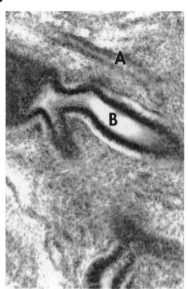

Stage 22

Figure 12. Low **(left)** and high **(right)** magnification views of a sagittally sectioned human embryo. The segmental pulmonary arteries (A) accompany the airways (B), but end as blind solid cords proximal to the distal end of the airway. An extensive vascular network exists in the intervening mesenchyme between airways.

56 ¹/₂ days

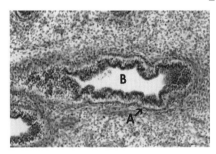
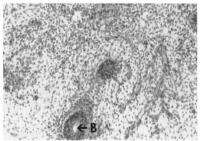

Stage 23

Figure 13. Photomicrographs of human embryonic lung. The pulmonary artery (A) accompanies the airway (B) to its distal tip. The arborizing network within the mesenchyme surrounding the most peripheral airway branches is separated from the airway by intervening mesenchyme.

12 weeks   **16 weeks**

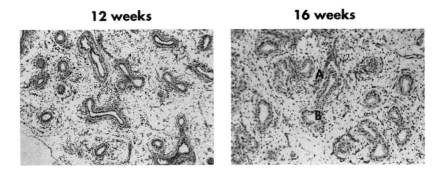

Figure 14. Photomicrographs of human fetal lung. At 12 weeks, the pleura is seen at the lower left corner. The subpleural airway buds are not accompanied by a pulmonary artery and are widely separated by intervening mesenchyme containing a vast network of vessels. By 16 weeks, the pulmonary artery (A) accompanies the airway but has still not reached the distal end. The mesenchyme between airways is significantly reduced.

22 weeks   **23 weeks**

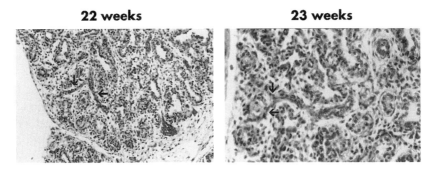

Figure 15. Photomicrographs of human fetal lung. At 22 weeks, the pleura is seen at the lower left corner, and the pulmonary artery (arrows) accompanies the airways up to the distal subpleural tip. At 23 weeks, the distal end of the pulmonary artery (arrows) encircles the end of the airway.

Late Fetal Vascular Development

Arteries

The full complement of preacinar vessels is present by the end of the 16th week. Subsequently, up to birth, there is a change in size only,[2] reflecting most likely matrix adaptation. Intra-acinar arterial branching occurs as respiratory bronchioli and saccules develop. Conventional and supernumerary arteries are identified here. A sphincter-like structure is present at the opening of many supernumerary arteries; it protrudes into the lumen of the axial or conventional artery.[8] More recently, Bunton et al[9] have elaborated on the structure of this valve, describing it as a "baffle valve." This site is heavily innervated by aminergic and adrenergic fibers, supporting the concept that valve function and, consequently, blood flow to the supernumerary artery is tightly controlled. This is further supported by the demonstration that the supernumerary and conventional arteries have a different response to pharmacological agents: the conventionals are more sensitive to constrictive agents, and the response of the supernumeraries to vasoconstrictors is potentiated by nitric oxide, whereas the conventionals are unaffected.[10] Variable diameters of the supernumerary arteries may provide for different opening pressures and thus progressive recruitment with demand. They also provide a means for collateral blood flow from a site proximal to the block in the axial artery to a capillary bed distal to the block, forming an "arcade" between the pulmonary arteries. The plexiform lesions of pulmonary occlusive vascular disease are formed at the origin of supernumerary branches.

Wall Structure

Elastin

The structure of the arterial wall changes from proximal to distal vessels in terms of elastic laminae thickness and number and layers of smooth muscle cells.[1,11] The main pulmonary artery has a structure similar to the aorta; ie, it is an elastic artery, with more than 7 elastic laminae, up to the seventh generation in the 19-week-old fetus. More peripherally, there is a transitional structure with 4–7 elastic laminae. Distal to this level the structure is muscular, with less than 4 elastic laminae and, finally, in small peripheral arteries, only an internal and external elastic lamina is present.

Smooth Muscle

Along any arterial pathway, a wholly muscular wall becomes partially muscular (3000 μm in diameter down to 30 μm), and then non-muscular (up to 150 μm in diameter).[1,11-14] At birth, no muscle is present in arterial walls beyond the level of the terminal bronchiolus.

Wall Thickness

Fetal vessel wall thickness is higher relative to external diameter, roughly double that in the adult.

Veins

The ratio of conventional and supernumerary veins is the same throughout fetal life, childhood, and in the adult.[4]

Structure

In early fetal life veins are free of muscle, which first appears in the wall at 28-weeks gestation, and is a continuous coat at term.

Bronchial Arteries

The bronchial arteries appear between 9 and 12 weeks as outgrowths from the descending aorta, and supply the walls of the bronchial tree and large pulmonary vessels as far as the cartilage plate extends.[15] The peripheral portion of the lung is supplied only by the pulmonary arteries at this time but, by birth, the bronchial arteries extend as far as the bronchioli. Pulmonary artery to bronchial artery anastomoses exist in vessels 35–100 μm in diameter.[3]

Transitional Circulation

At birth, as the lung expands with air, adaptation by the pulmonary arteries causes a rapid drop in pulmonary artery pressure. There are structural changes in the resistance segment of the pulmonary arterial tree resulting in changes in the external diameter and wall thickness of this precapillary segment.

In the Rabbit

Perinatal Adaptation, Normal and in Hypoxia

In the newborn rabbit, within the first 6 hours of birth, there is a fluctuation in the percentage of medial thickness which first decreases and then partially recovers. By 48–72 hours, the medial thickness decreases while the external diameter increases. This pattern of vascular change is not affected by cesarean delivery or by delivery into 10% hypobaric hypoxia.[16] Ultrastructurally, in the newborn rabbit, the resistance segment comprises a complete muscle coat one to four cell layers thick. The adaptation process is reflected by ultrastructural changes in the endothelial and smooth muscle cells of these vessels. Within an hour of birth, the endothelial cells become attenuated and there is a shift in caveolae from the luminal to the abluminal membrane. Between 6 and 72 hours, the numbers of caveolae within the smooth muscle cells of the media increase while the cells become slender and attenuated. Whereas hypoxia does not alter this pattern of change, evidence of cell injury is present.[17] In the pig, within 5 minutes of birth, there is dilatation and recruitment of small intra-acinar arteries associated with a "loss of arterial muscle."[18-20] Between 24 hours and 2 weeks, further loss of arterial muscle occurs. Presumably the "loss" of muscle is a consequence of the vascular dilatation and thinning that occurs as part of the adaptation process.

Tropoelastin

Elastin, the building block for elastic laminae, is an important component of the vessel wall. In preparation for extrauterine existence, the distribution of tropoelastin (TE) changes in the different segments of the rat fetal arteries and veins. In the rat, tropoelastin is produced in each of the three coats of the vessel: the intima, media, and adventitia (Figure 16).[21] In arteries and veins at different levels in the branching tree, the pattern of expression is different for each of the cell types and the timing of expression reflects changing hemodynamics and, hence, function. In the adult rat lung there is no detectable expression of TE in arteries, veins, or within the alveolar region.

Neonatal Vascular Development

Normal

In the newborn, development of new blood vessels is intra-acinar. A broad picture of intra-acinar lung growth is first provided as a framework within which to discuss vascular development.

Acinar Development

The acinus, the portion of the lung subtended by the terminal bronchiolus, is simple and small at birth. It generally comprises three to four generations of respiratory bronchioli and one or two alveolar ducts and saccules that make up the alveolar region. It is in this peripheral region that postnatal alveolar development occurs, increasing alveolar number from approximately 24 million at birth to approximately 300 million by 8 years.[22-26]

TROPOELASTIN - ISH

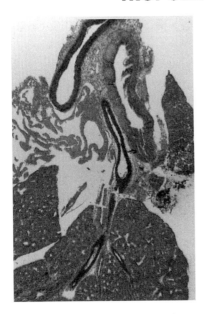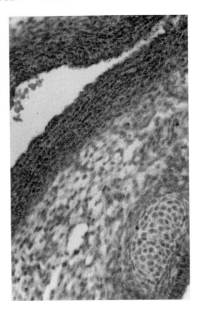

Figure 16. In situ hybridization for tropoelastin (TE) mRNA in a day 19 fetal rat lung. At **left**, an intense TE message is present in the pulmonary artery at the hilum (top) and in its segmental branches. The adjacent pulmonary vein shows no message for TE. At **right**, a TE message is seen within all three coats of the main pulmonary artery, intima, media, and adventitia, but not in luminal erythrocytes. (Reproduced with permission from Reference 21).

Intra-acinar Arterial Branching

With the growth of new alveoli there is an increase in the number of arterial branches within the acinus. Until 18 months of age, new conventional arteries appear, and supernumeraries develop for up to 8 years. Additional supernumeraries also appear in the preacinar region. The arteries increase in size, proximally more than distally. The ratio of alveoli to arteries remains constant throughout childhood at approximately 40:1. After age 10, when alveolar multiplication is complete and alveoli increase in size, the ratio of alveoli to arteries begins to drop.

Structure

The distribution of preacinar elastic and transitional arteries is unchanged during childhood, although the size range varies with age. However, in the small arteries, significant structural changes occur so that the appearance of medial smooth muscle in these intra-acinar vessels is delayed and muscle coats do not appear in alveolar wall arteries until about age 10. The larger arteries lose their fetal wall thickness by about 4 months, whereas in vessels less than 200 μm in diameter, wall thickness gradually increases.

Veins

During childhood, the veins also increase in size and there is an increase in the number of peripheral veins.[4] In a unit area of lung, the number of veins exceeds that of the arteries, presumably to accept the relatively greater blood flow.

In Disease

Developmental abnormalities of the pulmonary vasculature may affect the number of branches formed or the structure of the vessel wall. Structural alterations may be intrinsic or the result of an adaptational response to abnormal hemodynamics. In many types of congenital heart disease, for instance, the pulmonary circulation develops normally in utero, but adaptational changes occur after birth.[26-29] An exception is the systemic arteriovenous anastomosis in which high blood flow before birth gives rise to an abnormal vascular structure at birth. Congenital diaphragmatic hernia—the restricted space available for lung growth—produces hypoplastic lungs with a reduced number of airways and alveoli. Because the pulmonary arteries travel and branch with the airways, their number is also reduced, and their size is small but appropriate for the smaller lung volume. Arterial structure is also altered so that the walls are thicker and muscle extends into smaller, more peripheral vessels.[30-32]

Idiopathic (Persistent) Pulmonary Hypertension of the Newborn

Idiopathic (persistent) pulmonary hypertension of the newborn (PPHN) occurs with or without meconium aspiration (also known as meconium aspiration syndrome). In both instances, the *pattern* of arterial growth is normal, but *structural* alterations are present at birth and these have significant functional effects.[33-37] The preacinar arteries are either small or of normal size, but they frequently have increased collagenous adventitia. The intra-acinar arteries have thicker walls because of excessive muscularization and there is peripheral or "precocious muscularization"—muscle coats within smaller, normally nonmuscularized arteries.

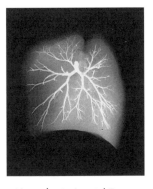 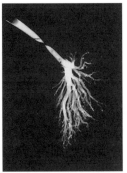 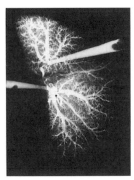

| Hypoplastic Arterial Tree
Maternal Cocaine Use | Osteogenesis
Imperfecta | Camptomelic
Dwarfism |

Figure 17. Postmortem barium angiograms of newborn human lungs, show a range of abnormal growth patterns for pre- and intra-acinar pulmonary arteries reflecting deranged angiogenesis: arterial hypoplasia **(left)** is reflected by the reduced branching and small caliber of the pulmonary arteries; in osteogenesis imperfecta **(center)**, there is tortuosity and crowding of the arteries in addition to reduced branching; in camptomelic dwarfism **(right)**, although lung volume is small, arterial size and branching are not severely affected.

Hypoplastic Vascular Bed

Here, the branching pattern is abnormal (reduced number) and vessel size is also reduced, resulting in an overall contracted vascular bed (Figure 17). Here also, hemodynamic responses produce excessive and precocious muscularization of intra-acinar arteries.[38,39]

Vicarious Experiments of Nature

The various abnormalities of pulmonary vascular development seen in the fetus and newborn can be regarded as experiments of nature. It is useful to attempt analysis of these recognized abnormalities in the context of the processes involved in early lung vascular development as outlined above.

Disordered Angiogenesis

Absence of the Main Pulmonary Artery or its Branches

In this condition, the central pulmonary artery to a lung is absent and the lung is supplied by a collateral vessel from the systemic circulation. The presumption is that central sprouting or angiogenesis fails, but that peripheral vasculogenesis is not affected and the systemic arteries assume the role of the pulmonary arterial tree.[40,41]

Misalignment of Blood Vessels

In this disorder, there is an anomalous relationship between the central pulmonary arteries and veins, with the veins sharing the same adventitial sheath as the arteries instead of traveling in their usual location within pulmonary septa. The abnormality, when restricted to misalignment of central vessels,[42] suggests disordered sprouting or angiogenesis. However, frequently there is abnormal development of the peripheral vascular bed as well, manifested as alveolar capillary dysplasia.[43-48] In this instance, there is an additional aberration in vasculogenesis (see below).

Dwarfism

In the skeletal dysplasias, the small thoracic cage is associated with small lungs. Analysis of airway, alveolar, and vascular development in fatal cases reveals a mixed pattern of disturbed growth; although all lungs are hypoplastic and have reduced airway and arterial branching, there is a wide range in the severity of alteration which cannot be explained by lung size alone.[49] For example, alveolar multiplication is sometimes paradoxically increased. Pulmonary vascular morphometry reveals a variety of structural features which, again, do not correlate with lung size.[50] We conclude that in some cases, the small thoracic cage results in a hypoplastic vascular bed. In others, however, there is a superadded direct metabolic effect, most likely related to the nature of the skeletal dysplasia which interferes with vascular development (Figure 17).

Disordered Vasculogenesis

Alveolar Capillary Dysplasia

In this rare and fatal disorder,[43-48] alveolar capillaries fail to form, with a consequent absence of formation of the normal air-blood barriers. When widespread throughout the lung, this condition is, of course, incompatible with independent air-breathing existence. It may, however, affect only one lobe or part of a lobe of the lung. When confined to the peripheral lung vasculature as alveolar capillary dysplasia, this condition reflects a disorder in vasculogenesis. It may be associated with misalignment of central vessels (see above) which points to a failure of a common control mechanism that governs both angiogenesis and vasculogenesis.

Fusion

The intrapulmonary arteriovenous malformation[51,52] may reflect a disorder of this third process—fusion—between the central angiogenic and peripheral vasculogenic components of early lung vascular development. Generally, this is a circumscribed lesion suggesting that overall angiogenesis and vasculogenesis has progressed normally, but that the mechanism that regulates fusion (? via chemotaxis) focally permits the faulty communication to be established. Rarely, the process is diffuse,[51] indicating a global failure of the fusion process.

Cellular and Molecular Events Involved in Lung Vascular Growth

The three processes involved in early lung vascular growth, angiogenesis, vasculogenesis, and fusion, were described in an earlier section in this chapter. Whereas these processes are distinct, it is likely that they share at least some regulatory mechanisms. Regulation may be effected through the actions of growth factors, the influence of genes, or through cell-cell interactions. The implication of factors or genes involved in vascular growth has arisen either from observing their expression within developing vessels, or from experiments in which overexpression or deprivation of select factors or genes has resulted in disordered vascular growth. A list, which is by no means complete, and subject to rapid expansion with advances in knowledge, is indicated in Table 1. This subject is discussed in greater detail later in this monograph (Chapters 6, 7, 9, 10, 12, and 17). Here, only select examples are mentioned by way of introduction.

Specific Factors

VEGF and VRP

Vascular endothelial growth factor (VEGF) is a potent mitogen and chemoattractant for endothelial cells.[53-55] In the human 16–22 week fetal lung, it is not present in vascular endothelial cells, although it is abundant in epithelial cells and myocytes. The tyrosine kinases flt-1 (VEGF-R1) and flk-1/KDR (VEGF-R2) are VEGF receptor proteins (VRP) and are expressed by endothelium.[56,57] In the mouse, VEGF is secreted by stromal

Table 1

Factors, Genes, and Receptors Involved in Vascular Growth

Factors	Genes	Receptors
VEGF and VRP	Flt	Tyrosine kinases:
PDGF	Tie	flt-4, flt-1, KDR(flk-1)
TNF	B-61	Angiotensin II Type 2
FGF	F-31	alk-1
Endothelin-1		
ACE		
Angiontensin type 1		
Laminin-α1, α5, β2		
NOS		
CD34		
HNF3β		
PlGF		
Interleukin-1		
TGF-β		
Angiopoietin		

VEGF = vascular endothelial growth factor; PDGF = platelet derived growth factor; FGF = fibroblast growth factor; VRP = VEGF receptor protein; ACE = angiotensin converting enzyme; NOS = nitric oxide synthase; HNF3β = hepatocyte nuclear factor 3; PlGF = placenta growth factor; TGF-β = transforming growth factor.

and mesenchymal cells and, during vascular development, there is coordinate expression of ligand and receptor. These studies suggest that VEGF and its receptors play an important role in both angiogenesis and vasculogenesis, and that a paracrine mechanism is involved.

Genetic Influence: Excess or Deprivation Experiments

VEGF, Flt-1, and Flk-1

The importance of VEGF in embryonic development is reflected by the fact that absence of even one allele (heterozygosity) results in death at E11-E12 with defects in vessel formation.[58,59] These studies also indicate a dose-dependent effect of VEGF on the developing vasculature. VEGF dose dependence was shown in avian embryo studies in which increased VEGF dosage, whether by microinjection or by VEGF-expressing retroviruses, resulted in an overgrowth of vessels.[60,61] Flt-1 null mice embryos die between E8.5 and E9.5 with abnormal vasculature, which suggests a defect in angiogenesis.[62] Flk-1 knockout mice embryos also die between E8.5 and E9.5 but these embryos almost totally lack vascular structures, pointing to a failure of formation of blood islands or vasculogenesis.[63]

TGF-β

Interactions between endothelial cells and undifferentiated mesenchymal cells, or between endothelial cells and smooth muscle cells or pericytes, lead to activation of transforming growth factor-β (TGF-β).[64,65] Activated TGF-β has been shown to inhibit endothelial and smooth muscle cell growth and migration,[66-70] and to induce differentiation of mesenchymal cells into smooth muscle cells and pericytes.[64] This would explain why approximately one-half of the TGF-β null mice and approximately one-quarter of the heterozygotes have defective hematopoiesis and vasculogenesis leading to in utero death.[71] In the human, it appears that disruptions in TGF-β signaling leads to abnormal vascular development. This is suggested by genetic studies in patients with hereditary hemorrhagic telangiectasia in whom mutations in genes encoding for endoglin[72] and activin receptor-like kinase 1[73] have been identified. These receptors are both expressed in endothelial cells.

Tie Receptor

These receptor tyrosine kinases appear to be specific for vascular endothelium. Preliminary evidence suggests that, with regard to the lung, this family of genes plays an important and differential role in the regulation of the processes of vasculogenesis and angiogenesis. In the mouse, expression of the tie-1 gene begins early in gestation (E8.5) in angioblasts, and continues throughout.[74] In the adult, however, expression is limited to capillaries within lung alveolar septa. Tie-1 null mice die shortly after birth of respiratory distress and reveal ultrastructural defects in the integrity of the endothelium, although overall vascular patterning is normal.[54] In murine chimeras, at E15.5, tie-1 deficient cells were present in the lung but, in the adult, there were reduced numbers in the lung vasculature.[75]

Conclusion

The early stages of lung vascular development involve three processes: angiogenesis, which contributes largely to the proximal vasculature; vasculogenesis, which contributes to the peripheral vasculature; and fusion between the proximal and peripheral systems, which establishes a circulation. Subsequently, and with increasing blood flow, proximal vessel growth involves an increase in size and a change in matrix components in the vessel wall. Peripherally, as alveoli multiply, angiogenesis occurs to expand the intra-acinar arterial and capillary bed. Hemodynamic changes resulting from increased blood flow lead to remodeling of the peripheral vascular tree as well. With identification of the molecules and genes involved in vessel growth, the regulatory mechanisms governing the processes of vascular cell differentiation, proliferation, migration, signal transduction, and remodeling will be elucidated. This, in turn, will explain the pathogenetic mechanisms at work in the variety of lung vascular anomalies encountered in the fetus and newborn.

Acknowledgment The author thanks Professor Lynne M. Reid for her helpful discussion and review of the manuscript.

References

1. Hislop A, Reid L. Growth and development of the respiratory system: Anatomical Development. In: Davis JA, Dobbing J, eds: *Scientific Foundations of Paediatrics*. 2nd ed. London: Heinemann Medical Publications; 1981:390–431.
2. Hislop A, Reid L. Intrapulmonary arterial development in fetal life-branching pattern and structure. *J Anat* 1972;113:35–48.
3. Robertson B. The normal intrapulmonary arterial pattern of the human late fetal and neonatal lung. *Acta Paediatr Scand* 1967;56:249.
4. Hislop A, Reid L. Fetal and childhood development of the intrapulmonary veins in man-branching pattern and structure. *Thorax* 1973;28:313–319.
5. Noden DM. Embryonic origins and assembly of blood vessels. *Am Rev Respir Dis* 1989;140:1097–1103.
6. deMello DE, Sawyer D, Galvin N, et al. Early fetal development of the mouse pulmonary vasculature. *Am J Respir Cell Mol Biol* 1997;16:568–581.
7. deMello DE, Reid LM. Embryonic and early fetal development of human lung vasculature and its functional implications. (Submitted for publication.)
8. Elliott FM, Reid L. Some new facts about the pulmonary artery and its branching pattern. *Clin Radiol* 1965;16:193–198.
9. Bunton, D, Fisher A, Shaw AM, et al. Musculoelastic structure at origin of pulmonary supernumerary artery resembles a baffle valve. *Br J Pharmacol* 1996;119:323P. Abstract.
10. Bunton D, Fisher A, MacDonald A, et al. Responses to agonists in bovine pulmonary conventional and supernumerary arteries: Effect of endogenous nitric oxide. *Br J Pharmacol* 1995;116:319P.
11. Hislop A, Reid L. Formation of the pulmonary vasculature. In: Hodson WA, ed: *Development of the Lung*. In: Lenfant C, ed: *Lung Biology in Health and Disease*. Vol 6. New York: Marcel Dekker; 1977;6:37–86.
12. deMello DE, Reid LM. Pre and post-natal development of the pulmonary circulation. In: Chernick V, Mellins RB, eds: *Basic Mechanisms of Pediatric Respiratory Disease: Cellular and Integrative*. Philadelphia: BC Decker Inc; 1991:36–54.
13. deMello DE, Reid LM. Arteries and veins. In: Crystal RG, West JB, Barnes PJ, et al, eds: *The Lung: Scientific Foundations*. 2nd ed. Philadelphia: Lippincott Raven Press; 1997:1117–1127.
14. Reid L. Structural remodeling of the pulmonary vasculature by environmental change and disease. In: Wagner WW Jr, Weir EK, eds: *The Pul-*

monary Circulation and Gas Exchange. Armonk, New York: Futura Publishing Co Inc; 1994:77–105.

15. Boyden EA. The developing bronchial arteries in a fetus of the 12th week. *Am J Anat* 1970;129:357–368.

16. deMello DE, Gashi-Luci L, Hu LM, et al. Effect of hypoxia on post-natal vascular adaption in the newborn rabbit. *FASEB J* 1988;2:A1181.

17. deMello DE, Thomas K, Heyman S, et al. Ultrastructural features of resistance arteries of newborn rabbits during perinatal adaptation in normoxia and hypoxia. *Lab Invest* 1992;(66):1:4P.

18. Haworth SG, Hislop AA. Adaptation of the pulmonary circulation to extra-uterine life in the pig and its relevance to the human infant. *Cardiovas Res* 1981;15(2):108–119.

19. Haworth SG, Hislop AA. Effect of hypoxia on adaptation of the pulmonary circulation to extra-uterine life in the pig. *Cardiovas Res* 1982;293–303.

20. Haworth SG, Hall SM, Chew M, et al. Thinning of fetal pulmonary arterial wall and postnatal remodeling: Ultrastructural studies on the respiratory unit arteries of the pig. *Virchows Arch* 1987;411:161–171.

21. Noguchi A, Samaha H, deMello DE. Tropoelastin gene expression in the rat pulmonary vasculature: A developmental study. *Ped Res* 1992;31(3):280–285.

22. deMello DE, Davies P, Reid LM. Lung growth and development. In: Simmons DH, ed. *Curr Pulmonol* 1989;10:159–208.

23. Hislop A, Reid L. Pulmonary arterial development during childhood: Branching pattern and structure. *Thorax* 1973;28:129–135.

24. Hislop A. The fetal and childhood development of the pulmonary circulation and its disturbance in certain types of congenital heart disease (dissertation). University of London, 1971.

25. Dunnill MS. Postnatal growth of the lung. *Thorax* 1962;17:329–333.

26. Davies G, Reid L. Growth of the alveoli and pulmonary arteries in childhood. *Thorax* 1970;25:669–681.

27. Hislop A, Haworth SG, Shinebourne EA, et al. Quantitative structural analysis of pulmonary vessels in isolated ventricular septal defect in infancy. *Br Heart J* 1975;37:1014–1021.

28. Haworth SG, Sauer U, Buhlmeyer K, et al. Development of the pulmonary circulation in ventricular septal defect: A quantitative structural study. *Am J Cardiol* 1977;40:781–788.

29. Rabinovitch MS, Haworth S, Vance Z, et al. Early pulmonary vascular changes in congenital heart disease studied in biopsy tissue. *Hum Pathol* 1980;11:499–509.

30. Beals DA, Schloo BL, Vacanti JP, et al. Pulmonary growth and remodeling in infants with high-risk congenital diaphragmatic hernia. *J Pediatr Surg* 1992;27(8):997–1001; discussion 1001–1002.

31. Geggel R, Murphy J, Langleben D, et al. Congenital diaphragmatic hernia: Arterial structural changes and persistent pulmonary hypertension after surgical repair. *J Pediatr* 1985;107:457–464.

32. Kittagawa N, Hislop A, Boyden EA, et al. Lung hypoplasia in congenital diaphragmatic hernia: A quantitative study of airway, artery and alveolar development. *Br J Surg* 1971;58:342–346.

33. Geggel RL, Reid L. The structural basis of PPHN. In: Philips JB III, ed: *Clinics in Perinatology*. Vol. II. Third Annual Symposium on Neonatal Pulmonary Hypertension. Philadelphia: WB Saunders; 1984:525–549.

34. Fox WW, Gewitz MH, Dinwiddie R, et al. Pulmonary hypertension in the perinatal aspiration syndromes. *J Pediatr* 1977;59:205–211.

35. Haworth SG, Reid L. Persistent fetal circulation: Newly recognized structural features. *J Pediatr* 1976;88:614–620.
36. Murphy JD, Rabinovitch M, Goldstein JD, et al. The structural basis of persistent pulmonary hypertension of the newborn infant. *J Pediatr* 1981;98: 962–967.
37. Murphy JD, Vawter, G, Reid L. Pulmonary vascular disease in fatal meconium aspiration. *J Pediatr* 1984;104:758–762.
38. Rendas A, Brown ER, Avery ME, et al. Prematurity, hypoplasia of the pulmonary vascular bed and hypertension: Fatal outcome in a ten-month-old infant. *Am Rev Respir Dis* 1980;121:873–880.
39. Haworth SG, Reid LM. Quantitative structural study of pulmonary circulation in the newborn with pulmonary atresia. *Thorax* 1977;32:129–133.
40. Hentrich F, Stoermer J, Wiesemann G. Unilateral proximal aplasia of the pulmonary artery: Studies on the clinical significance and embryologic interpretation. *Klinische Padiatrie* 1984;196:311–314.
41. Herraiz SI, Perez GW, Vergara RF, et al. Unilateral agenesis of the pulmonary artery: Experience with four cases. *Anales Espanoles de Pediatria* 1993;38:139–144.
42. Wagenvoort CA. Misalignment of lung vessels: A syndrome causing persistent neonatal pulmonary hypertension. *Hum Pathol* 1986;17:727–730.
43. Sirkin W, O'Hare BP, Cox PN, et al. Alveolar capillary dysplasia: Lung biopsy diagnosis, nitric oxide responsiveness, and bronchial generation count. *Pediatr Pathol Lab Med* 1997;17(1):125–132.
44. Janney CG, Askin FB, Kuhn C. Congenital alveolar capillary dysplasia: An unusual cause of respiratory distress in the newborn. *Am J Clin Pathol* 1981;76:722–727.
45. Langston C. Misalignment of pulmonary veins and alveolar capillary dysplasia. *Pediatr Pathol* 1991;11:163–170.
46. Cater G, Thibault DW, Beatty EC, et al. Misalignment of lung vessels and alveolar capillary dysplasia: A cause of persistent pulmonary hypertension. *J Pediatr* 1989;114:293–300.
47. Boggs S, Harris MC, Hoffman DJ, et al. Misalignment of pulmonary veins with alveolar capillary dysplasia: Affected siblings and variable phenotypic expression. *J Pediatr* 1994;124:125–128.
48. Cullinane C, Cox PN, Silver MM. Persistent pulmonary hypertension of the newborn due to alveolar capillary dysplasia. *Pediatr Pathol* 1992;12:499–514.
49. deMello DE, Reid L. Patterns of disturbed lung growth in newborns with skeletal dysplasia. *Mod Pathol* 1990;3(1):2P.
50. Sanford W, deMello D, Reid L. Patterns of pulmonary arterial growth in hypoplastic lungs of skeletal dysplasia. *Lab Invest* 1993;68(1):8P,#44.
51. Kapur S, Rome J, Chandra RS. Diffuse pulmonary arteriovenous malformation in a child with polysplenia syndrome. *Pediatr Pathol Lab Med* 1995;15:463–468.
52. Storck M, Mickley V, Abendroth D, et al. Pulmonary arteriovenous malformations: Aspects of surgical therapy. *Vasa* 1996;25:54–59.
53. Shifren JL, Doldi N, Ferrara N, et al. In the human fetus, vascular endothelial growth factor is expressed in epithelial cells and myocytes, but not vascular endothelium: Implications for mode of action. *J Clin Endocrinol Metab* 1994;79(1):316–322.
54. Beck L Jr, D'Amore PA. Vascular development: Cellular and molecular regulation. *FASEB J* 1997;11(5):365–373.

55. Stenmark KR, Mecham RP. Cellular and molecular mechanisms of pulmonary vascular remodeling. *Annu Rev Physiol* 1997;59:89–144.
56. Breier G, Clauss M, Risau W. Coordinate expression of vascular endothelial growth factor receptor-1 (flt-1) and its ligand suggests a paracrine regulation of murine vascular development. *Dev Dyn* 1995;204(3):228–239.
57. Kaipainen A, Korhonen J, Pajusola K, et al. The related flt4, flt1, and kdr receptor tyrosine kinases show distinct expression patterns in human fetal endothelial cells. *J Exp Med* 1993;178(6):2077–2088.
58. Carmeliet P, Ferreira V, Breier G, et al. Abnormal blood vessel development and lethality in embryos lacking a single VEGF allele. *Nature* 1996; 380:435–439.
59. Ferrara N, Carver-Moore K, Chen H, et al. Heterozygous embryonic lethality induced by targeted inactivation of the VEGF gene. *Nature* 1996; 380:439–442.
60. Drake CJ, Little CD. Exogenous vascular endothelial growth factor induces malformed and hyperfused vessels during embryonic neovascularization. *Proc Natl Acad Sci USA* 1995;92:7657–7661.
61. Flamme I, von Reutern M, Drexler HCA, et al. Overexpression of vascular endothelial growth factor in the avian embryo induces hypervascularization and increased vascular permeability without alterations of embryonic pattern formation. *Dev Biol* 1995;171:399–414.
62. Fong GH, Rossant J, Gertsenstein M, et al. Role of the flt-1 receptor tyrosine kinase in regulating the assembly of vascular endothelium. *Nature* 1995;376:66–70.
63. Shalaby F, Rossant J, Yamaguchi TP, et al. Failure of blood-island formation and vasculogenesis in Flk-1 deficient mice. *Nature* 1995;376:62–66.
64. Rohovsky SA, Hirschi KK, D'Amore PA. Growth factor effects on a model of vessel formation. *Surg Forum* 1996;47:390–391.
65. Antonelli-Orlidge A, Saunders KB, Smith SR, et al. An activated form of transforming growth factor β is produced by cocultures of endothelial cells and pericytes. *Proc Natl Acad Sci USA* 1989;86:4544–4548.
66. Orlidge A, D'Amore PA. Inhibition of capillary endothelial cell growth by pericytes and smooth muscle cells. *J Cell Biol* 1987;105:1455–1462.
67. Sato Y, Rifkin DB. Inhibition of endothelial cell movement by pericytes and smooth muscle cell: Activation of a latent transforming growth factor-β 1-like molecule by plasmin during co-culture. *J Cell Biol* 1989;109: 309–315.
68. D'Amore PA, Smith SR. Growth factor effects on cells of the vascular wall: A survey. *Growth Factors* 1993;8:61–75.
69. Heimark RL, Twardzik DR, Schwartz SM. Inhibition of endothelial regeneration by type-β transforming growth factor from platelets. *Science* 1986;233:1078–1080.
70. Battegay EJ, Raines EW, Seifert RA, et al. TGF-β induces bimodal proliferation of connective tissue cells via complex control of an autocrine PDGF loop. *Cell* 1991;63:515–524.
71. Dickson MC, Martin JS, Cousins FM, et al. Defective hematopoiesis and vasculogenesis in transforming growth factor-β 1 knock-out mice. *Development* 1995;121:1845–1854.
72. McAllister KA, Grogg KM, Johnson DW, et al. Endoglin, a TGF-βbinding protein of endothelial cells, is the gene for hereditary hemorrhagic telangiectasia type I. *Nature Genet* 1994;8:345–351.
73. Johnson DW, Berg JN, Baldwin MA, et al. Mutations in the activin recep-

tor-like kinase 1 gene in hereditary hemorrhagic telangiectasia type 2. *Nature Genet* 1996;13:189–195.

74. Korhonen J, Polvi A, Partanen J, et al. The mouse *tie* receptor tyrosine kinase gene: Expression during embryonic angiogenesis. *Oncogene* 1994;9: 395–403.

75. Partanen J, Puri MC, Schwartz L, et al. Cell autonomous functions of the receptor tyrosine kinase TIE in a late phase of angiogenic capillary growth and endothelial cell survival during murine development. *Development* 1996;122:3013–3021.

Section II

Vascular Cell Growth and Differentiation

Chapter 5

Contribution of the Adventitial Fibroblast to Pulmonary Vascular Disease

Kurt R. Stenmark, MD, Mita Das, PhD,
David Bouchey, PhD, and
Edward C. Dempsey, MD

Introduction

Vascular repair in response to injury or stress (often referred to as remodeling) is a common complication of many cardiovascular abnormalities, including pulmonary hypertension, systemic hypertension, atherosclerosis, vein graft remodeling, and restenosis following balloon dilatation of the coronary artery. It is not surprising that repair and remodeling occurs frequently in the vasculature, in that exposure of blood vessels to either excessive hemodynamic stress (eg, hypertension), noxious blood borne agents (eg, atherogenic lipids), locally released cytokines, or unusual environmental conditions (eg, hypoxia) requires readily available mechanisms to counteract these adverse stimuli and to preserve structure and function of the vessel wall. The responses, which presumably evolved developmentally for repair of injured tissue, often escape self-limiting control and can result, in the case of blood vessels, in luminal narrowing and obstruction to blood flow. Each cell (ie, endothelial cells, smooth muscle cells, and fibroblast) in the vascular wall plays a specific role in the response to injury. However, while the roles of the endothelial cell and smooth muscle cell (SMC) in vascular remodeling have been extensively studied, relatively little attention has been given to the adventitial fibroblast. Perhaps this is because the fibroblast is a relatively ill-defined cell which, at least compared to the SMC, exhibits

From: Weir EK, Archer SL, Reeves JT (eds). *The Fetal and Neonatal Pulmonary Circulations.*
Armonk, NY: Futura Publishing Company, Inc.; ©1999.

many undifferentiated properties. However, it has been well demonstrated that fibroblasts possess the capacity to develop several functions such as migration, rapid proliferation, synthesis of connective tissue components, contractility, and cytokine production in response to activation or stimulation. The myriad of functions performed by the fibroblast, especially in response to stimulation, suggest that these cells play a pivotal role in the repair of injury. This fact has been well documented in the setting of wound healing. As such, it is not surprising that fibroblasts may play an important role in the vascular response to injury. This chapter will provide a brief review of the changes that occur in the adventitial fibroblast in response to vascular stress, and the role the activated fibroblast then plays in pulmonary vascular disease.

Fibroblast Responses to Vascular Stress or Injury: In Vivo Studies

Hypoxia-induced pulmonary hypertension complicates the clinical course of many important pulmonary and cardiac diseases in children and adults.[1-3] The pulmonary hypertension and accompanying structural remodeling appear particularly severe in infants, and it is in this stage of life where adventitial changes often predominate. For instance, even the earliest pathological descriptions of persistent pulmonary hypertension of the newborn (PPHN) pointed out significant adventitial thickening.[4] Dramatic adventitial changes have also been observed in the lung vessels of young infants dying of high-altitude-induced pulmonary hypertension.[5] Similar, though less dramatic, changes are seen in the adventitial compartment of infants with cyanotic forms of congenital heart disease that are complicated by pulmonary hypertension.

In animal models, the earliest and most dramatic structural changes following hypoxic exposure are found in the adventitial compartment of the vessel wall.[1-3] Resident adventitial fibroblasts have been shown to exhibit early and sustained increases in proliferation that exceed those observed in endothelial cells or SMCs.[6,7] In addition, early and dramatic changes in extracellular matrix (ECM) protein synthesis occur.[8] These include early upregulation of collagen, fibronectin, and tropoelastin messenger RNAs (mRNAs) followed by a subsequent increased deposition of each of these proteins. These changes in the proliferative and matrix-producing phenotype of the fibroblast are accompanied by appearance of α-SM-actin, in at least some of the cells in the adventitial compartment, indicating a modulation of fibroblasts to myofibroblasts.[2] The fibroproliferative changes in the adventitia are ultimately associated with luminal narrowing and progressive decrease in the ability of the vessel wall to respond to vasodilating stimuli.[9]

The possibility that hypoxia acts directly or in unique ways on the adventitial fibroblast in the setting of chronic hypoxic pulmonary hypertension is raised by previously well-documented observations that reduced oxygen tension (anoxia/hypoxia) results in profound changes in fibroblast physiology and metabolism. Cellular anoxia represents a biochemical state distinct from hypoxia, yet still represents a normal physiological condition present during wound healing.[10] Since a response quite different from that seen with hypoxia is induced in anoxic fibroblasts, these cells must possess the unique ability to activate a different, possibly overlapping, set of genes to cope with these different environmental conditions.[11] The activity of several different transcription factors is known to be influenced by low oxygen tensions (Table 1). In cells that are stressed by oxygen deprivation, NF-κB activity increases as a result of phosphorylation and subsequent degradation of IκBα.[12] In other cells, low oxygen tensions induce the transcription of multiple members of the bZIP (basic/leucine zipper domain) superfamily,[13-15] result in nuclear accumulation of p53,[16] or induce the activity of hypoxia-inducible factor 1 (HIF-1).[17] Estes et al[18] demonstrated that one DNA-binding activity induced in hypoxic, anoxic, and cobalt-treated fibroblasts recognizes secondary anoxia-responsive element (SARE) and has electrophoretic mobility similar to that of HIF-1. It has also been demonstrated that a second, more prominent SARE-binding

Table 1

Gene Expression In Fibroblasts During Anoxic/Hypoxic Conditions

Gene	Anoxic	Hypoxic
Phosphoglycerokinase	+	+
Vascular endothelial growth factor (VEGF)	+	+
p21	+	+
p27	+	+
p53	+	+
Growth arrest and DNA-damage-inducible gene (GADDI53)	+	+
Procathepsin D	+	−
Cathepsin L	+	−
Hypoxia inducible factor	+	+
Anoxia inducible factor	+	−
NF-κB	+	+
Endonuclease	+	+

NF-κB = nuclear factor κB.

activity, termed the anoxia-inducible factor (AIF), is also induced in anoxic fibroblasts. Two-dimensional gel analysis indicated that AIF is a heterodimer comprised of 61- and 52-kD subunits and is likely to arise from post-translational modification of a heterodimeric SARE-binding complex present in aerobic cells. Identification of a mammalian anoxic response element has interesting implications. This element may prove useful in gene therapy regimens for targeting expression to physiological situations in which functional anaerobiosis exists, such as during wound healing. Interestingly, deregulation of genes normally expressed during anoxia is often also seen in cancer cells regardless of their state of oxygenation.[11] Thus, understanding the molecular basis of the mammalian anoxic regulatory pathway in fibroblasts and how similar genes become constitutively activated in malignancy may further lead to unique approaches to therapeutic intervention in settings of vascular disease complicated by hypoxia.

Based on the above, one might suspect that fibroblast changes in vascular disease may be unique to conditions or models of chronic hypoxia. However, recent observations in systemic models of vascular injury suggest that early activation and subsequent phenotypic modulation of the fibroblast is an important and perhaps ubiquitous response in the vascular remodeling that follows stress or injury. For example, it has been demonstrated that a sequence of events occurs in adventitial fibroblasts of the coronary vasculature following balloon catheter-induced injury which is similar to that seen in the skin wound healing process.[19-24] Cell proliferation is an early phenomenon and may involve the entire adventitia of the blood vessel.[20] The proliferation observed in the adventitia occurs earlier and is of greater magnitude than that seen in the coronary media. Subsequently, fibroblasts in the coronary artery adventitia have been shown to differentiate into a myofibroblast-like cells with the appearance of α-SM-actin in adventital cells beginning as early as 3 days and reaching a maximum at 14 days.[21] These changes in proliferation and contractile protein expression in adventitial cells are accompanied by the induction of procollagen α-1 mRNA and subsequent protein accumulation in the adventitial compartment.[22] Additionally, recent studies also suggest that these activated fibroblasts (? myofibroblasts) may migrate through the vessel wall and be at least partially responsible for the intimal thickening which ultimately characterizes the coronary vasculature following balloon injury.[23]

Adventitial fibroblasts have also been shown to be essential in the remodeling changes that venous grafts undergo after their placement in the arterial system.[24] Appearance of myofibroblasts and ultimately a collagenous scar may contribute to the failure of aortocoronary saphenous vein grafts to undergo compensatory dilatation when atherosclerotic lesions begin to compromise the lumen. Additionally, in hyper-

oxic models of lung injury, Jones et al have demonstrated that fibroblasts are activated, migrate, and acquire SMC-like characteristics in
the small pulmonary arteries.[3] Fibroblasts in this setting are strongly
suspected of being the "source" of cells in newly muscularized vessels.
Thus, observations in both the pulmonary and systemic circulations
suggest ubiquitous involvement of adventitial cells in the vascular repair process.

Fibroblast Interactions With Other Cell Types

A large body of experimental evidence demonstrates that fibroblasts may also exert significant phenotypic effects on other cell types,
raising the possibility that they contribute to the vascular remodeling
process in dynamic ways which are in addition to direct changes in their
phenotype. In fact, the idea that dynamic and reciprocal relationships
exist between fibroblasts and other cell types is well documented, especially in the developmental biology literature.[25] Interactions between
epithelium and mesenchyme have been shown to be critical for the morphogenesis of many different organs, including the lung (for a recent review, see Reference 26). Studies in both avian and mammalian species
have demonstrated that an interaction of the presumptive lung epithelium with lung mesenchyme is absolutely required for normal branching morphogenesis to proceed. Heterotypic recombination experiments
have indicated that the morphogenesis and cytodifferentiation of the epithelial component may be determined by the site of origin of the mesenchyme with which it is recombined. Conversely, epithelial cells may
influence various important aspects of fibroblast function such as matrix deposition and secretion of matrix-degrading enzymes.

The biochemical identity of the signal molecules mediating mes-
enchymal-epithelial interactions has been extensively investigated (for
review, see References 26 and 27). It has been established that matrix
proteins such as collagen, fibronectin, and proteoglycans play a prominent role. As suggested by many others, there is continuous feedback of
information between cell and matrix (see Figure 1). Interaction of specific matrix molecules with their receptors at the cell surface is involved
in a diverse array of cell behaviors. Fibroblasts also produce a number
of soluble factors that function as paracrine regulators of neighboring
cell (endothelial cells, SMC, epithelial) proliferation, migration, and
biosynthetic activity. The biological activity of the soluble factors and
the nature of the ECM in contact with the cells are mutually interde-
pendent in that soluble factors (eg, TGF-β, EGF, IGF) exert effects on matrix biosynthesis, and the response of cells to these factors is modulated
by the nature of the matrix.[27,28] Thus, fibroblasts, not surprisingly, may

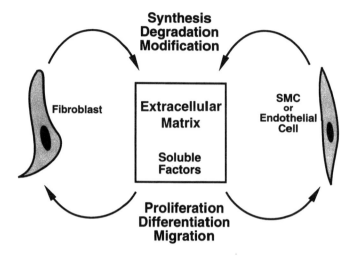

Figure 1. Dynamic reciprocity in vascular wall cell interactions. Changes in the production of extracellular matrix or soluble factors by one cell type may have profound effects on the phenotype of other cells in the vascular wall.

have significant effects on neighboring vascular wall cells and could contribute in unique ways to the vascular remodeling process.

Recent experiments have demonstrated the importance of fibroblast communication in vascular injury models. For instance, application of the inflammatory cytokine interleukin-1β to the adventitia induces coronary vasospasm and neointimal formation even without endoluminal manipulations.[29] These findings have relevance to clinical settings since the accumulation of mast cells and an inflammatory reaction are notable in patients with coronary vasospasm and fatal unstable coronary syndromes, respectively.[30,31] Similarly, molecules that can inhibit cellular proliferation applied to the adventitia have been shown to decrease the development of intimal thickening in response to luminal injury.[32-34] Thus, a substantial body of in vivo and in vitro evidence suggests a dynamic reciprocity in the interaction between adventitial fibroblasts and other vascular walls that is similar to the well-documented dynamic interaction between mesenchymal cells and epithelium during development.

Developmentally Regulated Changes in Fibroblast Growth Potential

The observation that developing blood vessels exhibit unique responses to injurious stimuli compared to mature vessels is supported by in vitro studies demonstrating that SMC and fibroblasts isolated at different developmental stages in life exhibit unique biochemical and functional characteristics. Several studies have demonstrated that SMC derived from embryonic, neonatal, and adult animals exhibit remarkably different growth potential.[1,2,35,36] In general, a high growth potential has been associated with SMC derived from the developing vasculature. Similarly, fetal fibroblasts have been shown to display a number of behavioral and biochemical characteristics not normally expressed by their adult counterparts. These include elevated production of unique soluble growth and transforming peptide factors, the synthesis of particular species and/or isoforms of matrix macromolecules, the presence of fetal-specific antigenic determinants, and production of several migration-stimulating factors (for review, see Reference 37). Programmed fetal to adult transitions in these many characteristics occur at various times during development, including the neonatal period, and appear to play an important role in the control of both the normal developmental process and the response to injury. Importantly, reexpression of fetal or neonatal-like characteristics and genes have been observed in SMC and fibroblasts following vascular injury in adult animals.[36]

Within the pulmonary circulation, we wanted to determine whether there were differences in the growth capacity of fibroblasts isolated from the pulmonary artery at different stages during development. We therefore measured the rate of fetal, neonatal, and adult fibroblast proliferation in 10% serum containing media. We found that fetal and neonatal fibroblasts had increased DNA synthesis, grew faster, and reached higher plateau densities than adult cells (Figure 2).[38] The earlier during gestation the fetal fibroblasts were harvested, the more rapid the growth that was observed. Serum-deprived fetal fibroblasts had increased DNA synthesis in response to a panel of potentially relevant mitogens, including PMA, IGF-1, PDGF, and the combination of PMA+IGF-1 compared with adult cells.

Little is known regarding the cellular mechanisms that might confer unique growth and differentiation properties to fibroblasts at various developmental stages. Protein kinase C (PKC) is a signaling pathway that has been shown to be important for both pulmonary and nonpulmonary vascular cell growth (for review, see References 39 and 40). This pathway is known to be developmentally regulated and has been shown to contribute specifically to the enhanced growth properties previously described for fetal and neonatal pulmonary artery SMC.[35] Increased expression of PKC has also been associated with enhanced growth capabilities of nonvascular fibroblasts. We therefore investigated the possibility that the augmented growth response to serum and peptide mitogens of fetal and neonatal fibroblasts compared with adults would be in some way related to changes in PKC signaling. We

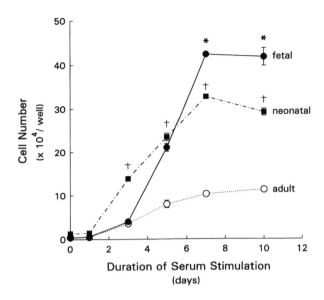

Figure 2. Serum-stimulated fetal and neonatal pulmonary artery adventitial fibroblasts grow faster and reach higher plateau densities than adult cells. Values are mean ± SE, n = 4 replicate wells. *p < 0.05 compared with day 0 result and matched neonatal and adult result at the same time. †p < 0.05 compared with day 0 result and matched adult result at same time. (Reproduced from Reference 38.)

established first that the rapidly growing fetal fibroblast had increased whole cellular PKC catalytic activity compared with adult cells.[38] Using three different PKC inhibitor strategies, we also documented that high rates of growth in fetal cells were associated with the PKC pathway by showing that three different PKC inhibitor strategies (dihydrosphengosine, chronic PMA treatment, and heparin) slowed the growth of fetal and neonatal fibroblast to a greater extent than adult cells.[38]

The PKC signaling pathway, however is a complex one, with 11 isozymes of PKC having been identified and divided into three distinct categories: (1) conventional (α, βI, βII, and γ); (2) novel (δ, ϵ, η, θ); and (3) atypical (ζ, ι, μ).[39,40] Conventional isozymes are calcium dependent, whereas novel and atypical isozymes are calcium independent. Developmental changes in the expression of individual isozymes have been observed and increased expression of selected PKC isozymes has been linked to augmented growth capacity. We therefore sought to determine specifically the isozymes of PKC that might be contributing to the developmental differences in growth exhibited by pulmonary artery adventitial fibroblasts. We detected seven PKC isozymes, three calcium-dependent (α, βI, βII) and four calcium-independent (δ, ϵ, ζ, μ),

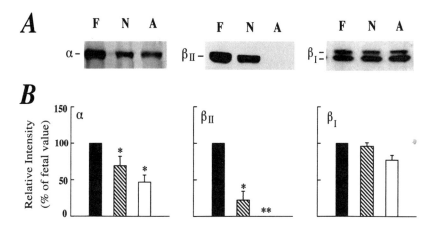

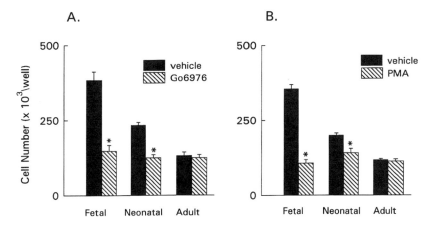

Figure 3. Expression of the Ca^{2+}-dependent α and βII isozymes of PKC is higher in immature pulmonary artery (PA) adventitial fibroblasts than in adult cells. A: Representative immunoblots for each Ca^{2+}-dependent isozyme. Whole cell lysates of fetal (F), neonatal (N), and adult (A) PA adventitial fibroblasts were resolved by SDS-PAGE, transferred to nitrocellulose, probed with PKC-α, -βI, and -βII antibodies. B: Quantitative analysis of expression pattern for each Ca^{2+}-dependent isozyme. Values are expressed as percent of the fetal value. *$p < 0.05$ compared with fetal cells and **$p < 0.05$ compared with fetal and neonatal cells. (Reproduced from Reference 41.)

Figure 4. Ca^{2+}-dependent α and βII isozymes of PKC contribute to the augmented growth of immature pulmonary artery adventitial fibroblasts. A: Go6976, a specific inhibitor of the Ca^{2+}-dependent isozymes of PKC, inhibits growth of immature pulmonary artery adventitial fibroblasts; n = 4 replicate wells. DMSO was used as the vehicle. *$p < 0.05$ compared with control cells. B: Pretreatment with 1 μM phorbol 12-myristate 13-acetate (PMA) for 24 hours (downregulates PKC-α and -βII, but not PKC-βI) has the same selective antiproliferative effect as Go6976; n = 4 replicate wells. *$p < 0.05$ compared with control cells. (Reproduced from Reference 41.)

in fibroblasts derived from the neonatal pulmonary artery.[41] We then demonstrated a selective increase in the expression of two calcium-dependent isozymes of PKC, α and βII, but not βI, in immature fibroblasts which paralleled the developmental differences in growth and PKC catalytic activity of immature pulmonary artery fibroblasts (Figure 3). Then, again using pharmacological antagonist strategies, we demonstrated that these same two isozymes, PKCα and βII, were involved in the enhanced growth of fetal and neonatal fibroblasts (Figure 4).

Hypoxia Stimulates Fibroblast Proliferation

PKC has many important downstream effectors. One important target, perhaps crucial for proliferation, is the mitogen-activated protein (MAP) kinase family of enzymes. Many studies have demonstrated that the MAP kinases p44 (Erk 1) and p42 (Erk 2) are crucial to proliferation in response to growth factors in a variety of cell types.[42,43] The growth factors, via their cell surface receptors, initiate a series of events culminating in the phosphorylation of Ras-GDP to the active form Ras-GTP. In turn, Ras then activates Raf which activates MEK (MAPKK/Erk kinase). MEK very specifically activates Erk 1 and Erk 2 by tyrosine and threonine phosphorylation. Active Erks are proline directed, serine-threonine kinases which then can: (1) phosphorylate cytoplasmic proteins, and (2) translocate to the nucleus where they activate transcription factors such as Elk-1, and activate genes involved in proliferation such as *c-fos*.

Recent work from the laboratories of Rhoades[44] and Hershenson[45] has shown that Erk-mediated signaling is also important in stress-induced proliferation via H_2O_2 in pulmonary arterial SMC and airway SMC, respectively. This response appears to be PKC dependent. We therefore sought to determine whether Erk 1 and Erk 2 mediate proliferation in pulmonary arterial adventitial fibroblasts induced by hypoxic stress. In order to separate the proliferative effects of hypoxia from those of growth factors and cytokines, we performed experiments in growth arrested, serum-deprived cells. Under these conditions, hypoxia induced an increase in DNA synthesis above normoxic levels, as measured by $[^3H]$-thymidine incorporation, in pulmonary artery adventitial fibroblasts as early as 24 hours after exposure. Continued exposure to hypoxia for 3 days resulted in increased cell density compared with cultures maintained in normoxic atmosphere.[46] Thus, the proliferative stimulus of hypoxia is both early and sustained. Interestingly, we found that when systemic adventitial fibroblasts, isolated from the aortas of the same animals, were assayed for hypoxic induction of DNA synthesis, only 25% of the cultures demonstrated hypoxia-induced increases in DNA synthesis.

We also wanted to determine whether the proliferative effect of hypoxia on adventitial fibroblasts was dependent on oxygen concentration. We compared levels of DNA synthesis under oxygen concentrations ranging from 1% to 20%. We found that 3% oxygen stimulated DNA synthesis maximally whereas 1% oxygen did not increase DNA synthesis. Hypoxic-induced proliferation was associated with an increase in Erk 1/Erk 2 activity, as measured by the ability of immunocomplexes to incorporate ^{32}P label onto EGF receptor peptides, a known substrate for Erk activity. Hypoxia induced a transient increase in Erk activity, peaking at 10 minutes and returning to basal levels at 30–45 minutes. The peak represented a 2.5-fold increase in activity which was 25% of the activity detected under maximal stimulation by serum. Transient increases in Erk activity have been reported with growth factor-induced proliferation of other cell types, usually peaking at 5 minutes and returning to basal at 15 minutes. Importantly, an increase in Erk activity was again noted at 24 and 72 hours in cells that remained exposed to hypoxic conditions. We also demonstrated that interruption of the Erk signaling pathway, by inhibition of Ras activation or inhibition of MEK activation, abrogated the ability of hypoxia to stimulate DNA synthesis and also abolished the increase in cell density noted with sustained hypoxia under serum-deprived conditions. Thus, it appears that the ability of hypoxia to stimulate proliferation in adventitial fibroblasts under serum-deprived conditions is at least partially dependent on the Erk signaling pathway. At the moment, our findings demonstrate the role for Ca^{2+}-dependent isozymes of PKC (α and βII) in the augmented growth of immature fibroblasts.[41] Therefore, we believe hypoxia-stimulated Erk activity to be at least partially dependent on PKC, a finding similar to that reported from hypoxia-induced proliferation in cardiomyocytes.[47]

Acquired Changes in Fibroblast Phenotype

In addition to the developmentally regulated changes in the proliferative and matrix-producing potential of fibroblasts, an expanding body of experimental observations also supports the concept that significant changes in the phenotypic properties of resident fibroblasts can occur in the setting of fibroproliferative disease.[48-55] These phenotypically altered fibroblasts might contribute significantly to the generation and maintenance of the fibroproliferative scarring response observed in chronic vascular remodeling. For example, stable increases in the proliferative capacity of mesenchymal cells have been observed in the affected organs of patients with atherosclerosis, progressive systemic sclerosis, idiopathic pulmonary fibrosis, interstitial renal fibrosis, and hepatic fibrosis.[48-55] In animal models of lung and renal fibrosis, increased proliferative capacity of fibroblasts isolated from fibrotic tissue has also been demonstrated. The phenotype has been observed to be stable for many population doublings suggesting significant and persistent changes which become intrinsic to the cell itself (ie, not dependent on changes in the local environment from which the cell was isolated). Little is known, however, of the signaling pathways that confer enhanced proliferative capabilities to fibroblasts from fibrotic organs.

We therefore performed studies to address the hypothesis that fibroblasts isolated from the pulmonary artery of neonatal animals with severe hypoxia-induced fibroproliferative changes would exhibit excessive and unique proliferative capabilities compared to fibroblasts from normal age-matched animals. We found, on a very consistent basis, that fibroblasts isolated from hypoxic hypertensive calves exhibited augmented growth responses to serum, hypoxia, and purified peptide mitogens compared to those obtained from age-matched control animals.[56] Importantly, a synergistic interaction between hypoxia and purified peptide mitogens was observed in fibroblasts isolated from the hypertensive animals which was not observed in fibroblasts from the control animals (Figure 5). These proliferative attributes persisted through numerous cell passages in culture suggesting acquired differences in fibroblast populations which were not simply due to changes in the in vivo cellular milieu (ie, growth factor, cytokines, and matrix components).[56]

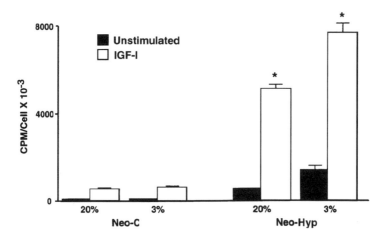

Figure 5. Pulmonary artery adventitial fibroblasts isolated from animals with hypoxic pulmonary hypertension demonstrate higher [^{3}H]-thymidine incorporation following stimulation with insulin-like growth factor-I (IGF-I) under both normoxic and hypoxic conditions compared with the cells isolated from control animals. Solid bars = unstimulated values; open bars = stimulated values. n = replicate wells. *$p < 0.05$ compared with results from control cells.

As might be expected from the developmental studies described above, changes in PKC isozyme expression also appear to participate in the unique hypoxic proliferation exhibited by cells from hypoxic pulmonary hypertensive animals. Studies utilizing both isozyme selective inhibitor strategies and immunoblot analysis demonstrated that the enhanced growth capabilities of fibroblasts from the hypertensive animals were related in part to increased levels of the PKC-βI and ζ-isozymes compared to fibroblasts from control animals. This is particularly interesting because the PKC-βI was not implicated in the enhanced growth capabilities of fetal versus adult cells. The finding supports the idea of an upregulation or switch to a new or different PKC signaling pathway. The PKC-βI isozyme appeared particularly important for the augmented growth capacity observed in fibroblasts from the hypertensive vessel wall under hypoxic conditions. Thus, the relative concentration and importance of specific PKC isozymes seems to change in fibroblasts during the development of fibroproliferative disease. The findings are compatible with those in nonvascular fibroblasts also demonstrating that PKC-βI and PKC-ζ are important in proliferative responses.

Contribution of Fibroblast Heterogeneity to Vascular Remodeling

Several possibilities must be considered in explaining how a stable phenotypic alteration of the adventitial fibroblast might develop. The first is that a large portion of resident fibroblasts are altered by changes that occur locally in the chronically hypoxic vascular wall. Hypoxia itself, a combination of hypoxia with subsequent hemodynamic changes, and ultimately the combination of hypoxia, hemodynamic changes, and changes in the local concentrations of cytokines, growth factors, and matrix proteins must be considered. Resident fibroblasts could be altered by these signals, which confer upon them a new stable phenotype that is manifested by intrinsically enhanced proliferative and matrix-producing capabilities. Another possibility is that selective expansion of a normally resident fibroblast population, with unusual or augmented growth properties, has occurred in vivo. This population could expand to the point where it is numerically the most important constituent of the activated or injured vessel wall. This population might then demonstrate selective advantage when cell cultures are done, and thus account for the apparent phenotypic change observed in fibroblast populations from the injured organ or vessel (Figure 6).

In addition to the developmentally regulated and site-specific differences in fibroblast phenotype that have been well documented, there is a growing body of literature that supports the existence of

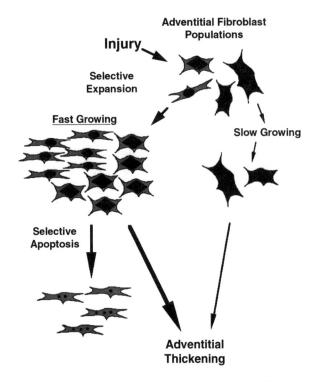

Figure 6. Hypothesis: Numerous heterogeneous adventitial fibroblast subpopulations exist. These cells have different intrinsic growth and matrix-producing capabilities. Fibroblast subpopulations with high growth potential may contribute selectively to adventitial thickening in response to injury. However, excessive proliferation is balanced by an increased rate of apoptosis in select fibroblast subpopulations.

phenotypic heterogeneity within the resident fibroblast population of a given tissue at a specified developmental stage. The extensive diversity of this intra-site heterogeneity includes differences in proliferative potential, synthesis of matrix molecules, production and response to growth factors, synthesis of matrix-degrading enzymes, phagocytic activity, and the presence of specific receptors and/or antigenic determinants at the cell surface (for review, see References 57 and 58).

To examine the possibility that several unique pulmonary artery adventitial fibroblast populations exist and thus contribute in unique ways to the vascular remodeling process, we used limited dilution and clonal expansion strategies to try to establish pure stable subpopulations of adventitial fibroblasts. We found that subpopulations of fibroblasts could be distinguished not only on the basis of their light microscopic appearance (ie, rounded or epitheloid vs. traditional elongated spindle shape), but also on the basis of their cytoskeletal protein expression. Subpopulations with a rounded appearance did not express SM-specific α-actin in culture.[59] In contrast, there was significantly brighter immunostaining with SM-specific α-actin antibody in fibroblast subpopulations demonstrating a spindle-like appearance. Marked differences in proliferative potential of different fibroblast clones were also documented. In general, cells exhibiting a spindle-like appearance tended to demonstrate far greater growth potential to serum or peptide mitogens than did the rounded cells. We also found that certain clones of fibroblasts expressed extremely high levels of type I and III collagen mRNA compared to other clones. In most, but not all instances, cells that exhibited a high growth potential also exhibited a high potential for collagen synthesis. On the other hand, elastin mRNA levels were significantly elevated in only one relatively slow growing clone of adventitial fibroblasts.

We also sought to determine if differences in the proliferative response of hypoxia existed between fibroblast clones. We found that there are subsets of fibroblasts that are highly sensitive to growth-promoting effects of hypoxia, and subsets that are resistant.[60] Susceptibility to the growth-promoting effects of hypoxia was not predictable on the basis of morphology or growth potential in serum. Collectively, these in vitro findings strongly support the idea that distinct subpopulations of fibroblasts exist within the pulmonary artery adventitia which may contribute selectively to the adventitial thickening observed in response to chronic hypoxia.

Changes in the relative proportion of different fibroblast subsets may have profound effects not only on the adventitial remodeling but also on the whole vessel wall. It is possible that alteration in the relative proportion of different fibroblast subsets with different capabilities for matrix protein and soluble growth factor production might be expected to influence the behavior of adjacent SMC or endothelial cells (dynamic reciprocity; see above). It is clear that there is continuous feedback of information between the cell and matrix such that the ECM in contact with the cells is itself a product of cellular activity (by virtue of biosynthesis, degradation, and modification of matrix macromolecules). In addition, the ECM influences various fundamental aspects of cell behavior such as the deposition of matrix itself, cell proliferation, and the pattern of gene expression and cell migration. Activation of a fibroblast subset secreting unique matrix molecules and soluble factors may thus have an influence on neighboring SMC or epithelial cells that is not exhibited under normal conditions.

Role of Apoptosis in Adventitial Remodeling

Within each cell line, cell number is determined by a balance between proliferation and death. Cell proliferation and death are highly regulated processes with numerous checks and balances. Apoptosis (programmed cell death) is a physiological form of cell death. Marked increases in the rate of apoptosis have been observed in SMC in vivo during the development of intimal thickening secondary to balloon injury.[61] In addition, SMC derived from human coronary atheromatous plaques have been shown to exhibit a markedly elevated rate of apoptosis in vitro. Interestingly, it has been demonstrated that hypoxia acts as a physiologically selective agent against apoptosis-competent cells in tumors, thus promoting the clonal expansion of the cells that acquire mutations in their apoptotic programs during tumor development.[62] Activation of JNK and p38 and concurrent inhibition of extracellular signal-regulated kinase (Erk) have been shown, at least in some cells, to be critical for induction of apoptosis.[63]

In preliminary studies, we found that different fibroblast subpopulations exhibit significant differences in their susceptibility to apoptosis upon serum withdrawal as well as in response to cytokines. Susceptibility to apoptosis upon serum withdrawal and in response to IFN-γ and IL-1α varies considerably among the cell subpopulations identified and appears not to be directly correlated to serum-stimulated growth rate. The fast growing subpopulation has significantly higher rate of apoptosis in response to serum withdrawal and cytokines than the slow growing population. It is not known whether hypoxia-sensitive subsets of fibroblasts have higher susceptibility to apoptosis or whether hypoxia can induce proliferation and apoptosis simultaneously in selective fibroblast subpopulations. The exact signaling mechanisms responsible for the induction of apoptosis in response to serum withdrawal, cytokines, and hypoxia in adventitial fibroblasts is also currently unknown.

Summary

Substantial experimental evidence supports the idea that the fibroblast may play a significant role in the vascular response to injury. The cell possesses the capability to rapidly respond to stress and to modulate its function to adapt rapidly to local vascular needs. It is also becoming clear that, as with SMC, numerous fibroblast subtypes exist in the vessel wall and each may serve special functions in response to injury. Future work is needed to determine more precisely the role of the fibroblast in the wide variety of vascular complications observed in many human diseases.

References

1. Stenmark KR, Mecham RP. Cellular and molecular mechanisms of pulmonary vascular remodeling. *Annu Rev Physiol* 1997;59:89–144.
2. Stenmark KR, Durmowicz AG, Dempsey EC. Modulation of vascular wall cell phenotype in pulmonary hypertension. In: Bishop JE, Reeves JJ, Laurent GJ, eds: *Pulmonary Vascular Remodeling*. London, UK: Portland Press; 1995.
3. Jones R, Reid L. Vascular remodelling in clinical and experimental pulmonary hypertensions. In: Bishop JE, Reeves JT, Laurent GJ, eds: *Pulmonary Vascular Remodelling*. London: Portland Press; 1995:47–115.
4. Murphy JD, Rabinovitch M, Goldstein JD, et al. The structural basis of persistent pulmonary hypertension of the newborn infant. *J Pediatr* 1981;98: 962–967.
5. Siu GJ, Liu YH, Chang XS, et al. Subacute infantile mountain sickness. *J Pathol* 1988;155:61–70.
6. Meyrick B, Reid L. Hypoxia and incorporation of [^{3}H]-thymidine by cells of the rat pulmonary arteries and alveolar wall. *Am J Pathol* 1979;96:51–70.
7. Belknap JK, Orton EC, Ensley B, et al. Hypoxia increases bromodeoxyuridine labeling indices in bovine neonatal pulmonary arteries. *Am J Respir Cell Mol Biol* 1997;16:366–371.
8. Durmowicz AG, Parks WC, Hyde DM, et al. Persistence, re-expression, and induction of pulmonary arterial fibronectin, tropoelastin and type I procollagen mRNA expression in neonatal hypoxic pulmonary hypertension. *Am J Pathol* 1994;145(6):1411–1420.
9. Durmowicz AG, Orton EC, Stenmark KR. Progressive loss of vasodilator responsive component of pulmonary hypertension in neonatal calves exposed to 4,570m. *Am J Physiol* 1993;265:H2175-H2183.
10. Anderson GR, Volpe CM, Russo CA, et al. The anoxic fibroblast response is an early stage wound healing program. *J Surg Res* 1995;59(6):666–674.
11. Anderson GR, Stoler DL, Scarcello LA. Normal fibroblasts responding to anoxia exhibit features of the malignant phenotype. *J Biol Chem* 1989;264: 14885-14892.
12. Koong AC, Chen EY, Giaccia AJ. Hypoxia causes the activation of nuclear factor kappa B through the phosphorylation of I kappa B alpha on tyrosine residues. *Cancer Res* 1994;54:1425–1430.
13. Ausserer WA, Bourrat-Floeck B, Green CJ, et al. Regulation of *c-jun* expression during hypoxic and low-glucose stress. *Mol Cell Biol* 1994;14:5032–5042.
14. Estes SD, Stoler DL, Anderson GR. Normal fibroblasts induce the c/EBPβ and ATF-4 bZIP transcription factors in response to anoxia. *Exp Cell Res* 1995;220(1):47–54.
15. Yao K-S, Xanthoudakis S, Curran T, et al. Activation of AP-1 and of a nuclear redox factor, Ref-1, in the response of HT29 colon cancer cells to hypoxia. *Mol Cell Biol* 1994;14:5997–6003.
16. Graeber TG, Peterson JF, Tsai M, et al. Hypoxia induces accumulation of p53 protein, but activation of a G_1-phase checkpoint by low-oxygen conditions is independent of p53 status. *Mol Cell Biol* 1994;14:6264–6277.
17. Semenza GL, Wang GL. A nuclear factor induced by hypoxia via de novo protein synthesis binds to the human erythropoietin gene enhancer at a site required for transcriptional activation. *Mol Cell Biol* 1992;12: 5447–5454.
18. Estes SD, Stoler DL, Anderson GR. Anoxic induction of a sarcoma virus-

related VL30 retrotransposon is mediated by a *cis*-acting element which binds hypoxia-inducible factor 1 and an anoxia inducible factor. *J Virol* 1995;69(10):6335–6341.

19. Scott NA, Cipolla GD, Ross CE, et al. Identification of a potential role for the adventitia in vascular lesion formation after balloon overstretch injury of porcine coronary arteries. *Circulation* 1996;93:2178–2187.

20. Shi Y, Pieniek M, Fard A, et al. Adventitial remodeling following coronary arterial injury. *Circulation* 1996;93:340–348.

21. Shi Y, O'Brien JE, Fard A, et al. Transforming growth factor β1 expression and myofibroblast formation during arterial repair. *Arterioscler Thromb Vasc Biol* 1996;16:1298–1305.

22. Shi Y, O'Brien JE, Ala-Kokko L, et al. Origin of extracellular matrix synthesis during coronary repair. *Circulation* 1997;95:997–1006.

23. Shi Y, O'Brien J, Fard A, et al. Adventitial myofibroblasts contribute to neointimal formation in injured porcine coronary arteries. *Circulation* 1996;94:1655–1664.

24. Shi Y, O'Brien JE, Mannion JD, et al. Remodeling of autologous saphenous vein grafts: The role of perivascular myofibroblasts. *Circulation* 1997;95 (12):2684–2693.

25. Wessells N. *Tissue Interactions and Development*. Menlo Park, CA: Benjamin; 1997.

26. Shannon JM, Deterding RR. Epithelial-mesenchymal interactions in lung development. In: McDonald JA, ed: *Lung Growth and Development*. New York: Marcel Dekker; 1997:81–118.

27. Minoo P, King RJ. Epithelial-mesenchymal interactions in lung development. *Annu Rev Physiol* 1994;56:13–45.

28. Cardoso WV. Transcription factors and pattern formation in the developing lung. *Am J Physiol* 1995;269:L429-L442.

29. Shimokawa H, Ito A, Fukumoto Y, et al. Chronic treatment with interleukin-1β induces coronary intimal lesions and vasopastic responses in pigs in vivo. *J Clin Invest* 1996;97:769–776.

30. Kolodgie FD, Virmani R, Cornhill F, et al. Increase in atherosclerosis and adventitial mast cells in cocaine abusers: An alternative mechanism of cocaine-associated coronary vasospasm and thrombosis. *J Am Coll Cardiol* 1991;17:1533–1560.

31. Kohchi K, Takebayashi S, Hiroki T, et al. Significance of adventitial inflammation of the coronary artery in patients with unstable angina: Results at autopsy. *Circulation* 1985;71:709–716.

32. Booth RGF, Martin JF, Honey AC, et al. Rapid development of atherosclerotic lesions in the rabbit carotid artery induced by perivascular manipulation. *Atherosclerosis* 1989;76:257–268.

33. Rogers C, Karnovsky MJ, Edelman ER. Inhibition of experimental neointimal hyperplasia and thrombosis depends on the type of vascular injury and the site of drug administration. *Circulation* 1993;88:1215–1221.

34. Andersen HR, Maeng M, Thorwest M, et al. Remodeling rather than neointimal formation explains luminal narrowing after deep vessel wall injury. *Circulation* 1996;93:1716–1724.

35. Dempsey EC, Badesch DB, Dobyns EL, et al. Enhanced growth capacity of neonatal pulmonary artery smooth muscle cells in vitro: Dependence on cell size, time from birth, insulin like growth factor I, and auto-activation of protein kinase C. *J Cell Physiol* 1994;160:469–481.

36. Xu Y, Stenmark KR, Das M, et al. Pulmonary artery smooth muscle cells

from chronically hypoxic neonatal calves retain fetal-like and acquire new growth properties. *Am J Physiol* 1997;273(17):L234-L245.

37. Schor SL, Schor AM. Clonal heterogeneity in fibroblast phenotype: Implications for the control of epithelial-mesenchymal interactions. *Bioessays* 1987;7(5):200–204.

38. Das M, Stenmark KR, Dempsey EC. Enhanced growth of fetal and neonatal pulmonary artery adventitial fibroblasts is dependent on protein kinase C. *Am J Physiol* 1995;269(13):L660-L667.

39. Nishizuka Y. Intracellular signaling by hydrolysis of phospholipids and activation of protein kinase C. *Science* 1992;258:607–614.

40. Johannes FJ, Prestle J, Dieterich S, et al. Characterization of activators and inhibitors of protein kinase C-µ. *Eur J Biochem* 1995;227:303–307.

41. Das M, Stenmark KR, Ruff LJ, et al. Selected isozymes of PKC contribute to augmented growth of fetal and neonatal bovine pulmonary artery fibroblasts. *Am J Physiol* 1997;273:L1276-L1284.

42. Waskiewicz AJ, Cooper JA. Mitogen and stress response pathways: MAP kinase cascades and phosphatase regulation in mammals and yeast. *Curr Opin Cell Biol* 1995;7:798–805.

43. Segal RA, Greenberg ME. Intracellular signalling pathways activated by neurotrophic factors. *Annu Rev Neurosci* 1996;19:463–489.

44. Zhang J, Jin N, Liu Y, et al. Hydrogen peroxide stimulates extracellular signal-regulated protein kinases in pulmonary arterial smooth muscle cells. *Am J Respir Cell Mol Biol* 1998;19:324–332.

45. Abe MK, Kartha S, Karpova AY, et al. Hydrogen peroxide activates extracelluar signal-regulated kinase via protein kinase C, Raf-1, and MEK1. *Am J Respir Cell Mol Biol* 1998;18:562–569.

46. Bouchey D, Nemenoff R, Stenmark KR. Hypoxia activates extracellular-signal regulated kinase (Erk) and induces proliferation in adventitial fibroblasts from the neonatal bovine main pulmonary artery (MPA-Fibs). *Mol Biol Cell* 1998;9S:1333. Abstract.

47. Seko Y, Tobe K, Takahashi N, et al. Hypoxia and hypoxia/reoxygenation activate Src family tyrosine kinases and p21 Ras in cultured rat cardiac myocytes. *Biochem Biophys Res Commun* 1996;226:530–535.

48. Jordana M, Kirpalani H, Gauldie J. Heterogeneity of human lung fibroblast proliferation in relation to disease expression. In: Phipps RP, ed: *Pulmonary Fibroblast Heterogeneity*. Boca Raton, FL: CRC Press, Inc; 1992:229–249.

49. Jordana M, Schulman J, McSharry C, et al. Heterogeneous proliferative characteristics of human adult lung fibroblast lines and clonally derived fibroblasts from control and fibrotic tissue. *Am Rev Respir Dis* 1988; 137:579–584.

50. Raghu G, Chen Y, Rusch V, et al. Differential proliferation of fibroblasts cultured from normal and fibrotic human lungs. *Am Rev Respir Dis* 1988; 138:703–708.

51. Chen B, Polunovsky V, White J, et al. Mesenchymal cells isolated after acute lung injury manifest an enhanced proliferative phenotype. *J Clin Invest* 1992;90:1778–1785

52. Torry DJ, Richards CD, Podor TJ, et al. Anchorage-independent colony growth of pulmonary fibroblasts derived from fibrotic human lung tissue. *J Clin Invest* 1994;93:1525–1532.

53. Krieg T, Meurer M. Systemic scleroderma. *J Am Acad Dermatol* 1988;18: 457–481.

54. Rodemann HP, Muller GA. Abnormal growth and clonal proliferation of

fibroblasts derived from kidneys with interstitial fibrosis. *Proc Soc Exp Biol Med* 1990;195(1):57–63.

55. Lukacs NW, Chensue SW, Smith RE, et al. Production of monocyte chemoattractant protein-1 and macrophage inflammatory protein-1 alpha by inflammatory granuloma fibroblasts. *Am J Pathol* 1994;144(4):711–718.

56. Das M, Dempsey EC, Bouchey D, et al. Chronic hypoxia induces exaggerated growth responses in pulmonary artery adventitial fibroblasts: Potential contribution of specific PKC isozymes. *Am J Resp Cell Mol Biol* 1999. In press.

57. Phipps RP. *Pulmonary Fibroblast Heterogeneity.* Boca Raton, FL: CRC Press, Inc; 1992:1–336.

58. Fries KM, Blieden T, Looney RJ, et al. Evidence of fibroblast heterogeneity and the role of fibroblast subpopulations in fibrosis. *Clin Immunol Immunopathol* 1994;72(3):283–292.

59. Das M, Dempsey EC, Stenmark KR. Selective subpopulations of pulmonary artery adventitial fibroblasts exhibit unique proliferative and apoptotic capabilities. *FASEB J* 1998;12(4):A339:1971.

60. Das M, Stenmark KR, Dempsey EC. Hypoxia stimulates growth of selective subsets of pulmonary artery adventitial fibroblasts. *FASEB J* 1997;11:A557.

61. Bennett MR, Evan GI, Schwartz SM. Apoptosis of human vascular smooth muscle cells derived from normal vessels and coronary atherosclerotic plaques. *J Clin Invest* 1995;95:2266–2274.

62. Graeber TG, Osmanian C, Jacks T, et al. Hypoxia-mediated selection of cells with diminished apoptotic potential in solid tumours. *Nature* 1996;379:88–91.

63. Xia Z, Dickens M, Raingeaud J, et al. Opposing effects of ERK and JNK-p38 MAP kinases on apoptosis. *Science* 1995;270:1326–1331.

Chapter 6

The Role of Thrombospondins 1 and 2 in Vascular Development

Lucas C. Armstrong, PhD,
Themis R. Kyriakides, PhD, and
Paul Bornstein, MD

Introduction

During vertebrate development, embryonic blood vessel formation begins, in a process termed vasculogenesis, with the differentiation of a population of mesodermal cells to form angioblasts, the precursors of endothelial cells (EC). The initial vascular network formed by vasculogenesis further expands by angiogenesis, in which sprouting or division of EC leads to the development of new capillaries.[1] The growth, migration, and differentiation of EC that, in the aggregate, constitute the mature vessel are directed and/or influenced by a complex array of extracellular molecules. The best appreciated angiogenic molecules are growth factors, such as vascular endothelial growth factor (VEGF), basic fibroblast growth factor (bFGF), and angiopoietins, which are soluble or transiently matrix-associated and potently stimulate growth by means of tyrosine kinase receptors.[2] Two soluble inhibitors of angiogenesis, angiostatin and endostatin, have been identified as fragments of plasminogen and type XVIII collagen, respectively, and were shown to be products of primary tumors that suppress the angiogenesis-dependent growth of metastases.[3,4] Structural extracellular matrix (ECM) molecules, including fibrillar collagens and basement membrane components, are also critical determinants in the development and maintenance of the vasculature.[5,6] Another class of extracellular proteins, termed matricellu-

The studies from the laboratory cited in this chapter were supported in part by National Institutes of Health Grants HL18645 and AR45418, and by National Science Foundation Grant EEC9529161.

From: Weir EK, Archer SL, Reeves JT (eds). *The Fetal and Neonatal Pulmonary Circulations.* Armonk, NY: Futura Publishing Company, Inc.; ©1999.

lar proteins, plays an important role in modulating cell-matrix interactions.[7] These proteins interact with the ECM but do not subserve primarily structural roles. Matricellular proteins include members of the thrombospondin, SPARC, and tenascin families, and osteopontin.[7] In this chapter, we will consider the evidence that two of these proteins, thrombospondin (TSP) 1 and 2, modulate angiogenesis in a complex fashion by means of multiple protein-protein interactions.

The thrombospondin protein family consists of five members that are encoded by separate genes and have distinct patterns of expression.[8] Each member of the family contains a divergent N-terminal domain, a short interchain disulfide-bonding sequence, three or four epidermal growth factor (EGF) -like repeats, seven Ca^{2+}-binding type III repeats and a conserved C-terminal domain (Figure 1). However, TSP1 and 2 are structurally distinct from TSP3–5/COMP, as TSP1 and 2 form 450 kD disulfide-bonded trimers with subunit molecular masses of 150 kD, while TSP3–5 form approximately 440–550 kD pentamers with predicted subunit molecular masses of 105–140 kD. The higher subunit molecular masses of TSP1 and 2 result from the presence in each of sev-

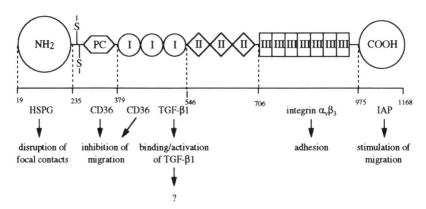

Figure 1. The domain organization, intermolecular interactions, and effects on endothelial cells (EC) of TSP1. TSP2 has a similar domain organization and is likely to engage in many of the same molecular interactions, but most of these remain undocumented. The domain organization of TSP1 and 2 consists of an N-terminal domain (NH$_2$), an interchain disulfide-bonding sequence ($-S-$), a type I procollagen-like domain (PC), three thrombospondin type I/properdin-like repeats (I), three EGF-like type II repeats (II), seven Ca^{2+}-binding type III repeats (III), and a C-terminal domain (COOH). Amino acid numbers demarcating domain boundaries are indicated. Proteins binding TSP1 and the resulting alterations in EC behavior are indicated beneath the interacting domain. The net effect of interactions of TSP1 with TGF-β1 on EC is unclear, as conflicting results regarding the effects of TGF-β1 on EC have been reported. IAP = integrin-associated protein; HSPG = heparan sulfate proteoglycan.

eral extra domains: a collagen propeptide-like domain and three properdin-like type I repeats between the N-terminal domain and the EGF-like repeats (Figure 1). By means of these different domains, TSP1 and 2 are capable of interacting with a diverse array of cell-surface receptors, matrix components, growth factors, and proteases. This complicated array of intermolecular interactions might explain the complex and sometime contradictory effects of TSP1 and 2 on cellular behavior, and points towards the ability of TSP1 and 2 to function as subtle modulators of multiple cellular processes.

Patterns of Expression of TSP1 and 2

TSP1 and 2 mRNA and protein are found in a wide spectrum of tissues, with overlapping patterns of expression in the developing and adult mouse.[9-13] TSP1 was first characterized as a component of platelet α-granules and has also been detected in megakaryocytes. Serum contains low levels of TSP1, which is perhaps platelet-derived. TSP2, on the other hand, is absent from platelets, and serum. TSP1 protein and mRNA have been found in epithelial layers, smooth and skeletal muscle, and connective tissue. TSP2 appears to be expressed more commonly in association with connective tissues, including reticular dermis, ligaments, meninges, and pericardium. Both proteins are found, in an overlapping pattern, within bone that develops by either intramembranous or endochondral ossification. Within lung, TSP1 mRNA is located largely in the bronchiolar epithelium, whereas TSP2 mRNA is concentrated in the region underlying the bronchioles.[12] A broad spectrum of cultured cells, including vascular smooth muscle cells (VSMC), EC, keratinocytes, osteoblasts, fibroblasts, and macrophages, secrete TSP1. Production of TSP2 by cultured cells has been less thoroughly characterized but has been observed in fibroblasts, adrenocortical cells, osteoblasts, and VSMC from several species. In the vasculature, TSP1 is found in the endothelium of developing and adult mice and in the intima and media of large vessels.[12,14] TSP2 mRNA is also associated with capillary and large vessel endothelium in developing chicken and mouse embryos.[12,15] However, by immunochemical methods, TSP2 is either undetectable[9] or detectable only in a subset of vessel endothelium.[11] TSP2 is absent from umbilical vein EC in culture, but expression by VSMC and fibroblasts in culture suggests that it may be a component of the vessel wall.[14,16]

The altered expression patterns of TSP1 and 2 in normal remodeling processes and pathological states suggest that TSP1 and 2 may play a role in modulating vascularization of tissues in disease states. However, the precise nature of the influence of TSP1 and 2 on vessel growth and maturation has been difficult to discern by correlation of the

expression patterns of TSPs with the extent of blood vessel proliferation. An antiangiogenic function for TSP1 has been inferred in the pro-
gesterone-dependent cycling of the human endometrium, since TSP1 is
produced at low levels during the angiogenic proliferative phase, and
at high levels during the secretory phase when blood vessel growth has
ceased.[17] During malignant progression of bladder epithelium, TSP1
expression varies inversely with the degree of angiogenesis, a finding
which is also consistent with an antiangiogenic function for TSP1.[18] A
positive role for TSP1 in pathological vascular smooth muscle growth
has been inferred from the observation that in atherosclerotic vessels
and in hypertensive pulmonary arteries, TSP1 is expressed in the neointimal layer and also, to a lesser degree, in the medial layer.[14,19,20] On the
other hand, in some pathological processes characterized by active angiogenesis, TSP1 has been found to be upregulated. During the early,
angiogenic stages of excisional wound healing, macrophages produce
abundant TSP1.[21] In angiogenic synovial tissues from patients with
rheumatoid arthritis, TSP1 is present in vascular EC, pericytes, and
macrophages.[22] Concordant with these observations, macrophages activated by LPS in vitro become highly angiogenic and produce elevated
levels of TSP1.[23] Assessment of the functional roles of TSP1 and 2 from
such observations must be made with the awareness that the balance of
positive and negative regulators of angiogenesis, rather than the mere
presence or absence of a given regulator, determines the rate and pattern of blood vessel growth.

Clarification of the roles of TSP1 and 2 has also been attempted by
the study of the effects of TSP1 and 2 in cultured cells, but the results of
such studies have not led to definitive conclusions. However, the examination of angiogenesis-dependent pathological processes, such as
wound healing and tumor growth, modeled in TSP1- and 2-null mice
(see below), has the exciting potential to enable a critical assessment of
the functional significance of such patterns of expression in vivo.

Effects of TSP1 and 2 on Endothelial Cells In Vitro

Angiogenesis occurs by at least two mechanisms, sprouting
angiogenesis and intussuception, each of which can be divided into a
series of distinct events involving a number of specialized EC functions.[1,2,24] Sprouting angiogenesis is the best understood process and
the only one in which the functions of TSP1 and 2 have been investigated. Initiation of sprouting angiogenesis involves budding of a
process from an EC in an existing vessel and invasion of the process
between adjacent cells and through the ECM. Proliferation of EC in the
direction of the neovessel occurs, and the ECs then differentiate to

form tubular structures with lumina. Mural cells, either pericytes in the microvasculature or smooth muscle cells in larger vessels, are recruited to provide stability and contractile properties to the neovessel, and in turn modulate EC growth.[25] Finally, EC deposit an abluminal basement membrane that further stabilizes the neovessel. The properties of EC that enable them to carry out angiogenesis can be modeled with EC in culture, and TSP1 and 2 have been shown to modulate many of these properties.

Adhesion of a variety of cell types to TSP1 has been well documented, but the ability of EC to adhere to TSP1 has been the focus of much controversy. A tenuous consensus has emerged that EC attach to surfaces coated with TSP1,[26-28] but that EC adhere less efficiently to TSP1 than to fibrinogen or fibronectin. Furthermore, TSP1 interferes with adhesion of EC to highly adhesive substrates such as fibronectin.[29] EC attachment to TSP1 appears to be mediated by the binding of $\alpha_v\beta_3$ integrin to an arginine-glycine-aspartic acid (RGD) sequence in the last type III repeat of TSP1.[27] A more consistent finding is that EC adhering to a TSP1-coated surface spread poorly. This interference with spreading is likely to result from the relative inability of EC to form focal contacts, structures that link the actin cytoskeleton to ECM-binding integrins at the cell surface, on a TSP1 substrate.[30] Soluble TSP1 disrupts focal adhesions of bovine aortic EC previously spread on a fibronectin substrate, but only slightly affects the state of spreading of the cells. Disruption of focal contacts by TSP1 does not necessarily impair the ability of a given cell type to spread; instead, cortical microspikes containing fascin, an actin-bundling protein, may mediate TSP1-dependent spreading, although this process has not been investigated in EC.[31] The ultimate consequences of such effects of TSP1 on adhesion are unclear. EC need to adhere to matrix to initiate migration, and TSP1 may inhibit this process, but cells must detach from a matrix to continue migration, a process that TSP1 may promote.

The effects of TSP1 on EC migration, as assayed in modified Boyden chambers, is similarly controversial. Several studies concluded that TSP1 inhibits bFGF-stimulated migration of bovine adrenal capillary EC and human microvascular EC.[32] Another study, however, demonstrated a positive migrational response of murine lung microvascular EC to TSP1.[26] One important variable that may explain such discordant results is the effect of increasing concentrations of TSP1 in the migrational assay, as low concentrations of TSP1 inhibit migration and high concentrations stimulate random migration.[32] These opposing effects appear to be mediated by separate domains of the TSP1 molecule. Interactions between the cell surface protein CD36 and sequences in the procollagen-like and first properdin domain of TSP1 mediate the inhibitory effects[32,33], whereas the stimulatory effects on chemotaxis are mediated by interaction between TSP1 and integrin-associated protein, IAP/CD47.[34]

Analyses of the effects of exogenous TSP1 are further complicated by the effects of endogenous synthesis of TSP1 by EC. Experimental inhibition of TSP1 production in bovine aortic EC by transfection with an antisense vector specific for TSP1 results in an exaggerated chemotactic response to bFGF.[35] A number of other factors are chemotactic for EC, and TSP1 or 2 inhibits migration induced by many of these factors, including VEGF, platelet-derived growth factor (PDGF), interleukin-8 (IL-8), prostaglandin E_1 (PGE$_1$), transforming growth factor-β1 (TGF-β1),[36] and scatter factor/hepatocyte growth factor (HGF).[37] However, TSP2 inhibits VEGF- and TGF-β1-induced migration less potently than does TSP1.[36] Two mechanisms could account for the abilities of TSP1 and 2 to inhibit a spectrum of chemotactic factors. First, TSP1 and 2 bind to EC directly; thus, an effect of this binding might be that EC are switched to a nonmigratory phenotype, as appears to be the case with the CD36-mediated inhibition by TSP1 of migration induced by bFGF, VEGF, and scatter factor.[33] Alternatively, TSP1 and 2 may bind to each of the growth factors and thereby block interaction with their cognate receptors. Remarkably, TSP1 has been shown to bind to PDGF[38], scatter factor[37], TGF-β1,[39,40] and bFGF.[41] However, TSP1 appears to bind bFGF too weakly to account for its inhibition of bFGF-induced migration (see below). Latent TGF-β1 binds to and is activated by a sequence in the type I repeats of TSP1.[39,40,42] TSP2 also binds to latent TGF-β1, but conflicting conclusions have been drawn regarding the ability of TSP2 to activate latent TGF-β1.[40,43] Although the reported differences in activation of TGF-β1 by TSP1 and 2[40] correlate well with the relative abilities of TSP1 and 2 to inhibit TGF-β1-induced migration, it is not clear whether such direct activation of TGF-β1 is sufficient to account for the inhibitory effect of TSP1 on migration. Further correlation of binding affinities between TSPs and growth factors and of the magnitude of migration with the concentration of growth factor is required to evaluate whether direct interaction between TSPs and growth factors influences migration.

TSP1 also appears to inhibit EC proliferation induced by bFGF, and this effect can be mimicked by heparin-binding fragments from the N-terminal domain and type I repeats of TSP1.[44] Different mechanisms operate in the inhibition by TSP1 of bFGF-induced migration and proliferation, as low picomolar concentrations of TSP1 inhibit chemotaxis, but high nanomolar concentrations of TSP1 are required to inhibit proliferation. Whereas TSP1 might inhibit bFGF-induced migration by interaction with cell-surface CD36, antagonism of bFGF-induced proliferation by TSP1 may result from direct binding of TSP1 to bFGF and the resulting interference with the interaction of the growth factor with its receptors on the EC surface.[41]

Effects of TSP1 and 2 on EC Morphogenesis In Vitro

Endothelial cells, when cultured in a three-dimensional collagen gel, organize into anastomosing cords in a process that recapitulates, to a degree, the formation of a vessel from invading EC. In addition, sparsely plated EC occasionally form cavities that resemble incipient vessel lumina.[45,46] In postconfluent cultures containing tubes, TSP1 appears to be associated preferentially with mature tubes, but its expression is down-regulated overall.[47,48] Several studies have demonstrated an inhibitory role for endogenous TSP1 in cord and lumen formation, as reduction of endogenous TSP1 by antibodies against TSP1 or by antisense oligonucleotides results in increased cord and lumen formation.[35,47,49,50] Another study found stimulatory effects of exogenous TSP1 on tubular network formation at low concentrations and inhibitory effects at higher concentrations.[51] The association of TSP1 with mature tubes and the inhibitory properties of TSP1 suggest that TSP1 serves as a feedback inhibitor to decrease the rate or extent of EC differentiation.

The study of TSP1 in transformed EC has led to some useful insights into the effects of TSP1 on EC growth and differentiation. EC transformed by expression of polyoma middle T antigen assume an aberrant phenotype in vitro, characterized by rapid growth rate, high saturation density, and inability to form cords.[52] When injected subcutaneously into mice, these transformed EC form cavernous hemangioendotheliomas. Interestingly, transformed EC are characterized by greatly reduced expression of TSP1, and stable transformation of these cells with a vector driving TSP1 expression reduces their tumorigenicity in vivo and restores normal growth characteristics in vitro.[52,53] TSP1 expression appears to be related reciprocally to that of platelet-endothelial cell adhesion molecule-1 (PECAM-1), which is highly expressed in transformed cells and contributes to the transformed cell phenotype.[54,55] Paradoxically, transformed EC with restored TSP1 expression form cords more readily than unaltered transformed EC[53], whereas normal EC, expressing endogenous TSP1, form cords more poorly than normal EC with experimentally reduced amounts of TSP1 (see above). As with migration, TSP1 may affect differentiation in a bimodal fashion, or TSP1 in concert with a transformation-dependent protein may elicit a response different from that resulting from expression of TSP1 in normal EC. These in vitro observations raise the possibility that TSP1 contributes to the maintenance of proper vessel growth and architecture in a complex manner in vivo.

Effects of TSP1 and 2 on Fibroblasts and VSMC In Vitro

Although TSP1 appears to have an overall inhibitory effect on EC at physiological concentrations, other cells of the vasculature are affected differently by TSP1. VSMC and fibroblasts, a subset of which are likely to be the precursors of the pericytes that contact the EC in the microvasculature, are induced to grow by TSP1.[56,57] VSMC stimulated by growth factors such as PDGF exhibit a synthetic phenotype and synthesize large amounts of TSP1, suggesting the existence of a positive autocrine loop.[57-59] The stimulatory effects of TSP1 may not extend to all responses of VSMC, as VSMC are inhibited by TSP1 in chemotaxis towards bFGF.[49] Synthesis of TSP1, but not TSP2, in NIH3T3 cells is also stimulated by mitogens,[60] a finding which points towards distinct functions for TSP1 and TSP2. As each of these cell types elaborates growth factors that may influence EC, these effects could result in an overall effect of TSP1 in vivo that differs from that observed in vitro. Inhibition of EC growth and stimulation of VSMC growth by TSP1 support a role for TSP1 in slowing vessel elongation and branching, and promoting vessel thickening. In addition, the presence of TSP1 at sites of neointimal formation implicates TSP1 as a potential modulatory molecule in the thickening of the smooth muscle layer seen in atherosclerosis and restenosis.

Effects of TSPs In Vivo

Angiogenesis in vivo is considerably more complex than the formation of cords and tubes by cultured EC, due to, eg, the interactions with neighboring cell types that exist in the animal. A number of methods have been developed in vivo to evaluate and/or quantify angiogenesis induced by experimental compounds.[24] Considerable evidence obtained with such assays points towards an overall antiangiogenic effect of TSP1 in vivo. By means of a rat corneal implant assay, in which an inert pellet containing the protein or extract of interest is placed under a flap of cornea, Bouck and colleagues identified tumor suppressor-dependent synthesis of an inhibitor of angiogenesis by a transformed baby hamster kidney cell line and found the inhibitor to be identical to the 140 kD C-terminal fragment of TSP1.[61,62] Peptides derived from TSP1 also inhibit vessel ingrowth into porous sponges implanted subcutaneously.[32] Human breast cancer cell lines stably transfected with TSP1 cDNA, when implanted subcutaneously into nude mice, display reduced angiogenesis relative to the parent cell line.[63] Furthermore, a human fibrosarcoma cell line, engineered to produce reduced amounts of TSP1 by transfection with antisense TSP1 cDNA, was found to have a decreased latency period when injected into nude mice. Interestingly, nude mice bearing subcutaneous tumors derived from the parent (high TSP1-producing) cell line exhibited decreased growth of lung metastases as a result of decreased systemic angiogenesis.[64] Therefore, TSP1 can inhibit angiogensis both locally and at locations distant from the site of production.

Exogenous TSP2 has also been demonstrated to inhibit angiogenesis in two experimental models in vivo. In the rat corneal implant assay, recombinant mouse and native bovine TSP2 inhibit neovascularization induced by bFGF. In addition, when applied to the surface of quail egg chorioallantoic membrane (CAM), recombinant TSP2 inhibits development of the CAM vasculature (preliminary evidence is cited in Reference 65).

Organ culture approaches to the study of angiogenesis are less frequently used, but allow for complex interactions between cell types to be studied in a fashion that is more amenable to analysis than are comparable experiments in a living animal. In one such assay, rat aortic explants in collagen gels developed more microvascular outgrowths in the presence of TSP1, implying an overall proangiogenic function for TSP1.[66] In this system, TSP1 appears to stimulate the growth of myofibroblasts which in turn stimulate the growth and migration of EC. This observation points towards the possibility that the net effect of TSP1 and 2 expression on angiogenesis may vary among tissues as a result of variable effects on local neighboring cells. For example, effects of TSP1 and 2 on large vessel and microvascular EC growth may differ as a result of the manner in which neighboring VSMC, pericytes, and fibroblasts respond to TSP1 and 2.

Vascular Development in TSP1- and TSP2-null Mice

A great deal has been learned about functions of angiogenic molecules in vivo by the analysis of mice with targeted disruptions of the corresponding genes, and one might expect that analysis of mice lacking TSP1 or 2 would clarify the roles of these proteins in vivo. Mice harboring targeted deletions of the genes encoding TSP1 or 2 have recently been generated.[67,68] Both strains are viable, fertile, and superficially appear quite healthy. However, both strains exhibit a broad range of subtle abnormalities, including features involving the vasculature, and many of the features are consistent with the variety of functions attributed to TSP1 and 2. The specific cellular and biochemical mechanisms by which TSP1 and 2 influence such diverse aspects of tissue homeostasis are currently unclear and pose a great challenge for future investigations.

The most prominent feature of mice lacking TSP1 is a chronic organizing pneumonia characterized by alveolar and perivascular edema and neutrophilic infiltration. Hyperplasia of the epithelium, including Clara cell, type II epithelial cell, and neuroendocrine cell populations, and the presence of hemosiderin-laden macrophages are prominent features of the TSP1-null mouse lung. Inflammation appears to occur in the absence of detectable pathogens, and it is currently unclear whether it is an abnormal response to normal pulmonary flora or dysregulation of the pulmonary immune system in the absence of an insult.[67] A second report on the same line of TSP1-null mouse lists a multitude of subtle alterations involving a variety of tissues.[69] Pulmonary involvement was noted as above, and thickening of the vascular smooth muscle layer of the bronchiolar arteries was also observed. Pancreatic islets exhibited hyperplasia, with a concomitant hypoplasia of the exocrine pancreas and the interstitial matrix. Increased vascularity of the pancreas was also evident, and preliminary evidence was provided for increased vascular density in skin[69] and retina.[70] Despite the fact that TSP1 is a prominent component of platelet α-granules and appears to be an important mediator of platelet function in vitro, TSP1-null mice have normal bleeding times and platelet function.

The pathology of the TSP1-null mouse was concluded to result from defective activation of TGF-β1 in the absence of TSP1, as: (1) TSP1-null mice had decreased amounts of active TGF-β1; (2) a TSP1-derived peptide, previously shown to activate TGF-β1, reversed lung and pancreatic pathologies when introduced systemically to TSP1-null mice; and (3) a latent TGF-β1-derived peptide, previously shown to block the activation of latent TGF-β1 by TSP1, caused lung and pancreatic pathologies similar to those of TSP1-null and TGF-β1-null mice when delivered systemically to wild-type mice.[69] The relationship between TGF-β1 activation and the increased vascular densities of skin, retina, and pancreatic islets is unclear. An essential role for TGF-β1 in vascular development is supported by the observation that a subset of TGF-β1-null mice exhibits defective development of yolk sac vasculature, which results in embryonic lethality at 10.5 days of gestation.[71] TGF-β1-null mice that survive this bottleneck do not exhibit vascular abnormalities. The partial angiogenic defect in TGF-β1-null mice and the observation that purified TGF-β1 is proangiogenic in vivo argue against lack of TGF-β1 as a mechanism for elevated angiogenesis in TSP1-null mice. TGF-β1 has complex effects on

EC in culture; it inhibits proliferation and migration of EC in subconflu-ent cultures and in coculture with VSMC or pericytes[72,73], but stimulates proliferation of EC in cords and tubes in postconfluent cultures.[74] This observation raises the possibility that the vascular phenotype may, un-der certain circumstances, be related to the lack of active TGF-β1. It is also possible that increased angiogenesis in TSP1-null mice occurs indepen-dently of TGF-β1. As TSP1 inhibits EC migration by binding directly to CD36 on the EC surface, lack of TSP1 may result in unliganded CD36 and relief from inhibition of migration. An experiment in which EC isolated from TSP1-null mice are examined for CD36- and TGF-β1-dependent mi-gration would resolve this issue.

TSP2-null mice also have a complex phenotype, but it is largely distinct from that of TSP1-null mice.[68] The most evident abnormalities of the TSP2-null mouse are skin fragility, tendon and ligament laxity, increased endosteal bone formation, a bleeding diathesis, and an ele-vated vascular density in certain tissues. The defect in tensile strength of the skin is correlated with disorganization of dermal collagen fibrils, and these fibrils are characterized by abnormal diameter and contour, as observed by electron microscopy. Tail tendon collagen fibrils are also unevenly contoured and larger in diameter than are wild-type fibrils. The formation of this abnormal matrix may result from defects in cell-cell interactions and adhesion to substrata by TSP2-null dermal fibro-blasts.[68] When plated onto bacteriologic plastic, dermal fibroblasts from wild-type mice attach in a well-dispersed fashion, whereas fibro-blasts from TSP2-null mice form aggregates. In addition, the mutant fi-broblasts display reduced adhesion to a variety of substrates, including tissue culture plastic, type I collagen, vitronectin, fibronectin, and TSP2. Such alterations in adhesive properties in TSP2-null fibroblasts are likely to be a consequence of dysregulated expression or activity of ad-hesion receptors on the cell surface.

TSP2-null mice have abnormally long bleeding times. The bleed-ing defect is not due to a clotting defect, as prothrombin and partial thromboplastin times are normal. Instead, a defect in platelet aggrega-tion and/or adhesion to the injured subendothelium are possible ex-planations. TSP2 is unlikely to play a direct role in platelet aggregation, as it is absent from blood and hematopoietic precursor cells.[12] In this re-spect it is paradoxical that TSP2-null mice display a bleeding defect, whereas TSP1-null mice appear to have normal hemostatic properties. Given that TSP2 is likely to be synthesized by bone marrow stromal cells, an abnormal marrow matrix in the TSP2-null mouse could hinder megakaryocyte precursor differentiation and subsequent platelet func-tion. Alternatively, TSP2 may be present in the normal subendothelial ECM, and function, along with von Willebrand factor and collagen, to induce platelet aggregation.

The observation of elevated vascular densities in some tissues of the TSP2-null mouse provides evidence for an antiangiogenic function for TSP2 in vivo, but also supports the idea that TSP2 is a modulating, rather than an essential, protein for vascular development. The excess of dermal microvasculature is relatively benign, with an approximately twofold increase in microvessel density and no apparent propensity for hemangioendothelioma or other vascular malformation. Several other tissues, such as embryonic thymus and subcutaneous adipose tissue, have similarly elevated vascular densities, but brain appears to have a normal microvessel density (unpublished observations). Subcutaneous implantation of foreign materials, such as polyvinyl alcohol (PVA) sponges or silicone rubber disks, stimulates formation of a foreign body reaction characterized by granulation tissue containing a marked excess of capillaries in TSP2-null mice (Figure 2 and unpublished observations). The mechanisms leading to increased vascular density in the TSP2-null mouse, and the relationship of such mechanisms to those responsible for the elevated vascular density in the TSP1-null mouse, are unclear. The simplest explanation for the vascular phenotypes in both lines of mice is that a deficiency of either TSP1 or 2 in the extracellular space relieves inhibition of EC growth and migration, either directly or due to a lack of sequestration of a growth factor(s). However, the observed alterations in the architecture of the collagenous matrix may influence angiogenesis, as cell-matrix interactions are critical for EC growth and differentiation. Finally, EC from TSP2-null mice may have intrinsic defects in cell-matrix and cell-cell interactions similar to those of TSP2-null dermal fibroblasts, and these defects may lead to increased growth and migration.

Conclusion

The results of experiments which test the effects of TSP1 and 2 in cultured cells, assays of angiogenesis in animals, and studies of mice lacking these proteins all indicate that TSP1 and 2 function as important modulators of multiple cellular functions. Through its interactions with TGF-β1 and perhaps other growth factors and cell surface receptors, TSP1 modulates the growth of a variety of immune, epithelial, and EC populations, and exerts a net antiangiogenic effect in vivo. TSP2 modulates cell-cell and cell-matrix interactions of fibroblasts and perhaps other cell types, and thereby influences the vascularization, mechanical properties, and structure of several connective tissues. Although the precise biochemical mechanism by which TSP2 affects such diverse cellular properties is unknown, it appears likely that the complex molecular structure of TSP2 allows for multiple intermolecular interactions and thereby influences multiple growth factor- and cell surface molecule-

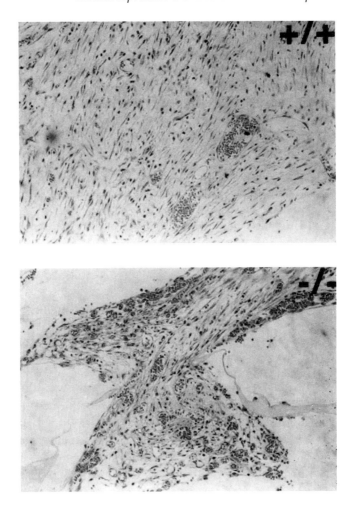

Figure 2. Vascularity of granulation tissue invading a polyvinyl alcohol (PVA) sponge implanted into wild-type and TSP2-null mice. PVA sponges (1 × 1 cm) were implanted subcutaneously into a control mouse (+/+) and a TSP2-null mouse (−/−), and were removed 14 days later. Sections were stained with hematoxylin and eosin. Substantial increases in fibroplasia and vascular invasion are evident in the sponge implanted into the TSP2-null mouse. Magnification: ×400.

mediated pathways. It is therefore appropriate to distinguish TSP1 and 2 from factors such as VEGF and angiopoietin family members, which act primarily upon the vasculature to direct its growth and assembly. Instead, TSP1 and 2 belong to a class of molecules that would appear to promote homeostasis at the tissue level by fine-tuning the growth and differentiation of the vasculature, and integrating vascular growth with the growth of other neighboring cell types.

References

1. Risau W. Mechanisms of angiogenesis. *Nature* 1997;386:671–674.
2. Hanahan D. Signaling vascular morphogenesis and maintenance. *Science* 1997;277:48–50.
3. O'Reilly MS, Boehm T, Shing Y, et al. Endostatin: An endogenous inhibitor of angiogenesis and tumor growth. *Cell* 1997;88:277–285.
4. O'Reilly MS, Holmgren L, Shing Y, et al. Angiostatin: A novel angiogenesis inhibitor that mediates the suppression of metastases by a Lewis lung carcinoma. *Cell* 1994;79:315–328.
5. Ingber DE, Folkman J. How does extracellular matrix control capillary morphogenesis? *Cell* 1989;58:803–805.
6. Vernon RB, Lara SL, Drake CJ, et al. Organized type I collagen influences endothelial patterns during "spontaneous angiogenesis in vitro": Planar cultures as models of vascular development. *In Vitro Cell Dev Biol Anim* 1995;31:120–131.
7. Bornstein P. Diversity of function is inherent in matricellular proteins: An appraisal of thrombospondin 1. *J Cell Biol* 1995;130:503–506.
8. Bornstein P, Sage EH. Thrombospondins. *Methods Enzymol* 1994;245:62–85.
9. Tooney PA, Sakai T, Sakai K, et al. Restricted localization of thrombospondin-2 protein during mouse embryogenesis: A comparison to thrombospondin-1. *Matrix Biol* 1998;17:131–143.
10. Corless CL, Mendoza A, Collins T, et al. Colocalization of thrombospondin and syndecan during murine development. *Dev Dyn* 1992;193:346–358.
11. Kyriakides TR, Zhu YH, Yang Z, et al. The distribution of the matricellular protein thrombospondin 2 in tissues of embryonic and adult mice. *J Histochem Cytochem* 1998;46:1007–1015.
12. Iruela-Arispe ML, Liska DJ, Sage EH, et al. Differential expression of thrombospondin 1, 2, and 3 during murine development. *Dev Dyn* 1993;197:40–56.
13. O'Shea KS, Dixit VM. Unique distribution of the extracellular matrix component thrombospondin in the developing mouse embryo. *J Cell Biol* 1988;107:2737–2748.
14. Reed MJ, Iruela-Arispe L, O'Brien ER, et al. Expression of thrombospondins by endothelial cells: Injury is correlated with TSP-1. *Am J Pathol* 1995;147:1068–1080.
15. Tucker RP. The in situ localization of tenascin splice variants and thrombospondin 2 mRNA in the avian embryo. *Development* 1993;117:347–358.
16. LaBell TL, Milewicz DJ, Disteche CM, et al. Thrombospondin II: Partial cDNA sequence, chromosome location, and expression of a second member of the thrombospondin gene family in humans. *Genomics* 1992;12:421–429.
17. Iruela-Arispe ML, Porter P, Bornstein P, et al. Thrombospondin-1, an inhibitor of angiogenesis, is regulated by progesterone in the human endometrium. *J Clin Invest* 1996;97:403–412.
18. Campbell SC, Volpert OV, Ivanovich M, et al. Molecular mediators of angiogenesis in bladder cancer. *Cancer Res* 1998;58:1298–1304.
19. Botney MD, Kaiser LR, Cooper JD, et al. Extracellular matrix protein gene expression in atherosclerotic hypertensive pulmonary arteries. *Am J Pathol* 1992;140:357–364.
20. Roth JJ, Gahtan V, Brown JL, et al. Thrombospondin-1 is elevated with both intimal hyperplasia and hypercholesterolemia. *J Surg Res* 1998;74:11–16.

21. DiPietro LA, Nissen NN, Gamelli RL, et al. Thrombospondin 1 synthesis and function in wound repair. *Am J Pathol* 1996;148:1851–1860.
22. Koch AE, Friedman J, Burrows JC, et al. Localization of the angiogenesis inhibitor thrombospondin in human synovial tissues. *Pathobiology* 1993; 61:1–6.
23. DiPietro LA, Polverini PJ. Angiogenic macrophages produce the angiogenic inhibitor thrombospondin 1. *Am J Pathol* 1993;143:678–684.
24. Jain RK, Schlenger K, Hockel M, et al. Quantitative angiogenesis assays: Progress and problems. *Nat Med* 1997;3:1203–1208.
25. Hirschi KK, D'Amore PA. Pericytes in the microvasculature. *Cardiovasc Res* 1996;32:687–698.
26. Taraboletti G, Roberts D, Liotta LA, et al. Platelet thrombospondin modulates endothelial cell adhesion, motility, and growth: A potential angiogenesis regulatory factor. *J Cell Biol* 1990;111:765–772.
27. Lawler J, Weinstein R, Hynes RO. Cell attachment to thrombospondin: The role of ARG-GLY-ASP, calcium, and integrin receptors. *J Cell Biol* 1988;107:2351–2361.
28. Tuszynski GP, Rothman V, Murphy A, et al. Thrombospondin promotes cell-substratum adhesion. *Science* 1987;236:1570–1573.
29. Lahav J. Thrombospondin inhibits adhesion of endothelial cells. *Exp Cell Res* 1988;177:199–204.
30. Murphy-Ullrich JE, Höök M. Thrombospondin modulates focal adhesions in endothelial cells. *J Cell Biol* 1989;109:1309–1319.
31. Adams JC. Characterization of cell-matrix adhesion requirements for the formation of fascin microspikes. *Mol Biol Cell* 1997;8:2345–2363.
32. Tolsma SS, Volpert OV, Good DJ, et al. Peptides derived from two separate domains of the matrix protein thrombospondin-1 have anti-angiogenic activity. *J Cell Biol* 1993;122:497–511.
33. Dawson DW, Pearce SF, Zhong R, et al. CD36 mediates the in vitro inhibitory effects of thrombospondin-1 on endothelial cells. *J Cell Biol* 1997;138:707–717.
34. Gao AG, Lindberg FP, Finn MB, et al. Integrin-associated protein is a receptor for the C-terminal domain of thrombospondin. *J Biol Chem* 1996; 271:21–24.
35. DiPietro LA, Nebgen DR, Polverini PJ. Downregulation of endothelial cell thrombospondin 1 enhances in vitro angiogenesis. *J Vasc Res* 1994;31:178–185.
36. Volpert OV, Tolsma SS, Pellerin S, et al. Inhibition of angiogenesis by thrombospondin-2. *Biochem Biophys Res Commun* 1995;217:326–332.
37. Lamszus K, Joseph A, Jin L, et al. Scatter factor binds to thrombospondin and other extracellular matrix components. *Am J Pathol* 1996;149:805–819.
38. Hogg PJ, Hotchkiss KA, Jimenez BM, et al. Interaction of platelet-derived growth factor with thrombospondin 1. *Biochem J* 1997;326:709–716.
39. Schultz-Cherry S, Ribeiro S, Gentry L, et al. Thrombospondin binds and activates the small and large forms of latent transforming growth factor-β in a chemically defined system. *J Biol Chem* 1994;269:26775-26782.
40. Schultz-Cherry S, Chen H, Mosher DF, et al. Regulation of transforming growth factor-β activation by discrete sequences of thrombospondin 1. *J Biol Chem* 1995;270:7304–7310.
41. Taraboletti G, Belotti D, Borsotti P, et al. The 140-kilodalton antiangiogenic fragment of thrombospondin-1 binds to basic fibroblast growth factor. *Cell Growth Differ* 1997;8:471–479.

42. Schultz-Cherry S, Lawler J, Murphy-Ullrich JE. The type 1 repeats of thrombospondin 1 activate latent transforming growth factor-β. *J Biol Chem* 1994;269:26783-26788.
43. Souchelnitskiy S, Chambaz EM, Feige JJ. Thrombospondins selectively activate one of the two latent forms of transforming growth factor-beta present in adrenocortical cell-conditioned medium. *Endocrinology* 1995;136: 5118–5126.
44. Vogel T, Guo NH, Krutzsch HC, et al. Modulation of endothelial cell proliferation, adhesion, and motility by recombinant heparin-binding domain and synthetic peptides from the type I repeats of thrombospondin. *J Cell Biochem* 1993;53:74–84.
45. Folkman J, Haudenschild C. Angiogenesis in vitro. *Nature* 1980;288:551–556.
46. Davis GE, Camarillo CW. An α2β1 integrin-dependent pinocytic mechanism involving intracellular vacuole formation and coalescence regulates capillary lumen and tube formation in three-dimensional collagen matrix. *Exp Cell Res* 1996;224:39–51.
47. Iruela-Arispe ML, Bornstein P, Sage H. Thrombospondin exerts an antiangiogenic effect on cord formation by endothelial cells in vitro. *Proc Natl Acad Sci USA* 1991;88:5026–5030.
48. Canfield AE, Boot-Handford RP, Schor AM. Thrombospondin gene expression by endothelial cells in culture is modulated by cell proliferation, cell shape and the substratum. *Biochem J* 1990;268:225–230.
49. Tolsma SS, Stack MS, Bouck N. Lumen formation and other angiogenic activities of cultured capillary endothelial cells are inhibited by thrombospondin-1. *Microvasc Res* 1997;54:13–26.
50. Canfield AE, Schor AM. Evidence that tenascin and thrombospondin-1 modulate sprouting of endothelial cells. *J Cell Sci* 1995;108:797–809.
51. Qian X, Wang TN, Rothman VL, et al. Thrombospondin-1 modulates angiogenesis in vitro by up-regulation of matrix metalloproteinase-9 in endothelial cells. *Exp Cell Res* 1997;235:403–412.
52. RayChaudhury A, Frazier WA, D'Amore PA. Comparison of normal and tumorigenic endothelial cells: Differences in thrombospondin production and responses to transforming growth factor-β. *J Cell Sci* 1994;107:39–46.
53. Sheibani N, Frazier WA. Thrombospondin 1 expression in transformed endothelial cells restores a normal phenotype and suppresses their tumorigenesis. *Proc Natl Acad Sci USA* 1995;92:6788–6792.
54. Sheibani N, Newman PJ, Frazier WA. Thrombospondin-1, a natural inhibitor of angiogenesis, regulates platelet-endothelial cell adhesion molecule-1 expression and endothelial cell morphogenesis. *Mol Biol Cell* 1997; 8:1329–1341.
55. Sheibani N, Frazier WA. Down-regulation of platelet endothelial cell adhesion molecule-1 results in thrombospondin-1 expression and concerted regulation of endothelial cell phenotype. *Mol Biol Cell* 1998;9:701–713.
56. Phan SH, Dillon RG, McGarry BM, et al. Stimulation of fibroblast proliferation by thrombospondin. *Biochem Biophys Res Commun* 1989;163:56–63.
57. Majack RA, Cook SC, Bornstein P. Control of smooth muscle cell growth by components of the extracellular matrix: Autocrine role for thrombospondin. *Proc Natl Acad Sci USA* 1986;83:9050–9054.
58. Majack RA, Cook SC, Bornstein P. Platelet-derived growth factor and heparin-like glycosaminoglycans regulate thrombospondin synthesis and deposition in the matrix by smooth muscle cells. *J Cell Biol* 1985;101:1059–1070.

59. Majack RA, Goodman LV, Dixit VM. Cell surface thrombospondin is functionally essential for vascular smooth muscle cell proliferation. *J Cell Biol* 1988;106:415–422.
60. Bornstein P, Devarayalu S, Li P, et al. A second thrombospondin gene in the mouse is similar in organization to thrombospondin 1 but does not respond to serum. *Proc Natl Acad Sci USA* 1991;88:8636–8640.
61. Good DJ, Polverini PJ, Rastinejad F, et al. A tumor suppressor-dependent inhibitor of angiogenesis is immunologically and functionally indistinguishable from a fragment of thrombospondin. *Proc Natl Acad Sci USA* 1990;87:6624–6628.
62. Rastinejad F, Polverini PJ, Bouck NP. Regulation of the activity of a new inhibitor of angiogenesis by a cancer suppressor gene. *Cell* 1989;56:345–355.
63. Dey NB, Boerth NJ, Murphy-Ullrich JE, et al. Cyclic GMP-dependent protein kinase inhibits osteopontin and thrombospondin production in rat aortic smooth muscle cells. *Circ Res* 1998;82:139–146.
64. Volpert OV, Lawler J, Bouck NP. A human fibrosarcoma inhibits systemic angiogenesis and the growth of experimental metastases via thrombospondin-1. *Proc Natl Acad Sci USA* 1998;95:6343–6348.
65. Parsons-Wingerter P, Lwai B, Yang MC, et al. A novel assay of angiogenesis in the quail chorioallantoic membrane: Stimulation by bFGF and inhibition by angiostatin according to fractal dimension and grid intersection. *Microvasc Res* 1998;55:201–214.
66. Nicosia RF, Tuszynski GP. Matrix-bound thrombospondin promotes angiogenesis in vitro. *J Cell Biol* 1994;124:183–193.
67. Lawler J, Sunday M, Thibert V, et al. Thrombospondin-1 is required for normal murine pulmonary homeostasis and its absence causes pneumonia. *J Clin Invest* 1998;101:982–992.
68. Kyriakides TR, Zhu YH, Smith LT, et al. Mice that lack thrombospondin 2 display connective tissue abnormalities that are associated with disordered collagen fibrillogenesis, an increased vascular density, and a bleeding diathesis. *J Cell Biol* 1998;140:419–430.
69. Crawford SE, Stellmach V, Murphy-Ullrich JE, et al. Thrombospondin-1 is a major activator of TGF-β1 in vivo. *Cell* 1998;93:1159–1170.
70. Stellmach V, Volpert OV, Crawford SE, et al. Tumour suppressor genes and angiogenesis: The role of TP53 in fibroblasts. *Eur J Cancer* 1996;32A:2394–2400.
71. Dickson MC, Martin JS, Cousins FM, et al. Defective haematopoiesis and vasculogenesis in transforming growth factor-β1 knock out mice. *Development* 1995;121:1845–1854.
72. Antonelli-Orlidge A, Saunders KB, Smith SR, et al. An activated form of transforming growth factor β is produced by cocultures of endothelial cells and pericytes. *Proc Natl Acad Sci USA* 1989;86:4544–4548.
73. Muller G, Behrens J, Nussbaumer U, et al. Inhibitory action of transforming growth factor β on endothelial cells. *Proc Natl Acad Sci USA* 1987;84:5600–5604.
74. Iruela-Arispe ML, Sage EH. Endothelial cells exhibiting angiogenesis in vitro proliferate in response to TGF-β1. *J Cell Biochem* 1993;52:414–430.

Chapter 7

Elastic Fiber Proteins in Pulmonary Vascular Development

Jennifer M.W. Hausladen, MD, and
Robert P. Mecham, PhD

The severity of pulmonary hypertension is determined, at least in part, by the extent of structural changes in the cellular and connective tissue components of the pulmonary vascular wall. These changes include vascular smooth muscle cell (VSMC) proliferation, hypertrophy, and matrix protein deposition. Common to all forms of human pulmonary hypertension are increases in the thickness of the medial layer of normally muscular arteries and an extension of muscle into smaller and more peripheral vessels.[1] In primary pulmonary hypertension (PPH) in adults, smooth muscle and endothelial cells also migrate into the vascular lumen to form neointimal lesions in elastic and muscular pulmonary arteries.[2–4]

Injury-induced changes in cell phenotype are complex and depend on many factors, including the cell type and the differentiation state of the cell at the time of injury.[5] Further, cells of a similar type (eg, VSMCs) may exhibit unique characteristics at different locations and thus respond in unique ways to the pulmonary hypertensive stimulus. We, and others, have documented an extensive heterogeneity within the smooth muscle population of both normal and hypertensive pulmonary arteries.[6–10] This heterogeneity provoked a general rethinking of the possible cellular mechanisms contributing to the structural and functional changes that occur in hypertension-induced remodeling. The results of this work advanced the possibility that different smooth muscle cell (SMC) types make unique contributions to the disease processes associated with pulmonary hypertension. Although we have made significant progress

This work was supported by National Institutes of Health Grants HL29594, HL41926, and HL53325.

From: Weir EK, Archer SL, Reeves JT (eds). *The Fetal and Neonatal Pulmonary Circulations.* Armonk, NY: Futura Publishing Company, Inc.; ©1999.

in addressing this question by identifying specific subpopulations of cells within the vascular wall, there remains the problem of characterizing the function and developmental origin of the different cell groups. It is clear from our findings, as well as similar studies in the systemic circulation (reviewed in Reference 11), that VSMCs do not terminally differentiate into a single phenotype. To understand the origins of SMC diversity in the vessel wall, it is necessary to address two questions: (1) How does the pulmonary vasculature develop, and (2) What is the origin(s) of SMCs in the pulmonary vessels?

Pulmonary Vascular Development

There have been many excellent studies describing pulmonary vascular development in late fetal and postnatal stages,[12–15] but early mechanisms of vascular formation are less well understood. The lungs begin as a ventral outpouching on the foregut. By successive dichotomous divisions, the airway tree increases in complexity as it invades the surrounding mesenchyme. During development, the differentiation of the endodermally derived epithelial tubules is strongly influenced by the interaction with the mesenchymal structures that are of mesodermal origin.[16,17]

The pulmonary arteries and veins develop concurrently, and their development before birth is closely related to that of the bronchial tree.[14] There is a double arterial and double venous supply in the adult lung, with the pulmonary arteries supplying the respiratory units and most of the pleura, while the bronchial (systemic) arteries supply the airway walls and lung hilum, including pleura and large blood vessel walls. Recent studies by deMello et al[18] and Buck et al,[19] and our findings described below, show that the pulmonary circulation develops by both vasculogenesis and angiogenesis. Using PECAM-1 as a marker for endothelial cells, Buck et al[19] found that the precursors of the major bronchial vessels appeared to be initiated by an angiogenic process in which endothelial cells comprising the vestiges of the brachial arches and segmental arteries migrated into the mesenchyme surrounding the early lung buds. These invading cells organized into a plexus of endothelial cells that eventually coalesced into fully patent vessels. In peripheral regions of the developing lung, small vessels formed directly (vasculogenesis) in undifferentiated mesenchyme surround the growing airway buds. These vessels formed a vascular plexus which, through a process of fusion and coalescence, linked up with larger vessels that had sprouted and migrated from more differentiated arteries and veins in proximal regions of the lung. As mentioned above, branching of the airways and arteries is contemporaneous, although branching of the airways occurs in advance of the arteries. The pulmonary veins develop later than the arteries, and although the architecture of the venous system reflects the already present bronchial and arterial branching pattern, the veins tend to run in the mesenchyme that demarcates the boundary between segments and subsegments of the lung.[14]

Elastic Fibers and Vascular Elasticity

The elastic properties of both systemic and pulmonary vessels are contributed by elastic fibers, which are produced by all three major cell types in the vessel wall. The major elastic structures in the vessel are the elastic lamellae that form circumferential sheets of elastin between smooth muscle layers in the medial compartment. The internal elastic lamina (IEL) is the first elastic structure formed in the vessel wall, and endothelial cells, together with their adjacent layer of SMCs, play a critical role in its formation. Once the IEL is formed, endothelial cells no longer express elastin unless reactivated by vessel injury.

The functional form of elastin is a highly cross-linked polymer of the secreted tropoelastin molecule. Polymerization occurs in the extracellular matrix through the assistance of microfibrils, which serve to align tropoelastin monomers with each other so that cross-linking can occur (a process catalyzed by the enzyme lysyl oxidase).[20] Microfibrils, 10–12 nm filaments with a bead-like ultrastructure, consist of the proteins fibrillin-1 and -2, microfibril-associated glycoprotein, latent transforming growth factor (TGF-β) binding protein-2 (LTBP-2), and possibly small molecular weight proteoglycans.[21,22] How these components associate to make a microfibril, however, is still unknown.

The fibrillin and LTBP families are made up of repeating domains that have homology to epidermal growth factor and latent TGF-β-binding protein. In addition to their structural role in the extracellular matrix, all members of the LTBP family bind latent TGF-β. It is not yet known whether the same is true for the fibrillins. As with other proteins that influence vascular development, deletion or mutation of elastic fiber components has profound implications for vessel integrity and function. Mutations in fibrillin-1 have been linked to Marfan syndrome and result in a weakened vascular wall prone to aneurysm and rupture.[23,24] Supravalvular aortic stenosis has been associated with the complete deletion of one allele of the elastin gene (as occurs in Williams syndrome) or mutations that render the gene product of one allele nonfunctional.[25,26]

In developing arteries, we, and others,[27] have observed that expression of the tropoelastin gene occurs coincident with the accumulation and condensation of mesenchymal cells around the endothelial tube, indicating that tropoelastin production is an early differentiation marker for cells of the arterial wall. Moreover, the high levels of tropoelastin synthesis by these cells (tropoelastin mRNA as assessed by in situ hybridization) suggests that the activation of tropoelastin gene expression is an important part of their differentiation program. There is also increasing evidence that the onset of elastin production correlates with dramatic morphological events in the vessel wall. In blood vessels in the developing chick, for example, major morphological alterations were first seen with the onset of elastin deposition including a loss of actin expression and clear separation of medial cell layers into lamellae.[28,29] Elastin is also one of the first genes activated in response to injury.

Expression of Elastic Fiber Proteins in Developing Lung

To characterize the spatial and temporal expression of elastic fiber proteins in the developing pulmonary circulation, we used in situ hybridization to study the expression of elastin, fibrillin-1, and fibrillin-2 in

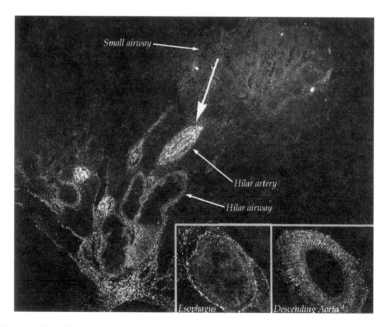

Figure 1. Darkfield in situ image of 70–90 day fetal bovine lung hybridized with a probe specific for fibrillin-1. Expression is strongest around the larger, well-differentiated hilar airways and in the medial and adventitial compartments of blood vessels. A similar pattern is evident in the descending aorta. The large arrow indicates a well-developed pulmonary artery.

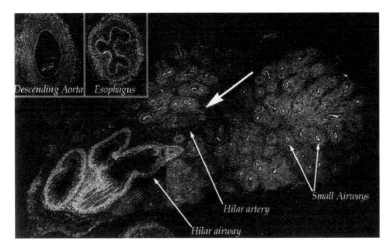

Figure 2. In situ hybridization showing fibrillin-2 expression in 70–90 day fetal bovine lung. Expression is strongest around the larger hilar airways and in respiratory epithelium in the more peripheral airways. There is little detectable signal in pulmonary arteries or veins, or in the descending aorta. In the esophagus, fibrillin-2 was expressed by cells immediately under the epithelial layer and near the outside of the structure (inset). The large arrow indicates a well-developed pulmonary artery.

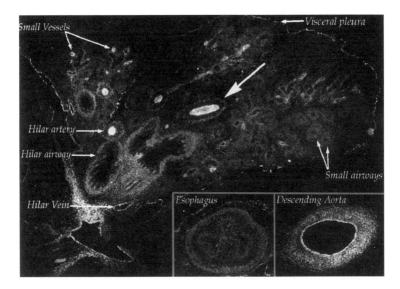

Figure 3. In situ hybridization showing elastin expression in 70–90 day fetal bovine lung. Intense signal is evident in the large and small vessels compared with the weaker expression found around the larger hilar airways. Endothelial cells in the descending aorta demonstrate a strong signal with a gradient of expression in the medial layer decreasing radially away from the lumen. No discernible signal was detected in the esophagus (inset). Large arrow indicates a well-developed pulmonary artery.

lungs from early bovine embryos. We chose to study the bovine lung be-cause of its relatively large size (even at embryonic stages) and because timing of bovine gestation and lung development is similar to humans. As the lung forms, both arteries and veins branch with the developing airways into undifferentiated mesenchyme, providing an excellent ex-perimental system for the study of elastic fiber gene expression in multi-ple cell types. Based on the accepted paradigm that microfibrils function to organize tropoelastin prior to cross-linking, we expected to find coex-pression of tropoelastin with microfibrillar proteins. To our surprise, we found unique and divergent patterns, suggesting that the function of elastic fiber proteins is more complex than initially anticipated.

Figures 1–3 show 10-week bovine lung hybridized with probes for fibrillin-1, fibrillin-2, and tropoelastin. At this stage of development, hi-lar regions of the lung show large, well-differentiated airways, arteries, and veins that branch within the enclosing mesenchyme. Regions of the lung around the large airways (lower left region in each figure) are more differentiated than areas where branching is still occurring (up-per right region).

Fibrillin-1

Fibrillin-1 was expressed in the loose connective tissue that sus-pends the hilar region of the lung and, to a lesser extent, in the periph-eral mesenchyme separating the branching segments (Figure 1). Ex-pression was also evident in well-differentiated blood vessels with highest levels in the intimal and adventitial compartments (Figure 4). There was no detectable expression in the condensed mesenchyme around the branching epithelium or in the epithelium itself. Also, fib-rillin-1 was not detected in the forming blood vessels in the less-differ-entiated, peripheral regions of the lung.

Fibrillin-2

Expression of fibrillin-2 was essentially opposite that of fibrillin-1 (Figure 2). Highest expression was evident in airway epithelium in both hilar and peripheral regions of the lung where polarization of the protein synthetic machinery to the luminal aspect of the cell resulted in a band-like expression pattern. Strong signal was also detected in the forming bronchial smooth muscle layer in the more differentiated air-ways. No signal was detected in the regions separating the branching segments, but low signal was evident in the condensed mesenchyme around the branching epithelium. Interestingly, fibrillin-2 expression was not detected in either large or small pulmonary vessels (Figure 4).

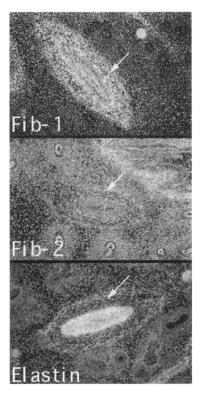

Figure 4. Expression of elastin and fibrillins in pulmonary artery detected by in situ hybridization. The location of the pulmonary artery in the lung is indicated by the large arrow in Figures 1–3.

Tropoelastin

Tropoelastin expression was first detected in the visceral pleura where it remained high throughout lung development. At early stages of blood vessel formation, tropoelastin expression was confined exclusively to endothelial cells. At later stages, after the vessel had developed a layered structure, SMCs in the media also expressed elastin, although at lower levels than endothelial cells (Figure 3). There was relatively little tropoelastin expression in the adventitia except possibly for the outermost rim of cells (Figure 4). Interestingly, tropoelastin was the only probe that clearly hybridized with the smaller, less-differentiated vessels in peripheral regions of the lung. There was no tropoelastin expression by epithelial cells in any region of the lung at this stage of development.

Elastin is a marker for early vascular development in peripheral regions of the lung.

Expression of elastin by endothelial cells proved to be a reliable marker of newly developing vessels in the peripheral lung. Figure 5 shows in situ hybridization of bovine lung demonstrating the close approximation of vascular structures with branching airways. In the more terminal regions (Figure 5, c-f), the bronchial tubules are embedded in a condensed bundle of mesenchyme. Here, tropoelastin signal was associated with a restricted subset of cells that, in many instances, could be identified as vascular cells by the presence of an intracellular space that occasionally contained a hematopoietic cell. Occasionally, mesenchymal cells began to show a concentric orientation around the developing vessel, suggestive of the pattern assumed by SMCs in the medial layer. Our evidence suggests that the cells that

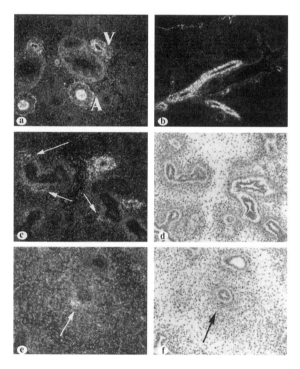

Figure 5. In situ hybridization showing elastin expression by SMCs and endothelial cells in developing arteries (A) and veins (V) around airways (a and b). In peripheral, less differentiated regions of the lung where airway branching is still ongoing, elastin expression occurs within discrete clusters of cells that represent forming blood vessels (c and e, arrows). Panels d and f are light microscopy images of c and e.

express elastin in the mesenchymal clusters are vascular cells in the process of vasculogenesis or angiogenesis. Interestingly, none of the known microfibrillar proteins are expressed with elastin, suggesting that tropoelastin is not being organized into elastic fibers at these sites.

Fibrillin-2 antibody detects smooth muscle cells in the bronchial but not pulmonary circulation.

A closer inspection of the fibrillin-2 in situ expression pattern around large bronchi in proximal, more differentiated regions of the 10-week bovine lung shown in Figure 2 suggests strong expression by the developing bronchial smooth muscle layer, as well as by cells in submucosal regions corresponding to the bronchial microvasculature. This vascular plexus, consisting of both capillaries and postcapillary venules, has its origins in the systemic circulation and, in contrast to the pulmonary circulation, is a high-pressure system in the mature lung. To determine which cells in this bronchial region produce fibrillin-2, an antibody specific for this protein was used in immunostaining of embryonic bovine lung sections. Vascular cells in arteries and veins around the highly developed bronchial airways stained positively with the fibrillin-2 antibody (not shown). Cells in the epithelial layer also stained, in agreement with the in situ results. Cells in adjacent pulmonary vessel, however, did not stain.

To determine whether the cells that were positive for fibrillin-2 were SMCs, we used the smooth muscle-specific 1E12 antibody[23,24] to stain parallel sections. As expected, cells in the bronchial vessels stained positively with this antibody, confirming their SMC origin. This antibody also stained the bronchial smooth muscle layer and microvascular cells of the vasa vasorum found in the adventitia of the larger pulmonary vessels. The 1E12 antibody only detected a subset of SMCs within the media of large pulmonary arteries, however. This is interesting in light of our earlier demonstration of multiple smooth muscle phenotypes in the pulmonary circulation.[6]

Conclusion

The results from this study have the following implications for understanding pulmonary vascular development: (1) elastin expression is a sensitive marker for following the recruitment of vascular cells (both endothelial and smooth muscle) within the undifferentiated mesenchyme; (2) expression of fibrillin-2 can be used to specifically detect SMCs in the bronchial (ie, systemic) circulation in the developing lung; and (3) the 1E12 antibody reacts with cells in the bronchial circulation and vasa vasorum, and with a subset of cells within the wall of large pulmonary vessels. The differential expression of fibrillin-2 and the 1E12 antigen by the bronchial and pulmonary vessels implies that SMCs that make up these two vascular beds are phenotypically different. This may reflect the different embryological origins of the two cell groups. As mentioned earlier, data from Buck et al[19] suggest that the bronchial circulation arises through an angiogenic process in which endothelial cells comprising the vestiges of the branchial arches and segmental arteries migrate into the mesenchyme surrounding the early lung buds. In peripheral regions of the developing lung, small vessels form directly (vasculogenesis) in undifferentiated mesenchyme surrounding the growing airway buds. The elastin, fibrillin-2, and 1E12 antibodies are reagents that will allow us to explore this process more completely.

The ability of elastin to act as a signaling molecule for cells is now well established. Many cell types, including SMCs, have an elastin receptor that functions to alter gene expression, mobilization of intracellular ions, and cell adhesion and movement.[30–32] Furthermore, elastin peptides can influence vascular tone by interacting with the elastin receptor on cells in the intact vessel wall[33] and are chemoattractants for both interstitial and inflammatory cells.[34,35] The presence of a receptor for elastin on a wide variety of cells establishes the importance of elastin as a signaling molecule.

Fibrillin-1 and -2 have also been shown to interact with receptors on the cell surface. Studies in our laboratory have shown that both proteins contain RGD sequences that interact with the $\alpha_v\beta_3$ and $\alpha_5\beta_1$ integrin receptors.[36] We feel that this interaction may have important implications for vessel development since $\alpha_v\beta_3$ integrin appears to be critical for the formation and/or maintenance of newly formed vessels.[37] Some cell types recognize a second, non-RGD-binding site within the fibrillin molecule. The nature of this site has not been determined.

Together, these observations lend support to the possibility that elastic fiber proteins have a dual function. Early in vascular development, their expression by endothelial cells and presumptive SMCs suggests a signaling function that could influence either the recruitment or differentiation state of smooth muscle precursor cells. Later in development, during coexpression of microfibrillar proteins and tropoelastin, the elastic fiber's mechanical properties are apparent when tropoelastin becomes cross-linked to form the elastic polymer.

References

1. Meyrick BO, Perkett EA. The sequence of cellular and hemodynamic changes of chronic pulmonary hypertension induced by hypoxia and other stimuli. *Am Rev Respir Dis* 1989;140:1486–1489.
2. Botney MD, Kaiser LR, Cooper JD, et al. Extracellular matrix protein gene expression in atherosclerotic hypertensive pulmonary arteries. *Am J Pathol* 1992;140:357–364.
3. Tuder RM, Groves B, Badesch DB, et al. Exuberant endothelial cell growth and elements of inflammation are present in plexiform lesions of pulmonary hypertension. *Am J Pathol* 1994;144:275–285.
4. Voelkel NF, Tuder RM. Cellular and molecular mechanisms in the pathogenesis of severe pulmonary hypertension. *Eur Resp J* 1995;8:2129–2138.
5. Stenmark KR, Dempsey EC, Badesch DB, et al. Regulation of pulmonary vascular wall cell growth: Developmental and site-specific heterogeneity. *Eur Respir Rev* 1993;3(review #16):629–637.
6. Prosser IW, Stenmark KR, Suthar M, et al. Regional heterogeneity of elastin and collagen gene expression in intralobar arteries in response to hypoxic pulmonary hypertension as demonstrated by in situ hybridization. *Am J Pathol* 1989;135:1073–1088.
7. Mecham RP, Stenmark KR, Parks WC. Connective tissue production by vascular smooth muscle in development and disease. *Chest* 1991;99:43S47S.
8. Stenmark KR, Durmowicz AG, Roby JD, et al. Persistence of the fetal pattern of tropoelastin gene expression in severe neonatal bovine pulmonary hypertension. *J Clin Invest* 1994;93:1234–1242.
9. Frid MG, Moiseeva EP, Stenmark KR. Multiple phenotypically distinct smooth muscle cell populations exist in the adult and developing bovine pulmonary arterial media in vivo. *Circ Res* 1994;75:669–681.
10. Wohrley JD, Frid MG, Moiseeva EP, et al. Hypoxia selectively induces proliferation in a specific subpopulation of smooth muscle cells in the bovine neonatal pulmonary arterial media. *J Clin Invest* 1995;96:273–281.
11. Owens GK. Regulation of differentiation of vascular smooth muscle cells. *Physiol Rev* 1995;75:487–517.
12. Burri PH, Weibel ER. Ultrastructure and morphometry of the developing lung. In: Hodson WA, ed: *Development of the Lung*. New York: Marcel Dekker; 1977:215–268.
13. Burri PH. Structural aspects of prenatal and postnatal development and growth of the lung. In: McDonald JA, ed: *Lung Growth and Development*. New York: Marcel Dekker; 1997:1–35.
14. Hislop A, Reid LM. Formation of the pulmonary vasculature. In: Hodson WA, ed: *Development of the Lung*. New York: Marcel Dekker; 1977:37–86.
15. O'Rahilly R. The early prenatal development of the human respiratory system. In: Nelson GE, ed: *Pulmonary Development*. New York: Marcel Dekker; 1985:3–18.
16. Wessells NK. Mammalian lung development: Interactions in formation and morphogenesis of tracheal buds. *J Exp Zool* 1970;175:455–466.
17. Spooner BS, Wessell NK. Mammalian lung development: Interactions in primordium formation and bronchial morphogenesis. *J Exp Zool* 1970;175:445–454.
18. deMello DE, Sawyer D, Galvin N, et al. Early fetal development of lung vasculature. *Am J Respir Cell Mol Biol* 1997;16:568–581.

19. Buck CA, Edelman JM, Buck CE, et al. Expression patterns of adhesion receptors in the developing mouse lung: Functional implications. *Cell Adhes Commun* 1996;4:69–87.
20. Mecham RP, Davis EC. Elastic fiber structure and assembly. In: Yurchenko PD, Birk DE, Mecham RP, eds: *Extracellular Matrix Assembly and Structure*. San Diego: Academic Press; 1994:281–314.
21. Gibson MA, Kumaratilake JS, Cleary EG. The protein components of the 12-nanometer microfibrils of elastic and non-elastic tissues. *J Biol Chem* 1989;264:4590–4598.
22. Cleary EG, Gibson MA. Elastin-associated microfibrils and microfibrillar proteins. *Int Rev Connect Tiss Res* 1983;10:97–209.
23. Hungerford JE, Owens GK, Argraves WS, et al. Development of the aortic vessel wall as defined by vascular smooth muscle and extracellular matrix markers. *Dev Biol* 1996;178:375–392.
24. Hungerford JE, Hoeffler JP, Bowers CW, et al. Identification of a novel marker for primordial smooth muscle and its differential expression pattern in contractile vs noncontractile cells. *J Cell Biol* 1997;137:925–937.
25. Curran ME, Atkinson DL, Ewart AK, et al. The elastin gene is disrupted by a translocation associated with supravalvular aortic-stenosis. *Cell* 1993; 73:159–168.
26. Ewart AK, Morris CA, Atkinson D, et al. Hemizygosity at the elastin locus in a developmental disorder, Williams syndrome. *Nat Genet* 1993;5: 11–16.
27. Selmin O, Volpin D, Bressan GM. Changes of cellular expression of mRNA for tropoelastin in the intraembryonic arterial vessels of developing chick revealed by *in situ* hybridization. *Matrix* 1991;11:347–358.
28. Bergwerff M, DeRuiter MC, Poelmann RE, et al. Onset of elastogenesis and downregulation of smooth muscle actin as distinguishing phenomena in artery differentiation in the chick embryo. *Anat Embryol* 1996;194:545–557.
29. Rosenquist TH, McCoy JR, Waldo KL, et al. Origin and propagation of elastogenesis in the developing cardiovascular system. *Anat Rec* 1988;221: 860–871.
30. Hinek A, Wrenn DS, Mecham RP, et al. The elastin receptor is a galactoside binding protein. *Science* 1988;239:1539–1541.
31. Mecham RP, Hinek A, Entwistle R, et al. Elastin binds to a multifunctional 67 kD peripheral membrane protein. *Biochemistry* 1989;28:3716–3722.
32. Blood CH, Sasse J, Brodt P, et al. Identification of a tumor cell receptor for VGVAPG, an elastin-derived chemotactic peptide. *J Cell Biol* 1988;107: 1987–1993.
33. Faury G, Chabaud A, Ristori MT, et al. Effect of age on the vasodilatory action of elastin peptides. *Mech Ageing Dev* 1997;95:31–42.
34. Senior RM, Griffin GL, Mecham RP, et al. Val-Gly-Val-Ala-Pro-Gly, a repeating peptide in elastin, is chemotactic for fibroblasts and monocytes. *J Cell Biol* 1984;99:870–874.
35. Senior RM, Griffin GL, Mecham RP. Chemotactic activity of elastin-derived peptides. *J Clin Invest* 1980;66:859–862.
36. Sakamoto H, Broekelmann T, Cheresh DA, et al. Cell-type specific recognition of RGD- and non-RGD-containing cell binding domains in fibrillin-1. *J Biol Chem* 1996;271:4916–4922.
37. Brooks PC, Clark RAF, Cheresh DA. Requirement of vascular integrin $\alpha v \beta 3$ for angiogenesis. *Science* 1994;264:569–571.

Chapter 8

Proteolytic Modulation of the Extracellular Matrix

Marlene Rabinovitch, MD

Introduction

Vascular cells, like other cells, take cues from changes in the extracellular matrix (ECM). These cues can result in cellular differentiation, proliferation in response to growth factors, or migration in response to chemotactic stimuli. The normal pulmonary circulation is under the tight regulation of this dynamic process. It assures that pulmonary arteries will dilate appropriately and that pulmonary vascular resistance will decrease when the lungs are inflated in the postnatal period. Changes in the ECM also ensure that the ductus arteriosus closes completely in the postnatal period. The understanding of how the ECM is modulated in a dynamic way would appear critical in being able to manipulate cell phenotype and, specifically, to reverse pathological changes that occur in disease. This chapter will address how proteinases, specifically endogenous vascular elastase and other serine elastases, matrix metalloproteinases, and a newly described chymase modulate the ECM. A review will be provided of work related to proteinase regulation of the glycoprotein tenascin, which alters cell shape and amplifies the proliferative response to growth factors. The ductus arteriosus has been an ideal model within which to study how, in the absence of increased proteolytic activity, impaired assembly of elastin and the consequent production of elastin peptides

This work was supported by Grant PG13920 from the Medical Research Council and by Grant T2229 from the Heart and Stroke Foundation of Ontario. The author is a Research Endowed Chair of the Heart and Stroke Foundation of Ontario.

From: Weir EK, Archer SL, Reeves JT (eds). *The Fetal and Neonatal Pulmonary Circulations.* Armonk, NY: Futura Publishing Company, Inc.; ©1999.

leads to the upregulation of fibronectin. Fibronectin is critical in switching smooth muscle cells (SMCs) from the contractile to the migratory mode, which accounts for the subsequent development of the intimal cushion. The molecular mechanisms involved in this process and the consequences for the development of the intimal cushion will be addressed. In addition, new work on a chymase that was recently cloned from vascular SMCs will be presented. This chymase can potentially activate matrix metalloproteinases and also serves as an angiotensin II-converting enzyme as well as an endothelin-converting enzyme.

Elastases in Pulmonary Vascular Remodeling

Endogenous vascular elastase appears to be an initiator of the structural remodeling that occurs in response to a pulmonary hypertension producing stimulus (Figure 1). In lung biopsies in children with congenital heart defects, fragmentation of elastin is an early structural change in those with pulmonary hypertension.[1] We also confirmed fragmentation and showed high turnover of elastin in pulmonary ar-

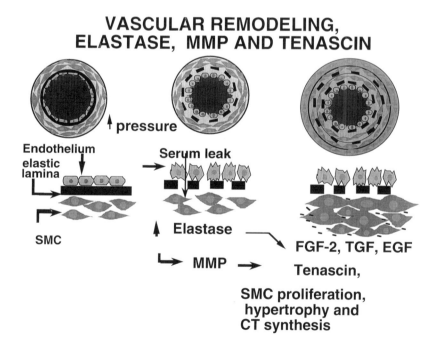

Figure 1. Schema showing how an elastase can induce changes in matrix proteins resulting in smooth muscle cell (SMC) proliferation and migration.

REGULATION OF
ENDOGENOUS VASCULAR ELASTASE

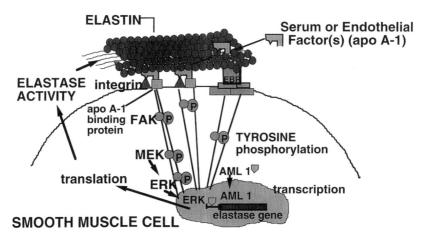

Figure 2. A proposed schema indicating how serum factor(s) or endothelial factors, ie, Apo A1, tethers elastin to the smooth muscle cell surface, permitting engagement of the elastin-binding protein (EBP) and perhaps cooperative interaction with integrin receptors resulting in tyrosine kinase activity. The subsequent promotion of DNA transcription and mRNA translation culminates in the induction of vascular elastase.

teries of experimental rats in which pulmonary hypertension was induced by the toxin monocrotaline.[2] A subsequent study reported that, in the adult rat with progressive pulmonary vascular disease following an injection of the toxin monocrotaline, there was an early increase in elastase activity at 2 days, and a more sustained elevated level between 16 and 28 days following injection of the toxin, ie, associated both with the initiation and with the progression of pulmonary vascular disease.[3] This enzyme is a serine elastase that we later documented as approximately 23 kD in molecular weight, localized to SMCs of the vessel wall, and which appeared to be immunologically related to the serine proteinase adipsin.[4] A cause and effect relationship between increased elastase activity and the development and progression of vascular disease was later shown in two experimental models: (1) rats subjected to chronic hypobaric hypoxia,[5] and (2) rats injected with the toxin monocrotaline.[6] In the latter study, we were able to show that even preventing the elevation in elastase activity at 2 weeks was effective in slowing the progression of pulmonary vascular disease.

Subsequent cell culture studies have tried to address how the elastase might be induced and how it might regulate the structural changes in the vessel wall. Serum factors which include apolipoprotein A1 tether elastin to the smooth muscle wall surface.[7,8] This invokes a tyrosine kinase signaling mechanism resulting in phosphorylation of focal adhesion kinase (FAK) and the mitogen-activated protein (MAP) kinase family members, Erk 1 and Erk 2 (Erk 1/2). The phosphorylation of Erk appears to be related to nuclear expression of the transcription factor AML 1 (Figure 2). AML 1 is upregulated following induction of SMCs to produce elastase.[9] It has been implicated in the regulation of the neutrophil elastase gene. In recent studies (as yet unpublished), we have shown that the modulation of elastase appears to be regulated by nitric oxide—nitric oxide suppresses elastase activity and also the pathway, resulting in AML 1 nuclear expression.

Elastase and Smooth Muscle Cell Proliferation

Induction of SMC proliferation by increased activity of elastase was further elucidated through cell culture study.[10] We showed that induction of endogenous vascular elastase or administration of leukocyte elastase released fibroblast growth factor FGF-2 from its associated proteoglycans in a biologically active form. It appeared, however, that elastase activity was concurrently mediating further changes in the compositon of the ECM which amplify the proliferative response.

Tenascin and Smooth Muscle Cell Proliferation

When collagen is degraded by elastases or by matrix metalloproteinases, cryptic RGD sites are exposed which associate with the β_3 integrins on SMC surfaces.[11] This results in the induction of a phosphorylation signal involving MAP kinase (Erk 1/2), which culminates in an increased transcription of the tenascin gene through a critical promoter element that appears in region 122 base pairs upstream from the start site of the coding region. Increased expression of tenascin clusters β_3 integrins, leading to the formation of focal adhesion contacts and subsequent clustering of growth factor (specifically epidermal growth factor [EGF]) receptors. The clustering of EGF receptors results in their rapid phosphorylation upon ligation (Figure 3). In fact, we have shown that tenascin appears to be a prerequisite for SMC proliferation in response to EGF.[12] It also amplifies the proliferative response to bFGF (Figure 4).

While these studies were performed in cell culture, the role of tenascin in progression of pulmonary vascular disease has been elucidated in experimental models as well as in biopsy tissue. We made the

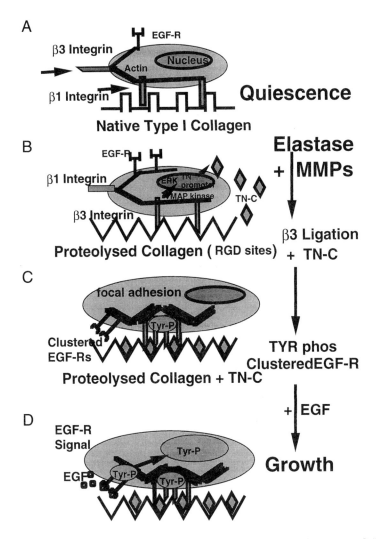

Figure 3. Hypothetical model for the regulation and function of tenascin-C (TN-C) in vascular smooth muscle cells. **A:** Vascular smooth muscle cells attach and spread on native type I collagen using β1 integrins. Under serum-free conditions, the cells withdraw from the cell cycle and become quiescent. **B:** Degradation of native type I collagen by matrix metalloproteinases (MMPs) leads to exposure of cryptic RGD sites that preferentially bind β3 subunit-containing integrins. In turn, occupancy and activation of β3 integrins signals the production of TN-C. **C:** Incorporation of multivalent TN-C protein into the underlying substrate leads to further aggregation and activation of β3-containing integrins (αβ3), and to the accumulation of tyrosine-phosphorylated (Tyr-P) signaling molecules and actin into a focal adhesion complex. Note that even in the absence of the EGF ligand, the TN-C-dependent reorganization of the cytoskeleton leads to clustering of actin-associated EGF-Rs. **D:** Addition of EGF ligand to clustered EGF-Rs results in rapid and substantial tyrosine phosphorylation of the EGF-R and activation of downstream pathways culminating in the generation of nuclear signals leading to cell proliferation.

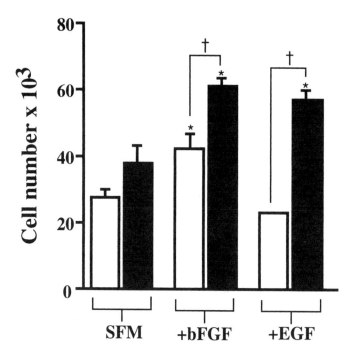

Figure 4. Smooth muscle cell growth in serum-free medium (SFM) was unaffected by addition of exogenous TN-C. In contrast, addition of basic fibroblast growth factor (bFGF) or epidermal growth factor (EGF) to TN-C-treated cultures resulted in a significant increase in cell number. Values represent mean ±SEM. *p < 0.05 vs corresponding SFM level; †p < 0.05 for difference related to TN-C.

observation that tenascin mRNA is upregulated in rat lungs within 14 days after injection of the toxin, monocrotaline, and this is associated with an induction of tenascin protein expression beginning in the medial-adventitial border but progressing to the subendothelial region of the vessel wall. Tenascin codistributes with proliferating cells as judged by BrDU labeling. In lung biopsy tissue from patients with pulmonary hypertension, tenascin is seen codistributing with proliferating cells and heightened growth factor expression in the neointima of thickened pulmonary arteries.[13]

   In cell culture we observed that not only was tenascin important as a proliferative factor, but also that tenascin was a cell survival factor in that its withdrawal, associated with suppression of matrix metalloproteinases, led to apoptosis.[11] We have now shown that hypertrophied pulmonary arteries can be made to regress when incubated with elastase or matrix metalloproteinase inhibitors or by suppressing tenascin mRNA translation by antisense.[14]

Vascular Smooth Muscle Chymase

Our group has just cloned a novel chymase from rat SMCs. This enzyme has the ability to convert angiotensin I to angiotensin II and may also be important in the regulation of endothelin and in the activation of matrix metalloproteinases. It appears to be induced in the early neonatal period.[15]

Fibronectin and Smooth Muscle Cell Migration

To understand mechanisms leading to SMC migration, which culminate in the development of neointimal formation, our group has studied the biology of intimal cushion formation in the ductus arteriosus.[16–23] Intimal cushions develop in the ductus arteriosus, ensuring that this vessel will close completely when it constricts in the postnatal period. Incomplete formation of intimal cushions results in patency of the ductus arteriosus.[24] Studies in our laboratory have investigated how changes in the ECM regulate endothelial and SMC behavior in the ductus arteriosus. We showed that, under the regulation of transforming growth factor-β (TGF-β), there is increased production of hyaluronan by endothelial cells of the ductus relative to other vascular sites, ie, pulmonary artery or aorta (Figure 5).[16] An endothelial factor, which is likely also TGF-β, stimulates SMCs to upregulate production of chondroitin sulfate. Chon-

INTIMAL CUSHION FORMATION IN THE DUCTUS ARTERIOSUS

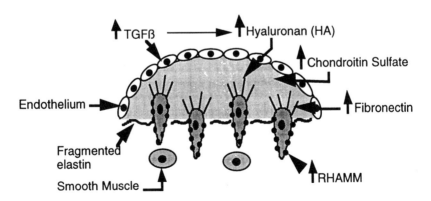

Figure 5. Schema showing changes in the extracellular matrix in the ductus arteriosus. RHAMM = receptor for hyaluronan-mediated motility.

droitin sulfate releases the elastin-binding protein from SMC surfaces,[20] resulting in impaired elastin assembly. This elastin-binding protein functions as an elastin chaperone intracellularly; lack of this protein results in inadequate protection of the elastin molecule from intracellular degradation.[23] A 52-kD truncated post-translational form of elastin, which lacks the C-terminal, is generated, and this molecule cannot be assembled or cross-linked properly.[22] Elastin peptides also appear to upregulate fibronectin at a post-transcriptional level.[19,21]

Our group has noted that ductus SMCs, despite their increased production of fibronectin do not show an increase in fibronectin mRNA levels or in mRNA transcription or stability. We therefore, directed our attention to mechanisms that may control post-transcriptional regulation of fibronectin at the level of mRNA translation. We identified an interaction between light chain 3 (LC3), of microtubule-associated protein 1A and 1B, and a sequence rich in A+U bases (ARE) in the fibronectin 3′untranslated region (UTR). Increased production of LC3 was observed in ductus relative to aortic SMCs, and transfection of LC3 into aortic cells changed their phenotype from contractile to migratory[25] (Figure 6). More recent work suggests that this increase in production of LC3 is under the regulation of nitric oxide.[26] Increased LC3 appears to recruit the mRNA to the polysomes .[27] This process is also dependent on an intact microtubule system (Figure 7) and appears to involve the ability of LC3 to sort or to initiate translation of mRNA by recruiting ribosomes (Figure 8).

Having identified the molecular mechanism that regulates increased efficiency of translation of fibronectin mRNA, we next addressed whether the system could be manipulated to advantage. We had observed that when transfecting ductus SMCs in culture with a construct bearing the fibronectin 3′UTR and the choramphenicol transferase (CAT) reporter sequence upstream, fibronectin synthesis was suppressed and the phenotype of the ductus cells switched from elongated or migratory to contractile. This suggested that the LC3 was being sequestered away from the endogenous fibronectin mRNA, and that the construct was acting as a decoy RNA.

To exploit this further, we conducted studies in which the ductus arteriosus in the fetal lamb was transfected using the HVJ (hemagglutinating virus of Japan)-liposome technique[28] and the DNA constructs with the ARE (LC3 sequestering sequence) intact (wild-type) or mutated (non-LC3 sequestering). At term, a patent ductus with no or minimal intimal cushions was observed in lambs transfected with the fibronectin 3′UTR decoy RNA, whereas when the mutant (non-LC3 sequestering) vector was transfected, intimal cushion formation was similar to that in nontransfected control twins.[29] We further confirmed that we had inter-

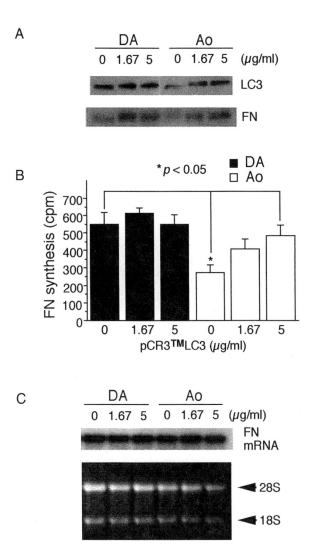

Figure 6. Overexpression of light chain 3 (LC3) in aortic (Ao) smooth muscle cells enhances fibronectin (FN) mRNA translation. **A:** A representative western blot shows that transfection of LC3 by the adenovirus component system (see methods) increased LC3 production in a dose-dependent manner in Ao but only partially in ductus arteriosus (DA) cells (top). The overexpression of LC3 in Ao cells also augmented FN synthesis to the levels observed in the DA cells, whereas this was not associated with a significant increase in FN synthesis in DA cells (bottom). The concentration of plasmid, pCR-LC3, used in the transfection is indicated at the top. **B:** Graph of quantitative assessment of FN synthesis from four different experiments showing that there is a significant decrease in the basal level of newly synthesized FN in Ao (white bars) compared with DA cells (black bars). *p < 0.05, superANOVA and Duncan's test of multiple comparisons. However, the newly synthesized FN in Ao cells is increased significantly after transfection with pCR-LC3 (p<0.05) in a dose-dependent manner. **C:** Northern blot analysis indicating that there is no change in the level of FN mRNA after LC3 transfection compared with controls in either DA or Ao cells. The loading condition is demonstrated by ethidium bromide staining of 18S and 28S.

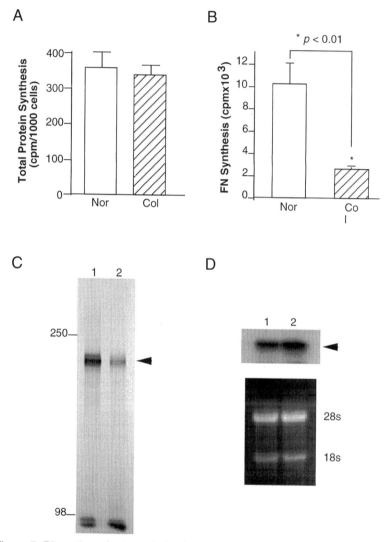

Figure 7. Disruption of microtubules by colchicine inhibits fibronectin synthesis. **A:** A quantitative study of total protein synthesis shows similar values in normal and colchicine-treated cultures from three different experiments. **B:** A quantitative analysis from four different experiments shows that fibronectin synthesis was significantly decreased in cells treated with colchicine compared to normal cultured cells (*p < 0.01, by Student *t* test). **C:** A representative autoradiograph of newly synthesized fibronectin (arrow) extracted from conditioned media of normal cultures (lane 1) or colchicine-treated cultures (lane 2). Equal amounts of total secreted proteins, as judged by trichloroacetic acid (TCA) precipitated counts, were used for fibronectin extraction. **D:** A representative northern blot analysis shows that the steady-state level of fibronectin mRNA (arrow) remains the same when normal (lane 1) and colchicine-treated (lane 2) smooth muscle cells are compared. 28s and 18s RNA are shown to confirm equal loading conditions. Three different experiments showed similar results.

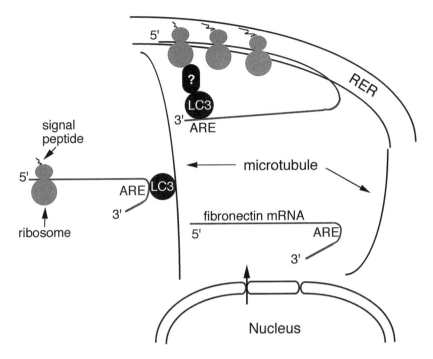

Figure 8. Proposed model of translational control of fibronectin expression by mRNA sorting. Fibronectin mRNA is sorted onto rough endoplasmic reticulum (RER) by nascent signal peptide, and translation is then initiated. The dual function of LC3, ie, binding of LC3 to fibronectin mRNA through the AU-rich element (ARE) at the 3'UTR and to microtubules, may facilitate sorting of fibronectin mRNA onto RER via microtubules. Alternatively, LC3 may dissociate from microtubules and link fibronectin mRNA to the ribosomal complex by binding to the ARE and to an unknown factor (designated "?") in the 60s ribosomal subunit.

fered with fibronectin synthesis at a critical time in the development of the ductus when the upregulation of fibronectin switches its SMCs from a contractile to a migratory phenotype.

This process appears to also be modulated by nitric oxide. That is, we showed in cell culture studies that ductus SMCs produce more nitric oxide than aortic cells, and that a decrease in nitric oxide prevents the production and the phosphorylation of LC3[27] and the induction of fibronectin.

References

1. Rabinovitch M, Bothwell T, Hayakawa BN, et al. Pulmonary artery endothelial abnormalities in patients with congenital heart defects and pulmonary hypertension: A correlation of light with scanning electron microscopy and transmission electron microscopy. *Lab Invest* 1986;55:632–653.

2. Todorovich-Hunter L, Ranger P, Johnson D, et al. Altered elastin and collagen synthesis associated with progressive pulmonary hypertension induced by monocrotaline: A biochemical and ultrastructural study. *Lab Invest* 1988;58:184–195.

3. Todorovich-Hunter L, Dodo H, McCready L, et al. Increased pulmonary artery elastolytic activity and monocrotaline-induced progressive hypertensive pulmonary vascular disease in adult rats compared to infant rats with non-progressive disease. *Am Rev Resp Dis* 1992;146:213–223.

4. Zhu L, Wigle D, Hinek A, et al. The endogenous vascular elastase which governs development and progression of monocrotaline-induced pulmonary hypertension in rats is a novel enzyme related to the serine proteinase adipsin. *J Clin Invest* 1994;94:1163–1171.

5. Maruyama K, Ye C, Woo M, et al. Chronic hypoxic pulmonary hypertension in rats and increased elastolytic activity. *Am J Physiol* 1991;261:H1716-H1726.

6. Ye C, Rabinovitch M. Inhibition of elastolysis by SC-37698® reduces development and progression of monocrotaline pulmonary hypertension. *Am J Physiol* 1991;261:H1255-H1267.

7. Kobayashi J, Wigle D, Childs T, et al. Serum-induced vascular smooth muscle cell elastolytic activity through tyrosine kinase intracellular signalling. *J Cell Physiol* 1994;160:121–131.

8. Thompson K, Kobayashi J, Childs T, et al. Endothelial and serum factors which include apolipoprotein A1 tether elastin to smooth muscle cells inducing serine elastase activity via tyrosine kinase-mediated transcription and translation. *J Cell Physiol* 1998;174:78–89.

9. Wigle D, Thompson K, Yablonsky S, et al. AML1-like transcription factor induces serine elastase activity in ovine pulmonary artery smooth muscle cells. *Circ Res* 1998;83:252–263.

10. Thompson K, Rabinovitch M. Exogenous leukocyte and endogenous elastases can mediate mitogenic activity in pulmonary artery smooth muscle cells by release of extracellular matrix-bound basic fibroblast growth factor. *J Cell Physiol* 1996;166(3):495–505.

11. Jones PL, Crack J, Rabinovitch M. Regulation of Tenascin-C, a vascular smooth muscle cell survival factor that interacts with the alpha v beta 3 integrin to promote epidermal growth factor receptor phosphorylation and growth. *J Cell Biol* 1997;139:279–293.

12. Jones PL, Rabinovitch M. Tenascin-C is induced with progressive pulmonary vascular disease in rats is functionally related to increased smooth muscle cell proliferation. *Circ Res* 1996;79:1131–1142.

13. Jones PL, Cowan KN, Rabinovitch M. Tenascin-C, proliferation and subendothelial fibronectin in progressive pulmonary vascular disease. *Am J Pathol* 1997;150:1349–1360.

14. Cowan K, Jones PL, Rabinovitch M. Regression of hypertrophied rat pulmonary arteries in organ culture is associated with suppression of proteolytic activity, inhibition of tenascin-C and smooth muscle cell apoptosis. *Circ Res* (in press).

15. Guo C, Rabinovitch M. A novel chymase cDNA cloned from rat pulmonary artery smooth muscle cells with increased vascular expression in spontaneously hypertensive rats. *Circulation* 1998;98(suppl):1–746.

16. Boudreau N, Rabinovitch M. Developmentally regulated changes in extracellular matrix in endothelial and smooth muscle cells in the ductus arteriosus may be related to intimal proliferation. *Lab Invest* 1991;64:187–199.

17. Boudreau N, Clausell N, Boyle J, et al. Transforming growth factor β regulates increased ductus arteriosus endothelial glycosaminoglycan synthesis and a post-transcriptional mechanism controls increased smooth muscle fibronectin, features associated with intimal proliferation. *Lab Invest* 1992;67:350–359.

18. Boudreau N, Turley E, Rabinovitch M. Fibronectin, hyaluronan, and a hyaluronan binding protein contribute to increased ductus arteriosus smooth muscle cell migration. *Dev Biol* 1991;143:235–247.

19. Hinek A, Molossi S, Rabinovitch M. Fibronectin synthesis is related to a reciprocal interplay between the 67-kD elastin binding protein and the IL-1β receptor on coronary smooth muscle cells. *Exp Cell Res* 1996;225:122–131.

20. Hinek A, Mecham RP, Keeley FW, et al. Impaired elastin fibre assembly related to reduced 67-kD elastin-binding protein in fetal lamb ductus arteriosus and in cultured aortic smooth muscle cells treated with chondroitin sulfate. *J Clin Invest* 1991;88:2083–2094.

21. Hinek A, Boyle J, Rabinovitch M. Vascular smooth muscle cell detachment from elastin and migration through elastic laminae is promoted by chondroitin sulfate-induced 'shedding' of the 67-kD cell surface elastin binding protein. *Exp Cell Res* 1992;203:344–353.

22. Hinek A, Rabinovitch M. The ductus arteriosus migratory smooth muscle cell phenotype processes tropoelastin to a 52-kDa product associated with impaired assembly of elastic laminae. *J Biol Chem* 1993;268:1405–1413.

23. Hinek A, Rabinovitch M. 67-kD elastin binding protein is a protective "companion" of extracellular insoluble elastin and intracellular tropoelastin. *J Cell Biol* 1994;126:563–574.

24. Gittenberger de Groot AGD, Strengers J, Mettnick M, et al. Histologic studies on normal and persistent ductus arteriosus in the dog. *J Am Coll Cardiol* 1985;6:394–404.

25. Zhou B, Boudreau N, Coulber C, et al. Microtubule-associated protein 1 light chain 3 is a fibronectin mRNA-binding protein linked to mRNA translation in lamb vascular smooth muscle cells. *J Clin Invest* 1997;100:3070–3082.

26. Mason C, Rabinovitch M. TNF-α induction of fibronectin synthesis is mediated by nitric oxide by a post-transcriptional mechanism involving increased expression and binding of LC3 to an ARE in the 3'UTR of FN mRNA. *FASEB J* 1998;12(Part 1):955.

27. Zhou B, Rabinovitch M. Microtubule involvement in translational regulation of fibronectin expression by light chain 3 of microtubule-associated protein 1 in vascular smooth muscle cells. *Circ Res* 1998;83:481–489.

28. Morishita R, Gibbons GH, Horiuchi M, et al. A gene therapy strategy using a transcription factor decoy of the E2F binding site inhibits smooth muscle proliferation in vivo. *Proc Natl Acad Sci USA* 1995;92:5855–5859.

29. Mason C, Bigras J-L, Zhou B, et al. Bioengineering patent ductus arteriosus in post-natal lambs. *Circulation* 1997;96:I-484.

Chapter 9

Signal Transduction Kinases in the Regulation of Matrix Metalloproteinase-9 Expression in Vascular Smooth Muscle Cells

Aesim Cho, PhD, and Michael A. Reidy, PhD

Introduction

Degradation of the extracellular matrix is a critical event required for cell migration during angiogenesis, and for remodeling of vessels during vascular injury such as atherosclerosis, restenosis, and plaque rupture. Matrix metalloproteinases (MMPs) are thought to play an important role in the extracellular proteolysis. MMPs constitute a family of 14 or more enzymes which includes collagenases, gelatinases, stromelysins, metalloelastase, and membrane-type MMP. The MMPs are secreted in a latent form containing zinc in the active site and require activation before they can degrade matrix components such as collagen, fibronectin, elastin, and laminin. In vascular tissues, both smooth muscle cells (SMCs) and macrophages can produce a variety of MMPs. MMP-1 (interstitial collagenase), MMP-3 (stromelysin), and MMP-9 (type IV collagenase) have been identified in human atherosclerotic lesions, and the enhanced expression of MMP-9 at the shoulders of these lesions has been linked to plaque rupture.[1] In experimental animal models, MMPs are also shown to be important for SMC migration into the intima. In a rat arterial injury model, after the initial medial SMC replication, medial SMCs migrate and first appear in the intima 4 days after injury, and then the subsequent proliferation of migrated cells leads to

This work was supported by National Institutes of Health Grants HL-03174 and HL-41103.

From: Weir EK, Archer SL, Reeves JT (eds). *The Fetal and Neonatal Pulmonary Circulations.* Armonk, NY: Futura Publishing Company, Inc.; ©1999.

the formation of neointima.[2] MMP-9 is expressed within 6 hours after injury and continues to be expressed for up to 6 days after injury, and MMP-2 (type IV collagenase) activity is markedly increased after 4 days.[3] Administration of an MMP inhibitor almost completely inhibited the number of SMCs migrating into the intima, implicating the importance of these MMPs in the migration of SMCs.[3] MMPs can therefore play important roles in lesion growth; however, little is known about the factors and the regulatory mechanism involved in the expression of MMPs in vascular smooth muscle cells (VSMCs).

Several growth factors and cytokines can modulate extracellular matrix synthesis and degradation. Some of these factors, such as basic fibroblast growth factor (bFGF), platelet-derived growth factor (PDGF), tumor necrosis factor-α (TNF-α), and interleukin-1 (IL-1), have been shown to induce MMPs, including MMP-1, MMP-2, MMP-3, and MMP-9 in a variety of cell types.[4-6] These growth factors and cytokines elicit intracellular signals via the mitogen-activated protein (MAP) kinase pathway. In mammalian cells, there are three distinct groups of MAP kinases: extracellular-regulated kinase (Erk), c-Jun N-terminal kinase (Jnk), and p38. The Erk pathway is mainly activated by growth factors leading to cell proliferation and cell growth, whereas the activation of Jnk and p38 pathways can lead to apoptosis and inhibition of cell growth.[7] Both Jnk and p38 are known as the members of the stress-activated protein kinase, since these kinases are strongly activated in response to stressful stimuli such as osmotic shock, UV light, and exposure to cytokines. Both Jnk and p38 phosphorylate the DNA-binding domain of activating transcription factor-1 (ATF-2), and Jnk can also phosphorylate c-Jun. c-Jun in combination with c-Fos binds to the activator protein-1 (AP-1) site; c-Jun can also dimerize with ATF-2 and binds to the tetradecanoyl phorbol acetate responsive (TRE) element of the promoter of many genes including *c-jun* and MMPs. p38 can also activate MAP kinase-activated protein kinase (MAPKAPK) 2 and 3 which phosphorylate the small heat shock proteins.[8]

Of interest to this study is the suggestion that these MAP kinases are important in the regulation of MMPs in various cell types. We investigated the signaling pathway involved in the regulation of MMP-9 expression in VSMCs and we demonstrated that activation of Jnk and p38 MAP kinase is important for induction of MMP-9 expression in VSMCs both in vitro and in vivo. This chapter will discuss the results of this investigation.

Growth Factors and Cytokines on MMP-9 Expression

Several growth factors and cytokines are expressed and active in the injured arteries which include bFGF, PDGF, TGF-β1 (transforming growth factor-β1), and TNF-α. In a previous study, our laboratory has shown that the rate of SMC migration in injured arteries is significantly increased by injection of bFGF, and that blocking antibody to FGF markedly reduced the cell migration.[9] Jawien et al demonstrated that PDGF promotes SMC migration and intimal thickening in rat arteries after injury.[10] A recent study by Jovinge et al showed that TNF-α is expressed in balloon-injured rat aorta and that TNF-α activates SMC migration in vitro.[11] bFGF and PDGF have been shown to upregulate collagenase and stromelysin production in human arterial SMCs and rat dermal papilla cells, respectively. Galis et al showed that TNF-α upregulated MMP-2 and MMP-9 expression in human saphenous vein SMCs.[1] We examined the effect of these factors, which are known to be expressed in injured artery, on MMP-9 activity and expression by zymography and northern blot analysis, respectively. TNF-α increased the MMP-9 activity and expression in a concentration-dependent manner whereas TGF-β1, PDGF-BB, or bFGF had little effect on MMP-9 expression. The gelatinolytic activity of MMP-2 was not affected by any of these growth factors and cytokines.

Activities of Mitogen-Activated Protein Kinases in Vascular Smooth Muscle Cells

The MAP kinase pathway is activated in response to growth factors and cytokines. To determine the signaling pathway involved in the activation of MMP-9 expression, we examined the activities of three MAP kinases—Erk, Jnk, and p38—in VSMCs using several kinase assays as described by Hibi et al and Graves et al.[12,13] Jnk and p38 MAP kinase activities in arterial SMCs were markedly increased with TNF-α treatment, with little effect on Erk activities. To examine whether direct activation of stress-activated protein (SAP) kinases can upregulate MMP-9 expression, SMCs were treated with anisomycin, which can activate both Jnk and p38. Anisomycin caused a potent activation of both Jnk and p38 activities, and significantly upregulated the MMP-9 mRNA level in VSMCs. These data suggest that activation of Jnk and p38 can induce MMP-9 expression.

Effect of Stress-Activated Protein Kinases on MMP-9 Expression in Arteries

Our laboratory previously showed that the activity of Jnk was increased immediately after balloon catheter injury.[14] We also observed that p38 MAP kinase activity increased immediately after injury. Thus, both Jnk and p38 are rapidly activated after injury and before the onset of transcriptional activation of MMP-9 gene. To examine whether the activation of Jnk and/or p38 MAP kinase can induce MMP-9 expression in vivo, anisomycin was administered (i.v.) to rats immediately following gentle denudation of the left carotid artery. The arterial MMP-9 mRNA level was markedly elevated with anisomycin treatment, suggesting that the activation of SAP kinases induces MMP-9 expression in vivo. Thus, the fact that activation of SAP kinases via anisomycin induces MMP-9 expression both in vitro and in vivo indicates that the SAP kinase pathway is important in the regulation of MMP-9 expression in vascular tissues.

Effect of Stress-Activated Protein Kinase Activity on MMP-9 Expression

To further examine the requirement of SAP kinase in the regulation of MMP-9 expression, cells were stimulated in the presence of a synthetic inhibitor of p38, SB203580. This inhibitor is a pyrimidazole compound and reversibly binds to active p38, thus preventing phosphorylation of its substrates.[15] When SMCs were pretreated with SB203580, TNF-α- and anisomycin-induced expression of MMP-9 was inhibited in a concentration-dependent manner.

Transcription Factors in the Regulation of MMP-9 in Smooth Muscle Cells

It is not clear how the activation of the SAP kinase pathway results in the induction of MMPs. Since inhibition of p38 MAP kinase blocked the transcription of the MMP-9 gene, we next examined the potential transcription factors involved in this process. Other DNA-binding sites of MMP-9 promoters such as AP-1, NF-κB, SP-1 and PEA3/Ets have been implicated in the regulation of MMP-9 gene transcription.[15] MAP kinases can modulate AP-1 activity by phosphorylation of c-Jun and c-Fos, and the AP-1 site has been implicated in the regulation of human MMP-9 promoter activity in nonvascular cells.[17,18] The SP-1-binding site has been implicated in the contact-mediated induction of the MMP-9 gene and in the TNF-α- and TPA (12-0-tetradecanoyl-phorbol-13-acetate)-induced expression of MMP-9 in tumor cells.[16,18] To examine for the potential DNA-binding elements involved in the p38 MAP kinase-mediated regulation of the MMP-9 gene in VSMCs, we performed electrophoretic mobility shift assays using several consensus oligonucleotides. We initially examined for AP-1-binding activity by an electrophoretic mobility shift experiment. Upon treatment with TNF-α or anisomycin, the binding activity of

AP-1 markedly increased; however, the binding of AP-1 site was not affected by pretreatment with SB203580, suggesting that this site is not involved in the p38 MAP kinase-mediated control of MMP-9 in VSMCs.

The electrophoretic mobility shift experiment with nuclear factor-κB (NF-κB) consensus oligonucleotide revealed multiple bands with the upper two bands specific for NF-κB. When cells were treated with TNF-α, the binding activity of p65 and p50 family of NF-κB was significantly increased; however, this increased binding was not affected by SB203580 treatment. In addition, anisomycin did not induce much NF-κB-binding activity, indicating that the activation of SAP kinases does not induce NF-κB binding in VSMCs. These results suggest that NF-κB transcription factors are unlikely to be involved in the transcriptional regulation of MMP-9 in VSMCs.

Next we incubated the nuclear extracts from VSMCs with SP-1 consensus oligonucleotide; the binding of SP-1 was only slightly increased with both TNF-α and anisomycin, and this binding was decreased when treated with p38 inhibitor. Interestingly this reduction in SP-1 binding with SB203580 treatment was markedly below the level observed in untreated cells, indicating that SB203580 somehow prevents the basal binding of SP-1 elements.

In summary, we showed that SAP kinases are involved in the TNF-α-induced regulation of MMP-9 in VSMCs, and that AP-1, NF-κB, and SP-1 elements are possibly important in the control of the MMP-9 gene, but they are not involved in the p38 MAP kinase-mediated activation of MMP-9 gene transcription.

References

1. Galis ZS, Sukhova GK, Lark MW, et al. Increased expression of matrix metalloproteinases and matrix degrading activity in vulnerable regions of human atherosclerotic plaques. *J Clin Invest* 1994;94:2493–2503.
2. Clowes AW, Reidy, MA, Clowes MM. Kinetics of cellular proliferation after arterial injury. I: Smooth muscle growth in the absence of endothelium. *Lab Invest* 1983;49:327–333.
3. Bendeck MP, Zempo N, Clowes AW, et al. Smooth muscle cell migration and matrix metalloproteinase expression after arterial injury in the rat. *Circ Res* 1994;75:539–545.
4. Kennedy SH, Qin H, Lin L, et al. Basic fibroblast growth regulates type I collagen and collagenase gene expression in human smooth muscle cells. *Am J Pathol* 1995;146:764–771.
5. Goodman LV, Ledbetter SR. Secretion of stromelysin by cultured dermal papilla cells: Differential regulation by growth factors and functional role in mitogen-induced cell proliferation. *J Cell Physiol* 1992;51:41–49.
6. Lee E, Vaughan DE, Parikh SH, et al. Regulation of matrix metalloproteinases and plasminogen activator inhibitor-1 synthesis by plasminogen in cultured human vascular smooth muscle cells. *Circ Res* 1996;78:44–49.

7. Robinson MJ, Cobb MH. Mitogen-activated protein kinase pathways. *Curr Opin Cell Biol* 1997;9:180–186.
8. Whitmarsh AJ, Davis RJ. Transcription factor AP-1 regulation by mitogen-activated protein kinase signal transduction pathways. *J Mol Med* 1996;74:589–607.
9. Jackson CL, Reidy MA. Basic fibroblast growth factor: Its role in the control of smooth muscle cell migration. *Am J Pathol* 1993;143:1031–1042.
10. Jawien A, Bowen-Pope DF, Lindner V, et al. Platelet-derived growth factor promotes smooth muscle cell migration and intimal thickening in a rat model of balloon angioplasty. *J Clin Invest* 1992;89:507–511.
11. Jovinge S, Hultgardh-Nilsson A, Regnstrom J, et al. Tumor necrosis factor-alpha activated smooth muscle cell migration in culture and is expressed in the balloon-injured rat aorta. *Arterioscler Thromb Vasc Biol* 1997;17:490–497.
12. Hibi M, Lin A, Minden ST, et al. Identification of an oncoprotein- and UV-responsive protein kinase that binds and potentiates the c-Jun activation domain. *Genes Dev* 1993;7:2135–2148.
13. Graves JD, Draves KE, Craxton A, et al. A comparison of signaling requirements for apoptosis of human B lymphocytes induced by the B cell receptor and CD95/Fas. *J Immunol* 1998;161:168–174.
14. Koyama H, Olson NE, Dastvan FF, et al. Cell replication in the arterial wall: Activation of signaling pathway following in vivo injury. *Circ Res* 1998;82:713–721.
15. Cuenda A, Rouse J, Doza YN, et al. SB 203580 is a specific inhibitor of a MAP kinase homologue which is stimulated by cellular stresses and interleukin-1. *FEBS Lett* 1995;364:229–233.
16. Himelstein BP, Lee EJ, Sato H, et al. Tumor cell contact mediated transcriptional activation of the fibroblast matrix metalloproteinase-9 gene: Involvement of multiple transcription factors including Ets and an alternating purine-pyrimidine repeat. *Clin Exp Metastasis* 1998;16:169–177.
17. Gum R, Wang H, Lengyel E, et al. Regulation of 92 kDa type IV collagenase expression by the jun aminoterminal kinase- and the extracellular signal-regulated kinase-dependent signaling cascades. *Oncogene* 1997;14:1481–1893.
18. Sato H, Seiki M. Regulatory mechanims of 92 kDa type IV collagenase gene expression which is associated with invasiveness of tumor cells. *Oncogene* 1993;8:395–405.

Chapter 10

Transcription Factors Controlling Cellular Proliferation During Vascular Repair

Roy C. Smith, PhD, Toshiaki Mano, MD, and Kenneth Walsh, PhD

Introduction

The proliferation of the smooth muscle cells of the vessel wall is a central feature of a number of cardiovascular disorders. Vascular smooth muscle cells (VSMCs) play a central role as the proliferative component of restenotic and atherosclerotic lesions. The peptide growth factors, their cognate receptors, and the intracellular signaling pathways activated by receptor occupancy have been extensively studied.[1] However, much less is known about how nuclear factors process these signals and regulate the downstream transcriptional events that determine whether proliferation or differentiation occurs. Here we review what is known about three transcriptional factors (*gax, GATA-6,* and *MEF2A*) that may function to control these processes, since a knowledge of these factors would have obvious utility in understanding vessel wall pathology and would aid in the design of therapeutic strategies.

Phenotypic modulation has been a useful concept for interpreting the responses of myocytes to vascular injury. In this model VSMCs exist in either a "contractile" or "synthetic" state.[2–5] Contractile state cells represent the VSMCs of the normal vessel wall, and are quiescent, nonmotile, and express high levels of contractile proteins, including smooth muscle-specific isoforms of actin and myosin, that are taken to be markers of a differentiated phenotype. Synthetic state VSMCs are associated with proliferative vessel wall lesions and express lower levels of the smooth mus-

From: Weir EK, Archer SL, Reeves JT (eds). *The Fetal and Neonatal Pulmonary Circulations.* Armonk, NY: Futura Publishing Company, Inc.; ©1999.

cle-specific contractile proteins, and higher levels of nonmuscle isoforms of myosin and actin.[6–12] These cells have considerably lower levels of cytoplasmic myofibrils,[4] secrete extracellular matrix components,[13] are motile,[3,4,14] and are responsive to growth factors.[1] By virtue of possessing these features, synthetic state VSMCs resemble the less differentiated precursors found in fetal blood vessels.[15–17] Synthetic VSMCs are associated with atherosclerotic lesions,[1,10,18–21] myointimal hyperplasia within prosthetic vascular grafts,[22–26] and the repair of arterial injury.[27,28] A consequence of phenotypic modulation is that a vascular myocyte must first return to a less differentiated state in order to proliferate, suggesting that a common set of nuclear factors may coordinate these processes.

Recent investigations have identified several transcription factors that regulate the expression of VSMC genes and thereby alter the VSMC phenotype. The expression of these factors is regulated by mitogens, indicating that they may function by controlling the expression of cell cycle regulators as well as VSMC-specific proteins.[29] In this chapter, we will briefly discuss several factors involved in VSMC transcriptional regulation and their involvement in modulating smooth muscle cell proliferation.

The Homeodomain Transcription Factor *Gax*

Homeobox genes are a class of transcription factors discovered by analysis of fruit fly homeotic mutations that give rise to abnormal body formation. These genes encode proteins that contain a characteristic 61 amino acid sequence, known as the homeodomain, which allows binding to a DNA sequence known as the homeobox.[30] In addition to being important in modeling body plan, members of this class of genes are involved in regulating the processes of organogenesis, cell growth, differentiation, and migration in a number of organisms including humans.[31–34] However, the functional significance of this class of genes is complex, since some homeobox genes can induce a less differentiated phenotype and promote uncontrolled cell proliferation,[35] while others promote a differentiated phenotype and inhibit proliferation.[36,37]

Vasuclar myocytes are capable of switching from a differentiated to a proliferative phenotype,[3] and since homeobox genes can function both as positive or negative regulators of cell growth, they may prove to be important determinants of the VSMC phenotype. When an adult rat aorta library was screened for the expression of homeobox genes, several were obtained, including a unique muscle-specific homoeobox gene, *gax* (growth arrest-specific homeobox).[38] In mouse embryos, *gax* is expressed in mesodermally derived tissues that give rise to the heart, the muscle of the gut, and the somites from which skeletal muscle is derived.[39] In addition, a neuroectodermal distribution of the *gax* protein was observed from the brain to the neural tube. Expression of *gax* mRNA is also observed in adult human tissue of the cardiovascular and pulmonary systems including the heart, lung, and aorta.[40]

The full-length human *gax* cDNA was obtained by an anchored polymerase chain reaction (PCR) approach and was mapped to the short arm of chromosome 7 at band p21 using fluorescence in situ hybridization.[41] The human and rat *gax* gene coding sequences are highly conserved (98%) at the protein level and, in addition to containing a homeodomain region, both contain trinucleotide repeat sequences encoding for 17 consecutive histidine or glutamine residues.

gax is expressed in quiescent VSMCs, both in vitro and in vivo, and the expression of its mRNA is rapidly downregulated by conditions that stimulate VSMC proliferation.[40,42] In rat VSMCs, *gax* mRNA levels are downregulated within 2 hours of growth factor stimulation. The reduced expression is transient and *gax* mRNA levels begin to rise between 8 and 24 hours after mitogen stimulation and return to near quiescent levels by 24 to 48 hours. This downregulation is dose-dependent and correlates with a mitogen's ability to stimulate DNA synthesis. Thus, the platelet-derived growth factor-AA (PDGF-AA) form, a weak VSMC mitogen, does not substantially alter *gax* transcript levels, while PDGF-BB, a potent mitogen, rapidly downregulates *gax* expression. In a different system, Yamashita et al[43] have recently shown that *gax* expression can be modulated by vasoactive peptides that function in the regulation of hemodynamic pressure. Angiotensin II, a vasoconstrictor that stimulates VSMC proliferation, downregulates *gax* expression while the vasodilator, C-type natriuretic peptide, induces *gax* expression, consistent with its ability to inhibit VSMC proliferation. This regulation of *gax* by mitogens and vasoactive peptides suggests that *gax* may have a regulatory function in controlling VSMC proliferation, possibly by governing the transition from the G0 to G1 phases of the cell cycle.

The mitogen-regulated *gax* expression observed in vitro led us to explore whether *gax* is regulated in a physiologically relevant manner. In a balloon-injured rat carotid artery, where VSMC proliferation is induced as a wound healing response, *gax* expression is rapidly downregulated.[44] The reduction in mRNA levels is transient and occurs in a manner similar to that seen with mitogen stimulation in vitro. Furthermore, the downregulation of *gax* coincided with the upregulation of early response genes such as c-*myc*. Collectively, these patterns of expression are consistent with *gax* functioning as a regulator of genes associated with the nonproliferative, contractile phenotype characteristic of VSMCs of the uninjured vessel wall.

The mitogen-regulated pattern of expression suggested the possibility that *gax* might also inhibit VSMC proliferation. Microinjection of recombinant *gax* protein into VSMCs significantly inhibited entry of VSMCs into the S phase.[45] The inhibition occurred only when *gax* was microinjected during the quiescent state (G0) or during early stages of the G1 phase of the cell cycle. The extent of growth inhibition was dose-dependent and similar to the levels of activity obtained with other strongly antiproliferative proteins, such as recombinant *MyoD* or anti-*ras* antibodies. When a replication-defective adenovirus vector encoding the *gax* cDNA (adeno-gax) was used to induce *gax* overexpression, VSMC proliferation was inhibited in the G1 phase of the cell cycle and the inhibition was correlated with increased expression of the cdk kinase inhibitor p21 and a decrease in cdk2 kinase activity.[45] The induction of p21 was also detected at the level of mRNA, and an ability of *gax* to transactivate the p21 promoter suggests a transcriptional link. Fibroblasts deficient in p21 are not susceptible to a reduction in cdk2 activity or growth inhibition by *gax* overexpression, emphasizing the interrelationship between *gax* and p21.

In addition to its ability to inhibit cell cycle progression, *gax* overexpression can also induce apoptosis in serum-stimulated, but not quiescent, VSMCs in a p21-independent manner.[46] Arrest in the G1 or S phase was not required to induce apoptosis of adeno-gax infected cultures indicating that *gax*-mediated apoptosis is independent of its ability to induce cell cycle arrest. Adeno-gax overexpression leads to down-regulation of the antiapoptotic protein *bcl-2* and upregulation of the apoptotic accelerator *bax*, indicating that *gax* functions by altering the balance of apoptotic regulatory proteins. These observations suggest that the homeostatic balance between cell growth and death, as influenced by *gax*, occurs via mitogen-dependent pathways that control the expression of *bcl-2* family proteins.

The high transduction efficiency obtained with adenoviral vectors has proven essential for in vivo studies of VSMC proliferation. Balloon-denuded rat carotid arteries exhibit excessive VSMC proliferation and neointima formation, but when exposed to a solution of adeno-gax virus immediately following injury, neointima formation and luminal narrowing were significantly reduced.[45] In another study, percutaneous angioplasty and adenovirus-mediated *gax* gene transfer were performed on rabbit iliac arteries, an animal model that has several features in common with clinical angioplasty procedures. In this system, adeno-gax treatment reduced the hyperproliferative response of VSMCs to balloon injury, as demonstrated by an increase in lumen diameter and a decrease in neointima formation.[47] The in vivo studies indicate that, consistent with its ability to influence VSMC proliferation, the *gax* homeodomain protein can ameliorate injury-induced changes in vessel wall morphology.

The GATA-Binding Transcription Factor *GATA-6*

The promoters of a number of genes expressed in VSMCs contain a *GATA*-binding transcription factor binding site, (A/T)*GATA*(A/G). This family of transcription factors is encoded by six genes that are characterized by the presence of two zinc-finger domains. *GATA-1, GATA-2,* and *GATA-3* are mainly expressed in hematopoietic-derived tissues while *GATA-4, GATA-5,* and *GATA-6* are expressed in mesoderm-derived tissues including heart and intestines.[48] Since VSMCs are derived from lateral plate mesoderm, like cardiomyocytes, and the *GATA* factors *4, 5,* and *6* are expressed in visceral muscle, it seemed highly probable that *GATA* factors may have important regulatory roles in vascular smooth muscle.

Recently, the human *GATA-6* gene was isolated from a human fetal heart cDNA library with a mixture of probes to portions of the Xenopus *GATA-5* and chicken *GATA-4* cDNAs.[49] The cDNA contained a single open reading frame predicted to encode a 45.3-kD protein, comprised of 449 amino acids, which contains two zinc-finger domains similar to those found in other members of the GATA-binding transcription factor family. *GATA-6* maps to human chromosome 18q11.1–11.2 by fluorescent in situ hybridization and is the predominant *GATA* isoform in the vasculature. *GATA-6* is expressed in cultures of both rat and human VSMCs and the transcript can be detected in cDNA derived from human aorta.[49] In other organs, *GATA-4* and *-6* transcripts are prominent in the heart, pancreas, and ovary, but only *GATA-6* mRNA is found in the lung and spleen.

In VSMCs, *GATA-6* transcripts are downregulated when quiescent cultures are stimulated to proliferate by mitogen activation.[49] These data demonstrate that *GATA-6* expression is both tissue-specific and mitogen-responsive. In a manner similar to *gax*, ectopic *GATA-6* expression inhibits the proliferation of rat VSMC and induces the expression of the general cdk inhibitor p21.[50] Of significance, p21-deficient fibroblasts expressing *GATA-6* are not inhibited and remain capable of cell cycle progression, suggesting that the upregulation of p21 expression largely accounts for the observed G1 cell cycle arrest. However, unlike *gax*, *GATA-6* does not transactivate the p21 promoter, suggesting that *GATA-6* acts either through a distant regulatory site or by increasing p21 stability via a post-transcriptional mechanism, as has recently been demonstrated for *C/EBP-α*.[51]

Since the mitogen-regulated expression of *GATA-6* was similar to that observed for *gax*, we investigated whether *GATA-6* could also modulate VSMC proliferation following ballgvboon injury. *GATA-6* transcript, protein, and DNA-binding activity are downregulated in rat carotid arteries upon balloon injury.[51a] An adenovirus vector expressing the *GATA-6* cDNA (adeno-GATA-6) inhibited cell growth in vitro, and adeno-GATA-6-mediated gene transfer to the vessel wall following balloon injury partially restored levels of *GATA-6* protein and activity to preinjury levels, significantly inhibiting neointima lesion formation. These data indicate that *GATA-6* downregulation following injury is an essential feature of the proliferative response to vessel wall injury.

In summary, *GATA-6* can regulate the expression of the p21 cdk inhibitor and inhibit S-phase entry. It seems reasonable to speculate that *GATA-6* functions in VSMCs, like *GATA-4* does in the heart, to activate the expression of contractile protein genes associated with the differentiated phenotype, though VSMC-specific gene targets for *GATA-6* are currently unknown. Therefore, *GATA-6* may serve multiple regulatory roles in VSMCs by functioning to coordinate VSMC proliferation and differentiation during normal vessel development.

The MADS Box Transcription Factor *MEF2A*

The *MEF2/RSRF* (myocyte-specific enhancer factor 2/related to serum response factor) family of transcription factors were first identified in skeletal myoblasts but are also expressed in VSMCs. The *MEF2/RSRF* genes are members of the MADS box family of transcriptional regulators and are encoded by four genes, *MEF2A, B, C, and D*.[52] *MEF2* proteins bind to a consensus A/T-rich sequence which is widely distributed in the promoter regions of muscle-specific and growth factor-induced genes. A functional *MEF2*-binding site also occurs in the promoter of the *gax* gene and *MEF2* can transactivate *gax* expression in a site-dependent manner.[53]

MEF2 family members have essential regulatory functions in the differentiation of striated muscle.[54,55] *MEF2* and other myogenic bHLH transcription factors exhibit cross-regulation during myogenesis, where they appear to be indispensable for terminal differentiation.[56,57] In contrast, the *MEF2* factors also regulate the expression of mitogen-inducible immediate-early genes, such as c-*jun*, that are critical for the initiation of cell proliferation.[58–60] While *MEF2* isoforms have been detected in VSMCs,[61,62] their role in VSMC proliferation and differentiation has not been determined. Recently, the regulation of *MEF2* expression in VSMCs has been examined both in vitro and in vivo.

MEF2A is the predominant *MEF2* isoform expressed in VSMCs and its importance is highlighted by the observation that *MEF2A* DNA-binding activity is upregulated 4 hours following mitogen stimulation of quiescent VSMCs.[63] The increased binding activity was maintained throughout the cell cycle and an increase in *MEF2A* protein levels, but not mRNA levels, was observed. This increase was not due to a difference in *MEF2A* protein since a difference in protein stability could not be detected by comparing quiescent and serum-induced cultures, indicating a mitogen-induced activation of *MEF2A* translation. The translational regulation of *MEF2A* may be confered by a highly conserved element located in the 3' untranslated region of the transcript.[64] More recently, it has been demonstrated that *MEF2* transcription factors are upregulated as VSMC proliferation is initiated in the vessel wall in response to injury.[65] Thus, while the data concerning *MEF2A* function in the vasculature is still limited, it may function by inducing VSMCs to adopt a less differentiated state, thereby assuming a phenotypic behavior similar to their embryonic precursors.

Conclusion

An understanding of the mechanisms by which tissue-specific transcriptional factors influence VSMC differentiation should aid in identifying the regulatory pathways functional in the maintenance of vascular homeostasis. In this chapter, we have described three mitogen-regulated transcriptional factors that may function in controlling VSMC phenotypic modulation, presumably by regulating the expression of VSMC-specific genes. For each of these factors, the mitogen-regulated pattern of expression observed in vitro was predictive of the expression observed in vivo when VSMCs were induced to proliferate following vascular injury. In addition, two of these factors, *gax* and *GATA-6,* inhibit VSMC proliferation when overexpressed in vitro and have similar antiproliferative properties in vivo where adenovirus-mediated expression limited the proliferation of VSMCs following vascular injury. Both of these antiproliferative transcriptional factors induce the expression of an inhibitor of cell cycle progression, the cdk kinase inhibitor p21. These studies represent a promising beginning in our understanding of the mechanisms by which endogenous factors induce VSMC differentiation and quiescence, and should identify new therapeutic targets for preventing the VSMC hyperproliferation that is characteristic of a number of vascular pathologies.

References

1. Ross R. The pathogenesis of atherosclerosis: A perspective for the 1990s. *Nature* 1993;362:801–809.
2. Chamley-Campbell J, Campbell GR, Ross R. The smooth muscle cell in culture. *Physiol Rev* 1979;59:1–61.
3. Campbell GR, Campbell JH. Phenotypic modulation of smooth muscle cells in primary culture. In: Campbell JH, Campbell GR, eds: *Vascular Smooth Muscle in Culture.* Boca Raton: CRC Press, Inc; 1987:39–55.

4. Campbell GR, Campbell JH, Manderson JA, et al. Arterial smooth muscle: a multifunctional mesenchymal cell. *Arch Pathol Lab Med* 1988;112:977–986.
5. Chamley-Campbell JH, Campbell GR. What controls smooth muscle phenotype? *Atherosclerosis* 1981;40:347–357.
6. Blank RS, Thompson MM, Owens GK. Cell cycle versus density dependence of smooth muscle alpha actin expression in cultured rat aortic smooth muscle cells. *J Cell Biol* 1988;107:299–306.
7. Simons M, Leclerc G, Safian RD, et al. Relation between activated smooth-muscle cells in coronary-artery lesions and restenosis after atherectomy. *N Engl J Med* 1993;328:608–613.
8. Leclerc G, Isner JM, Kearney M, et al. Evidence implicating nonmuscle myosin in restenosis. Use of in situ hybridization to analyze human vascular lesions obtained by directional atherectomy. *Circulation* 1992;85:543–553.
9. Desmoulière A, Rubbia-Brandt L, Gabbiani G. Modulation of actin isoform expression in cultured arterial smooth muscle cells by heparin and culture conditions. *Arterioscler Thromb* 1991;11:244–253.
10. Gabbiani G, Kocher O, Bloom WS, et al. Actin expression in smooth muscle cells of rat aortic intimal thickening, human atheromatous plaque, and cultured rat aortic media. *J Clin Invest* 1984;73:148–152.
11. Blank RS, Owens GK. Platelet-derived growth factor regulates actin isoform expression and growth state in cultured rat aortic smooth muscle cells. *J Cell Physiol* 1990;142:635–642.
12. Campbell JH, Kocher O, Skalli O, et al. Cytodifferentiation and expression of α-smooth muscle actin mRNA and protein during primary culture of aortic smooth muscle cells: Correlation with cell density and proliferative state. *Arteriosclerosis* 1989;9:633–643.
13. Majack RA, Bornstein P. Biosynthesis and modulation of extracellular matrix components by cultured vascular smooth muscle cells. In: Campbell JH, Campbell GR, eds: *Vascular Smooth Muscle in Culture.* Boca Raton: CRC Press, Inc; 1987:117–131.
14. Pickering JG, Weir L, Rosenfield K, et al. Smooth muscle cell outgrowth from human atherosclerotic plaque: Implications for the assessment of lesion biology. *J Am Coll Cardiol* 1992;20:1430–1439.
15. Glukhova MA, Frid MG, Koteliansky VE. Phenotypic changes of human aortic smooth muscle cells during development and in the adult vessel. *Am J Physiol* 1991(suppl);261:78–80.
16. Hultgårdh-Nilsson A, Krondahl U, Querol-Ferrer V, et al. Differences in growth factor response in smooth muscle cells isolated from adult and neonatal rats. *Differentiation* 1991;47:99–105.
17. Kocher O, Gabbiani G. Expression of actin mRNA in rat aortic smooth muscle cells during development, experimental intimal thickening, and culture. *Differentiation* 1986;32:245–251.
18. Birinyi LK, Warner SJ, Salomon RN, et al. Observations on human smooth muscle cell cultures from hyperplastic lesions of prosthetic bypass grafts: Production of a platelet-derived growth factor-like mitogen and expression of a gene for a platelet-derived growth factor receptor—a preliminary study. *J Vasc Surg* 1989;10:157–165.
19. Kuro-o M, Nagai R, Nakahara K, et al. cDNA cloning of a myosin heavy chain isoform in embryonic smooth muscle and its expression during vascular development and in arteriosclerosis. *J Biol Chem* 1991;266:3768–3773.
20. Schwartz SM, Heimark RL, Majesky MW. Developmental mechanisms underlying the pathology of arteries. *Physiol Rev* 1990;70:1177–1209.

21. Yoshida Y, Mitsumata M, Yamane T, et al. Morphology and increased growth rate of atherosclerotic intimal smooth muscle cells. *Arch Pathol Lab Med* 1988;112:987–996.
22. Clowes AW, Kirkman TR, Clowes MM. Mechanisms of arterial graft failure. II. Chronic endothelial and smooth muscle cell proliferation in healing polytetrafluoroethylene prostheses. *J Vasc Surg* 1986;3:877–884.
23. Graham LM, Fox PL. Growth factor production following prosthetic graft implantation. *J Vasc Surg* 1991;13:742–744.
24. Kanda K, Matsuda T, Miwa H, et al. Phenotypic modulation of smooth muscle cells in intima-media incorporated hybrid vascular prostheses. *ASAIO J* 1993;39:M278-M282.
25. Margolin DA, Kaufman BR, DeLuca DJ, et al. Increased platelet-derived growth factor production and intimal thickening during healing of Dacron grafts in a canine model. *J Vasc Surg* 1993;17:856–866.
26. Painter TA. Myointimal hyperplasia: Pathogenesis and implications. 1. In vitro characteristics. *Artif Organs* 1991;15:42–55.
27. Majesky MW, Giachelli CM, Reidy MA, et al. Rat carotid neointimal smooth muscle cells reexpress a developmentally regulated mRNA phenotype during repair of arterial injury. *Circ Res* 1992;71:759–768.
28. Manderson JA, Mosee PRL, Safstron JA, et al. Balloon catheter injury to rabbit carotid artery. I. Changes in smooth muscle phenotype. *Arteriosclerosis* 1989;9:289–298.
29. Gorski DH, Walsh K. Mitogen-responsive nuclear factors that mediate growth control signals in vascular myocytes. *Cardiovasc Res* 1995;30:585–592.
30. Scott MP. Vertebrate homeobox gene nomenclature. *Cell* 1992;71:551–553.
31. Chisaka O, Capecchi MR. Regionally restricted developmental defects resulting from targeted disruption of the mouse homeobox gene *Hox-1.5*. *Nature* 1991;350:473–479.
32. Chisaka O, Musci TS, Capecchi MR. Developmental defects of the ear, cranial nerves and hindbrain resulting from targeted disruption of the mouse homeobox gene *Hox-1.6*. *Nature* 1992;355:516–520.
33. Hoppler S, Bienz M. Specification of a single cell type by a *Drosophila* homeotic gene. *Cell* 1994;76:689–702.
34. Schummer M, Scheurlen I, Schaller C, et al. HOM/HOX homeobox genes are present in hydra (*Chlorohydra viridissima*) and are differentially expressed during regeneration. *EMBO J* 1992;11:1815–1823.
35. Song K, Wang Y, Sassoon D. Expression of *Hox-7.1* in myoblasts inhibits terminal differentiation and induces cell transformation. *Nature* 1992;360:477–481.
36. Muller MM, Ruppert S, Schaffner W, et al. A cloned octamer transcription factor stimulates transcription from lymphoid-specific promoters in non-B cells. *Nature* 1988;336:544–551.
37. Castrillo JL, Theill LE, Karin M. Function of the homeodomain protein GHF1 in pituitary cell proliferation. *Science* 1991;253:197–199.
38. Gorski DH, LePage DF, Walsh K. Cloning and sequence analysis of homeobox transcription factor cDNAs with an inosine-containing probe. *BioTech* 1994;16:856–865.
39. Skopicki HA, Lyons GE, Shatteman G, et al. Embryonic expression of the Gax homeodomain gene in cardiac, smooth and skeletal muscle. *Circ Res* 1997;80:452–462.
40. Gorski DH, Patel CV, Walsh K. Homeobox transcription factor regulation in the cardiovascular system. *Trends Cardiovasc Med* 1993;3:184–190.

41. LePage DF, Altomare DA, Testa JR, et al. Molecular cloning and localization of the human *GAX* gene to 7p21. *Genomics* 1994;24:535–540.

42. Gorski DH, LePage DF, Patel CV, et al. Molecular cloning of a diverged homeobox gene that is rapidly down-regulated during the G_0/G_1 transition in vascular smooth muscle cells. *Mol Cell Biol* 1993;13:3722–3733.

43. Yamashita J, Itoh H, Ogawa Y, et al. Opposite regulation of Gax homeobox expression by Angiotensin II and C-type natriuretic peptide. *Hypertension* 1997;29:381–387.

44. Weir L, Chen D, Pastore C, et al. Expression of GAX, a growth-arrest homeobox gene, is rapidly down-regulated in the rat carotid artery during the proliferative response to balloon injury. *J Biol Chem* 1995;270:5457–5461.

45. Smith RC, Branellec D, Gorski DH, et al. p21^{CIP1}-mediated inhibition of cell proliferation by overexpression of the *gax* homeodomain gene. *Genes Dev* 1997;11:1674–1689.

46. Perlman H, Sata M, Le Roux A, et al. Bax-mediated cell death by the Gax homeoprotein requires mitogen-activation but is independent of cell cycle activity. *EMBO J* 1998;17:3576–3586.

47. Maillard L, Van Belle E, Smith RC, et al. Percutaneous delivery of the *gax* gene inhibits vessel stenosis in a rabbit model of balloon angioplasty. *Cardiovasc Res* 1997;35:536–546.

48. Simon MC. Gotta have GATA. *Nat Genet* 1995;11:9–11.

49. Suzuki E, Evans T, Lowry J, et al. The human *GATA-6* gene: Structure, chromosomal location and regulation of expression by tissue-specific and mitogen-responsive signals. *Genomics* 1996;38:283–290.

50. Perlman HR, Suzuki E, Simonson M, et al. *GATA-6* induces p21CIP1 expression and G1 cell cycle arrest. *J Biol Chem* 1998;273:13713–13718.

51. Timchenko NA, Harris TE, Wilde M, et al. CCAAT/enhancer binding protein α regulates p21 protein and hepatocyte proliferation in newborn mice. *Mol Cell Biol* 1997;17:7353–7361.

51a. Mano T, Luo Z, Malendowicz SI, et al. Reversal of GATA-6 downregulation promotes smooth muscle differentiation and inhibits intimal hyperplasia in ballon-injured rat carotid artery. *Circ Res* 1999;84:647-654.

52. Breitbart RE, Liang C, Smoot LB, et al. A fourth human MEF2 transcription factor, hMEF2D, is an early marker of myogenic lineage. *Development* 1993;118:1095–1106.

53. Andrés V, Fisher S, Wearsch P, et al. Regulation of *Gax* homeobox gene transcription by a combination of positive factors including MEF2. *Mol Cell Biol* 1995;15:4272–4281.

54. Kaushal S, Schneider JW, Nadal-Ginard B, et al. Activation of the myogenic lineage by MEF2A, a factor that induces and cooperates with MyoD. *Science* 1994;266:1236–1240.

55. Molkentin JD, Black BL, Martin JF, et al. Cooperative activation of muscle gene expression by MEF2 and myogenic bHLH proteins. *Cell* 1995;83:1125–1136.

56. Cserjesi P, Olson EN. Myogenin induces the myocyte-specific enhancer binding factor MEF2 independently of other muscle-specific gene products. *Mol Cell Biol* 1991;11:4854–4862.

57. Buckingham M. Molecular biology of muscle development (meeting review). *Cell* 1994;78:15–21.

58. Han DKM, Liau G. Identification and characterization of developmentally regulated genes in vascular smooth muscle. *Circ Res* 1992;71:711–719.

59. Han T-H, Prywes R. Regulatory role of MEF2D in serum induction of the c-*jun* promoter. *Mol Cell Biol* 1995;15:2907–2915.

60. Pollock R, Treisman R. Human SRF-related proteins: DNA-binding properties and potential regulatory targets. *Genes Dev* 1991;5:2327–2341.
61. Martin JF, Miano JM, Hustad CM, et al. A MEF2 gene that generates a muscle-specific isoform via alternative splicing. *Mol Cell Biol* 1994;14:1647–1656.
62. Yu Y-T, Breitbart RE, Smoot LB, et al. Human myocyte-specific enhancer factor 2 comprises a group of tissue-restricted MADS box transcription factors. *Genes Dev* 1992;6:1783–1798.
63. Suzuki E, Guo K, Kolman M, et al. Serum-induction of MEF2/RSRF expression in vascular myocytes is mediated at the level of translation. *Mol Cell Biol* 1995;15:3415–3423.
64. Suzuki E, Lowry J, Sonoda G, et al. Structures and chromosome locations of the human MEF2A gene and a pseudogene MEF2AP. *Cytogenet Cell Genet* 1996;73:244–249.
65. Firulli AB, Miano JM, Bi W, et al. Myocyte enhancer binding factor-2 expression and activity in vascular smooth muscle cells. *Circ Res* 1996;78: 196–204.

Chapter 11

Perlecan Heparan Sulfates in the Control of Vascular Smooth Muscle Cell Proliferation

*Mary C.M. Weiser-Evans, PhD, and
Kurt R. Stenmark, MD*

The adult uninjured blood vessel wall is a remarkably quiescent tissue exhibiting a vascular smooth muscle cell (SMC) replication index of < 0.06% per day.[1,2] Significant proliferation of SMCs occurs only during development and after vascular injury. In the adult, excessive replication of SMCs is an important contributor to atherosclerosis, to the restenosis of vascular grafts and angioplasties, and to the maintenance of the hypertensive state (reviewed in Reference 3). In the neonate, SMC replication is an important component of the vascular remodeling commonly observed in persistent pulmonary hypertension of the newborn.[4,5] Because SMCs in diseased vessels have been shown to reexpress many characteristics of those observed in immature blood vessels, it has been hypothesized that vascular SMCs reiterate a developmental sequence of gene expression related to growth control during the process of injury repair.[6-8] Our research goals have been to elucidate the mechanisms that suppress SMC replication once vascular morphogenesis is complete, and to define the factors that maintain adult, contractile SMCs in a quiescent state in the normal, uninjured blood vessel. Since the unscheduled replication of SMCs plays such an important role in the development of many vascular disease states, an understanding of the normal growth suppressive mechanisms endogenous to the mature blood vessel wall may lead to the development of therapeutic agents capable of preventing such replication.

This work was supported by National Institutes of Health Grants HL-46481 and HL-47685 and by American Heart Association grant 95008610.

From: Weir EK, Archer SL, Reeves JT (eds). *The Fetal and Neonatal Pulmonary Circulations.* Armonk, NY: Futura Publishing Company, Inc.; ©1999.

SMC Replication Rates and Growth Potential Change Dramatically During Development and After Vascular Injury

Research from our laboratory has followed two convergent approaches to identify the factors that terminate SMC replication following development and injury repair. We believe that SMCs acquire various growth suppressive mechanisms during their normal developmental maturation into quiescent, contractile cells. The first approach we have taken is to elucidate the factors that drive aortic SMC replication during development, in order to determine how these stimulatory signals are lost or suppressed as the aorta matures into a quiescent, fully differentiated tissue. Using this approach, we have shown that one mechanism contributing to SMC growth suppression is the loss of the capacity for self-driven growth at intrauterine day 19 in the rat.

In our original studies related to this approach,[9] we documented the daily in vivo replication rates of aortic SMCs throughout development in the rat (Figure 1). Briefly, SMCs replicate at a very high rate

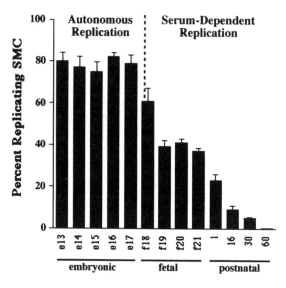

Figure 1. Aortic smooth muscle cells (SMC) demonstrate dramatic in vivo changes in replication rates during vascular development. In vivo SMC replication rates throughout aortic development (embryonic day 13 through postnatal day 60) were analyzed using bromodeoxyuridine (BrdU) immunohistochemistry. Aortic SMCs were isolated at the indicated time points and were assessed in vitro for their ability to sustain DNA replication and to increase cell number under mitogen-deprived conditions (ie, exhibit self-driven, autonomous replication).

(>80% per day) throughout embryonic life. At the embryonic-to-fetal transition (between embryonic day 17 and fetal day 19), the SMC replication rate dramatically declines to < 40% per day. During postnatal life, SMCs gradually acquire a quiescent phenotype, reaching a replication rate of < 0.06% per day in the adult. Aortic SMCs therefore undergo a > 2000-fold decrease in replication rate from embryonic to adult life.

Using the same techniques, we also established the pattern of in vivo SMC proliferation during normal pulmonary vascular development (data not shown).[10] We found dramatic differences in the rates of pulmonary artery (PA) SMC proliferation at specific times during the course of lung development. The observed pattern of PA SMC replication, consisting of rapid rates of replication during the embryonic period followed by a sharp decline in DNA synthesis after the embryonic-to-fetal transition, is strikingly similar to the developmental pattern of aortic SMC replication. These observations suggest that proliferation of vascular SMCs during the embryonic and early fetal periods of development may be controlled by intrinsic, developmentally timed cellular mechanisms, and that the pattern of aortic and PA SMC replication during development may be a characteristic feature of the developing vascular system.

To study the mechanisms regulating the proliferation of vascular SMCs during development in more detail, we cultured aortic SMCs from various developmental time points and characterized their growth phenotypes in more detail.[9] Embryonic aortic SMCs, which exhibited a very high in vivo replication rate, demonstrated in vitro a significant potential for self-driven, autonomous replication, as assessed by the ability to replicate DNA and increase cell number under serum-deprived conditions (Figure 1). Several lines of evidence suggested that the autonomous growth of embryonic SMCs was driven by a unique mechanism independent of known SMC mitogens, including: (1) data showing that embryonic SMC replication was not associated with the detectable secretion of mitogenic activity capable of stimulating adult SMCs; (2) data demonstrating no evidence of growth factor receptor autophosphorylation; and (3) data exhibiting no significant differences in the expression patterns of tyrosine phosphorylated proteins between adult and embryonic SMCs. The dramatic decline in in vivo proliferation observed between embryonic day 17 and fetal day 19 corresponds with the loss of autonomous growth capacity in SMCs cultured from fetal, neonatal, and adult SMCs (Figure 1). Loss of autonomous growth capacity in fetal life suggests that important changes in gene expression and phenotype occur in developing SMCs. Consistent with this, data from our laboratory suggest that the switch from autonomous to serum-dependent growth is due to the developmental acquisition of a transacting "adult"-specific factor capable of suppressing autonomous replication.[11] This as yet undefined inhibitory factor appears to be actively and continuously maintained in the adult, given that it remains present in adult SMCs long after self-driven replication is initially suppressed during development. Therefore, it is likely that the expression of this developmentally regulated "extinguisher" may be continuously essential for normal SMC growth control.

Similar to other adult tissues, the SMC response to injury appears to be associated with a reiteration of specific developmental processes. A variety of studies have shown that adult SMCs responding to injury express genes or gene products (such as tropoelastin, type I collagen, tenascin, H19, cytokeratin 8, and extradomain-A fibronectin) that are characteristic of earlier developmental states.[6,7,12–15] Conversely, genes such as smooth muscle-specific α-actin, tropomyosin, desmin, and myosin, which are expressed preferentially in adult SMCs in vivo, are downregulated when adult SMCs are stimulated to migrate and divide following injurious stimuli.[16,17] At present, it is not clear if all adult me-

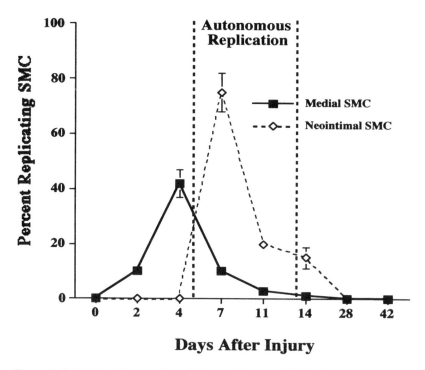

Days After Injury

Figure 2. Following injury to the adult carotid artery, SMCs demonstrate similar in vivo changes in replication rates as observed during vascular development. Adult rat carotid arteries were subjected to balloon catheter injury, and in vivo replication rates were analyzed preinjury and at the indicated time points after injury using BrdU immunohistochemistry. To assess their capacity for autonomous replication, carotid artery SMCs were isolated and analyzed in vitro for their ability to replicate (increase cell number and replicate DNA) under mitogen-deprived conditions.

dial SMCs are capable of responding to injury with changes in gene expression and replicative potential, or if the postinjury response is limited to a subset of SMCs.[18] Recent data demonstrate that the arterial wall is composed of several phenotypically distinct SMC populations, each of which exhibit different growth properties,[19,20] suggesting that the reiteration of a developmental program of SMC growth control is limited to a specific subset of SMCs. Despite this apparent diversity in SMC phenotype, the factors that regulate SMC proliferation during vascular development and following injury to the adult blood vessel remain poorly understood. However, recent studies from our laboratory have found that adult SMCs derived from injured vessels transiently reexpress certain "embryonic" growth characteristics, including a significant capacity for autonomous replication (Figure 2).[21] Reexpression of the autonomous growth phenotype occurs between day 7 (Neo7 SMC) and day 14 (Neo14 SMC) after injury and appears to be associated with the loss of "adult" suppressor function.[21] Such a mechanism may be particularly useful in cell types, like vascular SMCs, that do not undergo terminal differentiation and which are intricately involved in injury repair in the adult. These data therefore support the hypothesis that patterns and mechanisms of SMC replication, gene expression, and growth suppression that are present early in development are reiterated in adult SMCs following vascular injury. Injury to the adult blood vessel may result in the loss or inactivation of putative "adult"-specific suppressor factors resulting in the reexpression of the autonomous growth phenotype.

Perlecan Heparan Sulfates Regulate SMC Replication and Mitogen Responsiveness

In addition to being replicatively quiescent, adult SMCs in vivo appear to be relatively unresponsive to mitogens that markedly stimulate cultured SMCs. Exposure of SMCs to exogenous mitogens alone, either in vivo or in cultured tissue explants, does not appear sufficient to initiate DNA synthesis,[22–24] suggesting the presence of potent growth-suppressive mechanisms operative in the adult blood vessel wall. Our first approach to understanding the factors regulating SMC quiescence led to the identification of one mechanism as being the loss of autonomous growth capacity by the developmentally timed expression of an intrinsic suppressor of SMC replication (as described above). A second approach we have taken is to study fully quiescent, adult tissues and to identify molecular changes that occur as these differentiated cells "modulate" into more immature cells capable of replication. Using this approach, we have shown that the developmentally timed accumulation of growth inhibitory basement membrane components may contribute to the suppression of SMC replication during development, and to the relative unresponsiveness of these cells to mitogenic stimulation in the adult blood vessel wall (Figure 3).

Ample evidence exists that suggests that extracellular matrix (ECM) and basement membrane components are involved in the control of SMC differentiation and growth control. For example, fibronectin appears to facilitate the expression of a synthetic SMC phenotype,[25] while other matrix components may induce the expression of a "contractile" phenotype and inhibit SMC proliferation. Components of the ECM that have been reported to inhibit SMC replication include heparan sulfates, laminin, and collagen type IV.[26–30] Further, when actively replicating "synthetic" SMCs are cultured on intact basement membranes isolated from the Engelbreth-Holm-Swarm (EHS) mouse tumor, they become growth-inhibited, activate mitogen-activated protein (MAP) kinases less efficiently in response to mitogens, and exhibit more differentiated functions.[31,32] Others have extensively studied (in non-SMC systems) the role of extracellular matrices in the control of cellular differentiation and in the activation of tissue-specific gene expression, and a "matrix response element" has been postulated to exist in the promoters of genes whose expression is positively regulated by the matrix.[33,34]

To elucidate the role that basement membrane components may play in controlling SMC replication and SMC "activation," our laboratory has studied the expression of Oct-1, a prototype member of the POU-domain family of transcription factors and a protein believed essential for cell replication, in SMCs under various growth and differentiated states.[35] Oct-1 transcripts were readily detectable in growing sparse and confluent SMCs, in growth-inhibited sparse and confluent SMCs, and in sparse SMCs that were growth-arrested in the presence of heparin or transforming growth factor-β (TGF-β) (data not shown). However, Oct-1 transcripts could not be detected in RNA samples isolated from normal, uninjured (in vivo) adult rat aortas (Figure 4A). The

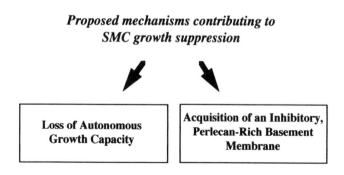

Figure 3. Hypothetical mechanisms regulating SMC growth suppression.

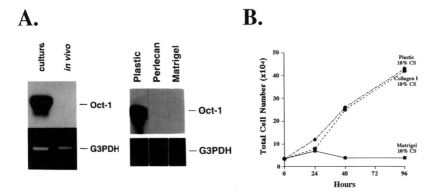

Figure 4. Perlecan-rich basement membranes suppress the expression of growth-essential transcription factors and mitogen-induced growth of adult SMCs. **A:** Combined RT-PCR/Southern blot analysis was used to examine the expression of Oct-1 mRNA in SMCs isolated from intact aortas (in vivo), or SMCs plated on plastic (in vitro), Matrigel basement membranes, or perlecan matrices. **B:** SMCs were plated on plastic, collagen gels, or Matrigel basement membranes and were stimulated with 10% calf serum (CS). Total cell numbers were determined at the indicated time points.

expression of Oct-1 by vascular SMCs therefore appears to be induced during the in vivo to in vitro transition, and may thereafter be constitutively expressed under culture conditions.

When the aortic media from adult rats was enzyme-dispersed (under mitogen-free conditions) into single cells, Oct-1 gene transcription was rapidly initiated even before plating, suggesting that disruption of cell:matrix interactions is sufficient to induce Oct-1 expression. When serially passaged SMCs (which constitutively expressed Oct-1 messenger RNA [mRNA]) were plated on EHS-derived basement membranes (commercially available as "Matrigel," Collaborative Biomedical Products, Bedford, MA), Oct-1 expression was inhibited within 24 hours (Figure 4A), and SMC replication effectively ceased even in the continued presence of 10% calf serum (Figure 4B). Transcripts for Oct-1 were rapidly reexpressed (within 60 minutes) following removal of cells from basement membranes; reexpression was dependent on gene transcription. Expression of c-*fos* mRNA by cultured SMCs was similarly controlled by intact basement membranes. The data suggest a model in which injury to the SMC basement membrane "activates" SMCs, in part by the derepressed expression of growth-essential transcription factors, through the removal of inhibitory influences to allow subsequent replication.

We next sought to determine which component(s) of basement membranes were responsible for the suppression of Oct-1 gene expression. SMCs were plated, for 48 hours, on uncoated bacteriological plastic, on plastic coated with intact basement membranes, or on individual matrices of laminin, type IV collagen, fibronectin, or perlecan, and then were examined morphologically and for the expression of Oct-1 mRNA. Only perlecan matrices mimicked intact basement membranes in causing morphological changes in SMCs (data not shown) and in suppressing Oct-1 gene expression (Figure 4A). The Oct-1-suppressing activity of intact basement membranes was found to be susceptible to degradation by purified heparinase, but not by chondroitinase or hyaluronidase. Since perlecan is the predominant heparan sulfate-containing component of basement membranes, we concluded that the heparan sulfate chains of perlecan are capable of suppressing Oct-1 gene expression. Based on the above data, we proposed that adult SMCs are surrounded by a perlecan-rich, growth-inhibitory ECM that may largely prevent SMC replication in the absence of matrix injury.

The In Vivo Pattern of Perlecan Expression is Consistent With a Potential Role for Perlecan Heparan Sulfates in SMC Growth Suppression

Given these results, we examined the pattern of expression of perlecan during rat aortic development using a combined perlecan in situ hybridization-bromodeoxyuridine (BrdU) immunohistochemistry technique (to correlate perlecan mRNA expression with SMC growth state).[36] We determined that perlecan gene expression in the developing rat aorta begins around fetal day 18, a developmental point marking the onset of the rapid and dramatic decrease in SMC replication (as described above), and remains readily detectable throughout postnatal life (Figure 5). This observation was supported by RT-PCR analysis of in vitro SMCs, which demonstrated that cultured embryonic day 17 SMCs do not express detectable perlecan message, in contrast to cultured and in vivo adult SMCs. Further, we showed that perlecan gene expression was largely limited to nonreplicative SMCs, ie, those cells which presumably have ceased replication during development (data not shown). Perlecan mRNA and protein therefore appear during aortic development in a pattern consistent with a role for this proteoglycan in the developmental inhibition of SMC replication, or as a component of a growth-suppressive basement membrane deposited following the cessation of replication.

We also analyzed the pattern of expression of perlecan mRNA in the developing rat lung and determined the correlation between perlecan expression and PA SMC replication (data not shown).[10] Similar to the aorta, perlecan mRNA was first detected in the lung vasculature at

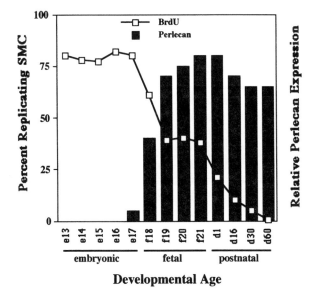

Developmental Age

Figure 5. Perlecan mRNA and protein are first significantly expressed in vivo at fetal day 19, following the dramatic decrease in SMC proliferation. In vivo SMC replication rates throughout aortic development (embryonic day 13 through postnatal day 60) were analyzed using BrdU immunohistochemistry. In situ hybridization and immunohistochemical analyses were used to detect perlecan mRNA and protein in the same tissue sections. The percent of BrdU-positive (replicating) SMCs is plotted on the left axis. The relative expression of perlecan (reported as arbitrary units; fold antisense signal over sense signal) is plotted on the right axis.

fetal day 18, continued to be expressed at high levels throughout fetal life, and remained detectable in adult PA SMCs. The expression of perlecan transcripts was limited almost entirely to nonreplicating SMCs. Taken together, the data emphatically support a variety of previous data suggesting that heparan sulfate proteoglycans may be physiologically important regulators of SMC function in vivo.

The in vivo developmental data suggested that perlecan may play a determinant role in the cessation of SMC replication during vascular morphogenesis, and may play a role in maintaining SMCs in a quiescent state in the adult blood vessel wall. The Oct-1 data suggested that matrix injury-induced expression of growth-essential transcription factors may be one of the earliest responses to vascular trauma and may therefore render SMCs competent to respond to subsequent mitogenic stimulation. We thus sought to determine if changes in perlecan expression occur following vascular injury in vivo and to determine their relationship to SMC replication. We studied two experimental injury processes in the adult rat: (1) stenosis resulting from carotid artery balloon catheter injury, and (2) pulmonary hypertension resulting from chronic hypoxia exposure.[37] In both instances, SMCs demonstrated large, but transient, increases in replication following the injurious stimulus, with replication rates peaking 7 days postinjury in both models (Figure 6). Using in situ hybridization analysis, in the carotid artery injury model we found that perlecan transcripts were expressed at low, but detectable, levels in uninjured carotid arteries, were initially downregulated in the carotid artery tunica media, and that downregulation corresponded to periods of increasing SMC replication. An upregulation of perlecan mRNA was observed by 7 days after injury, first in the arterial media and later in the developing neointima. Perlecan transcripts continued to be expressed at high levels 14 days after injury, but were markedly downregulated by 3 weeks after injury, demonstrating that perlecan is significantly expressed during periods of large in vivo decreases in SMC proliferation (Figure 6A).

In a model of chronic hypoxia-induced pulmonary hypertension, perlecan transcripts were found to be low, but detectable, during the phase of peak SMC replication. Significant increases in perlecan mRNA expression were detected between 7 and 14 days of hypoxic exposure,

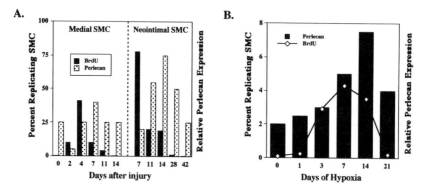

Figure 6. Following vascular injury, peak expression of perlecan occurs during periods of in vivo decreases in SMC replication. A: Carotid arteries of control or balloon-injured, BrdU-treated rats were harvested at the indicated times and were analyzed for replicating medial and/or neointimal SMCs using BrdU immunohistochemistry, and for perlecan mRNA expression using in situ hybridization. B: Adult rats were exposed to hypobaric hypoxia (380 mm Hg) for the indicated times. Animals were injected with BrdU 24 hours prior to sacrifice and lung tissue was harvested. Replicating PA SMC and PA SMC perlecan mRNA expression were analyzed as described above. The percent of BrdU-positive (replicating) SMCs is plotted on the left axis. The relative expression of perlecan (reported as arbitrary units; fold antisense signal over sense signal) is plotted on the right axis.

correlating with a noticeable decrease in SMC replication (Figure 6B). Perlecan mRNA continued to be expressed at high levels through 3 weeks of hypoxic exposure, suggesting that, in the presence of chronic injury, continuous production of perlecan may be compensatory in nature. In contrast, in the balloon-injury model, which consists of an acute insult to the vasculature, significant expression of perlecan is more tightly regulated temporally. In combination, these data suggest that vascular injury results in the disruption of an inhibitory perlecan-rich ECM and this disruption is associated with increasing rates of SMC replication. However, peak expression of perlecan mRNA correlates with significant decreases in SMC proliferation, suggesting that the re-expression of perlecan following vascular injury, similar to the expression pattern observed during vascular development, may play an important role in the postinjury suppression of SMC replication.

Intracellular Signaling Pathways Involved in Perlecan-Mediated SMC Growth Inhibition

The role of heparin-like molecules in the control of vascular SMC replication,[28–30,38–47] migration,[48] and differentiation[49] has been extensively studied. The available evidence indicates that a significant amount of inhibitory heparan sulfates are produced by both endothelial and smooth muscle cells,[27,29,30] exist normally within the tunica media of the adult blood vessel wall,[50] and may function as endogenous suppressors of cell replication.[29,30] Perlecan, the predominant basement membrane heparan sulfate proteoglycan,[51] has been identified as an important inhibitory species produced by vascular cells.[30,35,36] EHS-derived perlecan is a hybrid proteoglycan containing both heparan sulfate and chondroitin sulfate side chains.[52] Several recent reports[53,54] have indicated that certain cell types can interact directly with an RGD cell attachment sequence present in the perlecan core protein; however, most of the biological activity of perlecan is thought to reside in its constituent heparan sulfate side chains. Heparan sulfates are known to interact with a variety of ECM proteins, but no known heparan sulfate "receptor" capable of transmitting a growth-inhibitory signal has yet been described. A single report[55] has appeared describing the presence of an uncharacterized, 78-kD cell-surface protein which reportedly acts as a heparin-binding protein. A variety of mechanisms have been proposed to account for the ability of heparin-like molecules to inhibit SMC replication, including heparin-induced changes in ECM accumulation,[39,40,44] inhibition of binding of thrombospondin to the SMC surface,[46] activation of latent TGF-β,[47] downregulation of c-*myc* expression,[38] inhibition of protein kinase C-mediated responses,[41,42] and inhibition of mitogen-receptor interactions.[45] However, growth inhibition by heparin does not appear to be related to the activation of TGF-β or to the intracellular activation of p53- or pRB-mediated pathways, since SMCs transformed with the large T antigen of SV-40 (in which p53 and pRB are functionally absent) remain fully inhibitable by heparin[43] and are resistant to TGF-β-mediated inhibition (our unpublished observations). At present, the molecular mechanisms by which heparin-like molecules inhibit SMC replication remain unclear.

Little is known about intracellular signaling pathways induced by ECM ligands (see References 56 and 57 for reviews). The most intensely studied matrix-mediated signaling systems are those activated by integrins, a family of transmembrane matrix receptors. Activation of integrins by ligand occupation and clustering has been shown to result in changes in gene expression,[58] phosphorylation of the focal adhesion kinase p125[FAK],[59] elevation of intracellular Ca^{2+} levels,[60] increases in cellular pH,[61] and generation of phospholipid metabolites.[62] The cellular pathways activated by heparin-like molecules (as reviewed above) may or may not be due to integrin activation. Recently, however, the β_1 integrin was shown to mediate the adhesion of several cell lines to EHS-derived perlecan.[63] In this report, it was shown that both the core protein and the heparan sulfate side chains were required for maximal cell adhesion. A separate study has reported that heparan sulfate glycosaminoglycans can act as a ligand for the binding of Mac-1, a β_2 integrin found on hematopoetic cells.[64] Therefore, it is possible that perlecan-induced growth inhibition is mediated through integrin activation.

It is important to note, however, that a central signaling pathway for integrin receptors appears to be their ability to activate the Erk-type MAP kinase pathway, an intracellular signaling pathway involved in cell cycle progression.[65–67] It has been established that interactions between integrin cell adhesion receptors and their extracellular ligands are central to cell migration and growth.[65,66] Consistent with this, several recent reports have shown that, following vascular injury, injured SMCs increase their production of specific ECM components and this upregulation of ECM expression is associated with integrin activation and subsequent SMC replication.[67–70] Therefore, rather than activating an integrin-mediated, MAP kinase-dependent intracellular pathway, we hypothesized that perlecan-rich basement membranes inhibit SMC growth by actively inhibiting this pathway. To test this hypothesis, we first examined the expression and the activity levels of the MAP kinases, p44[Erk-1] and p42[Erk-2], in adult, serum-dependent SMCs (isolated from adult uninjured aortas) cultured on individual matrices of fibronectin, laminin, and type IV collagen, known integrin ligands, and on Matrigel basement membranes (Figure 7). Using Western blot analysis, we found that p44[Erk-1] protein was expressed at high levels by adult SMCs plated on fibronectin, laminin, and type IV collagen matrices, but was down-

A.

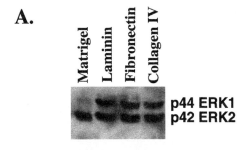

p44 ERK1
p42 ERK2

B.
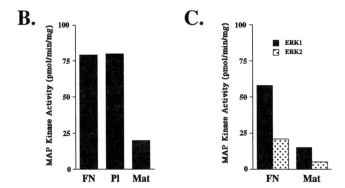

C.

Figure 7. p44^{Erk-1} is preferentially stimulated, and downregulated by Matrigel basement membranes, in adult SMCs. **A:** Adult aortic SMCs were plated on Matrigel basement membranes or on individual matrices of laminin, fibronectin, or type IV collagen in serum-free medium for 24 hours. Cell lysates were collected and analyzed for the expression of p44^{Erk-1} and p42^{Erk-2} proteins using Western blot analysis. **B:** Adult aortic SMCs were plated on Matrigel (Mat) basement membranes, on fibronectin (FN) matrices, or on plastic (Pl). Total Erk activity (analyzed as the ability of Erk 1 and Erk 2 immunoprecipitates to phosphorylate myelin basic protein) was measured following stimulation with 10% calf serum. **C:** Adult aortic SMCs were plated on Matrigel basement membranes or on fibronectin matrices. p44^{Erk-1} or p42^{Erk-2} activities (analyzed as the ability of p44^{Erk-1} or p42^{Erk-2} immunoprecipitates to phosphoylate myelin basic protein) were measured following stimulation with 10% calf serum.

regulated when adult SMCs were plated on Matrigel basement membranes (Figure 7A). p42^{Erk-2} protein, in contrast, was constitutively expressed by SMCs plated on all ECM matrices examined (Figure 7A). Mitogen-stimulated total (Erk 1 and Erk 2) MAP kinase activity (measured as the ability of Erk 1 and Erk 2 immunoprecipitates to phosphorylate myelin basic protein) was significantly increased in SMCs plated on fibronectin matrices or on plastic, but was inhibited in SMCs plated on Matrigel basement membranes (Figure 7B). Interestingly, however, we found that p44^{Erk-1} kinase activity was preferentially stimulated in adult SMCs, and downregulated by basement membranes, whereas p42^{Erk-2} serum-induced activity was barely detectable in all adult SMC cultures (Figure 7C) suggesting that the majority of MAP kinase activity in adult SMCs is derived from p44^{Erk-1}.

We also examined the expression and the activity levels of the Erk proteins by autonomously replicating embryonic day 17 (e17) and neointimal day 7 (Neo7) SMCs. In contrast to adult SMCs, in which mitogen-induced replication is suppressed by basement membranes, replication

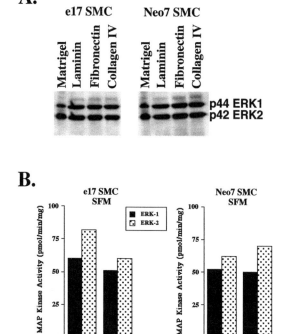

Figure 8. p44^{Erk-1} and p42^{Erk-2} are equally activated, and are uninhibitable by basement membranes, in mitogen-deprived, autonomously replicating SMCs. A: Western blot analysis was used to detect the expression of p44^{Erk-1} and p42^{Erk-2} proteins by embryonic day 17 (e17) and neointimal day 7 (Neo7) SMCs plated on the indicated matrices as described in Figure 7. B: e17 and Neo7 SMCs were plated on Matrigel (Mat) basement membranes and on fibronectin (FN) matrices in serum-free medium (SFM). Basal, mitogen-deprived p44^{Erk-1} and p42^{Erk-2} activities were measured (as described in Figure 7).

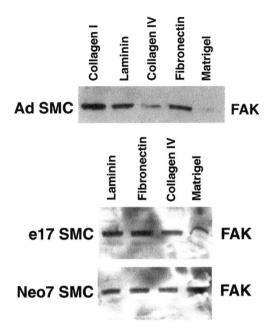

Figure 9. Activation of focal adhesion kinase is inhibited by plating adult (Ad) SMCs, but not e17 and Neo7 SMCs, on Matrigel basement membranes. Ad and e17 aortic and Neo7 carotid artery SMCs were plated on Matrigel basement membranes or on individual matrix protein matrices in serum-free medium. Cell lysates were collected and immunoprecipitated with an anti-FAK (focal adhesion kinase) antibody. Western blot analysis and an antiphosphotyrosine antibody were used to analyze FAK immunoprecipitates for activation.

of these cells on Matrigel basement membranes is not inhibited (data not shown), suggesting that this proliferation-associated signaling pathway may be constitutively active in autonomously replicating SMCs. Consistent with the lack of an inhibitory effect of basement membranes on growth, we found that both p44^{Erk-1} and p42^{Erk-2} proteins continue to be abundantly expressed when e17 and Neo7 SMCs are cultured on basement membranes (Figure 8A). Moreover, basal, mitogen-independent p44^{Erk-1} and p42^{Erk-2} kinase activities are equally activated, are significantly higher than activity measured in mitogen-stimulated adult SMCs, and are uninhibitable by basement membranes (Figure 8B), suggesting that autonomously replicating SMCs are constitutively activated and unresponsive to the inhibitory effects of basement membranes.

Focal adhesion kinase (FAK) is an integrin-activated intracellular tyrosine kinase linked to the MAP kinase (Erk) growth pathway. Engagement of ECM proteins to their integrin receptors results in tyrosine phosphorylation, and subsequent activation, of FAK. Since FAK is believed to be an intracellular substrate coupling ECM-induced integrin-mediated signals to the MAP kinase pathway, we next examined the effect of basement membranes on the activity level of FAK in serum- dependent adult SMCs and in serum-independent embryonic and neo-intimal SMCs. For these experiments, adult, e17, and Neo7 SMCs were plated on individual matrices of collagen type I, laminin, fibronectin, or collagen type IV or on Matrigel basement membranes under serum-free conditions. FAK immunoprecipitates were then analyzed by Western blot analysis for activation using an antiphosphotyrosine antibody. While FAK protein was constitutively expressed by all cell types examined under all culture conditions analyzed (data not shown), activation of FAK (ie, tyrosine phosphorylation) was inhibited by plating adult SMCs on Matrigel basement membranes (Figure 9). In contrast, FAK was constitutively activated in

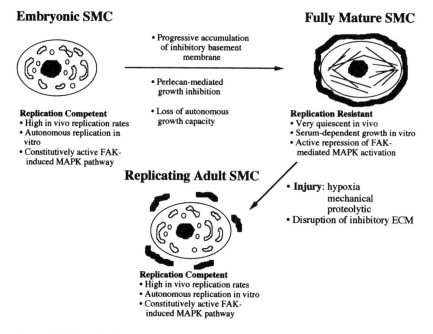

Embryonic SMC   **Fully Mature SMC**

• Progressive accumulation
  of inhibitory basement
  membrane

• Perlecan-mediated
  growth inhibition

Replication Competent   • Loss of autonomous   **Replication Resistant**
• High in vivo replication rates   growth capacity   • Very quiescent in vivo
• Autonomous replication in   • Serum-dependent growth in vitro
  vitro   • Active repression of FAK-
• Constitutively active FAK-   mediated MAPK activation
  induced MAPK pathway

Replicating Adult SMC
                                                        • **Injury:** hypoxia
                                                            mechanical
                                                            proteolytic
                                                        • Disruption of inhibitory ECM

Replication Competent
• High in vivo replication rates
• Autonomous replication in vitro
• Constitutively active FAK-
  induced MAPK pathway

Figure 10. Hypothetical role for SMC perlecan heparan sulfate-enriched basement membranes in the control of SMC growth suppression. We propose that a major component of blood vessel maturation involves the deposition, by SMCs, of basement membrane components (in particular, perlecan) which: (1) promote cellular differentiation; (2) inhibit the expression of growth-essential transcription factors; and (3) prevent SMCs from replicating in the absence of prior matrix injury. Perlecan-rich basement membranes actively suppress SMC growth by inhibiting an integrin-induced, focal adhesion kinase-dependent activation of the MAP kinase pathway. Induction of SMC mitogen responsiveness following vascular injury is, at least in part, due to the disruption of this inhibitory matrix.

autonomously replicating embryonic and neointimal SMCs (Figure 9). These data suggest that the ECM-mediated activation of FAK is a necessary prerequisite for the induction of replication competence in adult SMCs. However, it appears likely that autonomously replicating SMCs express a constitutively active FAK and MAP kinase signaling pathway which precludes the necessity for an ECM-mediated activation of these cell types.

In conclusion, we have presented data which support our hypothesis that SMCs acquire various growth-suppressive mechanisms during their transition into quiescent, contractile cells both during development and after vascular injury (Figure 10). One proposed mechanism which we believe renders SMCs unresponsive to mitogenic stimulation in the adult blood vessel wall is the acquisition of a perlecan-rich SMC basement membrane. We propose that in uninjured adult blood vessels, perlecan-rich basement membranes actively suppress SMC growth by inhibiting the integrin-induced, FAK-dependent activation of the MAP kinase signaling pathway. Therefore, activation of SMCs (ie, induction of mitogen responsiveness) following vascular injury is, at least in part, due to the disruption of an inhibitory basement membrane and subsequent activation of this signaling pathway. However, autonomously replicating embryonic and neointimal SMCs, which express a constitutively active FAK-induced MAP kinase pathway, are unresponsive to the inhibitory effects of basement membranes. Therefore, it appears likely that both proposed mechanisms, the loss of autonomous growth potential and the acquisition of an inhibitory ECM, must be in place for SMCs to be fully quiescent in uninjured adult blood vessels.

References

1. Clowes AW, Reidy MA, Clowes MM. Kinetics of cellular proliferation after arterial injury. *Lab Invest* 1983;49:327–333.
2. Lombardi DM, Reidy MA, Schwartz SM. Methodological considerations important in the accurate quantitation of aortic smooth muscle cell replication in the normal rat. *Am J Pathol* 1991;138:441–446.
3. Schwartz SM, deBlois D, O'Brien ERM. The intima: Soil for atherosclerosis and restenosis. *Circ Res* 1995;77:445–465.
4. Stenmark KR, Fasules J, Hyde DN, et al. Severe pulmonary hypertension and arterial adventitial changes in newborn calves at 4,300 meters. *J Appl Physiol* 1987;62:821–830.
5. Stenmark KR, Orton EC, Reeves JT, et al. Vascular remodeling in neonatal pulmonary hypertension: Role of the smooth muscle cell. *Chest* 1988; 93:127S-132S.
6. Majesky MW, Giachelli CM, Reidy MA, et al. Rat carotid neointimal smooth muscle cells reexpress a developmentally regulated mRNA phenotype during repair of arterial injury. *Circ Res* 1992;71:759–768.

7. Schwartz SM, Campbell GR, Campbell JH. Replication of smooth muscle cells in vascular disease. *Circ Res* 1986;58:427–444.

8. Gabbiani G, Kocher O, Bloom WS, et al. Actin expression in smooth muscle cells of rat aortic intimal thickening, human atheromatous plaque, and cultured rat aortic media. *J Clin Invest* 1984;73:148–152.

9. Cook CL, Weiser MCM, Schwartz PE, et al. Developmentally timed expression of an embryonic growth phenotype in vascular smooth muscle cells. *Circ Res* 1994;74:189–196.

10. Belknap JK, Weiser-Evans MCM, Grieshaber SS, et al. Relationship between perlecan and tropoelastin gene expression and cell replication in the developing rat pulmonary vasculature. *Am J Resp Cell Mol Biol* 1999;20:24–34.

11. Majack RA. Extinction of autonomous growth potential in embryonic: Adult vascular smooth muscle cell heterokaryons. *J Clin Invest* 1995;95:464–468.

12. Glukhova MA, Frid MG, Shekhonin BV, et al. Expression of fibronectin variants in vascular and visceral smooth muscle cells in development. *Dev Biol* 1990;141:193–202.

13. Hedin U, Holm J, Hansson GK. Induction of tenascin in rat arterial injury: Relationship to altered smooth muscle cell phenotype. *Am J Pathol* 1991;139:649–656.

14. Kim DK, Zhang L, Dzau VJ, et al. H19, a developmentally regulated gene, is reexpressed in rat vascular smooth muscle cells after injury. *J Clin Invest* 1994;93:355–360.

15. Jahn L, Kreuzer J, von Hodenberg E, et al. Cytokeratins 8 and 18 in smooth muscle cells: Detection in human coronary artery, peripheral vascular, and vein graft disease, and in transplantation-associated arteriosclerosis. *Arterioscler Thromb* 1993;13:1631–1639.

16. Kocher O, Gabbiani G. Expression of actin mRNA in rat aortic smooth muscle cells during development, experimental intimal thickening, and culture. *Differentiation* 1986;32:245–251.

17. Kocher O, Skalli O, Bloom WS, et al. Cytoskeleton of rat aortic smooth muscle cells: Normal conditions and experimental intimal thickening. *Lab Invest* 1984;50:645–652.

18. Schwartz SM. Biology of the neointima. *Exp Nephrol* 1994;2:63–67.

19. Topouzis S, Majesky MW. Smooth muscle lineage diversity in the chick embryo: Two types of aortic smooth muscle cells differ in growth and receptor-mediated transcriptional responses to transforming growth factor-beta. *Dev Biol* 1996;178(2):430–445.

20. Frid MG, Moiseeva E, Stemnark KR. Multiple phenotypically distinct smooth muscle cell populations exist in the adult and developing bovine pulmonary arterial media in vivo. *Circ Res* 1994;75:669–681.

21. Weiser-Evans MCM, Quinn BE, Michael R, et al. Transient reexpression of an "embryonic" autonomous growth phenotype by adult carotid artery smooth muscle cells following vascular injury. *J Cell Physiol*. In press.

22. Lindner V, Majack RA, Reidy MA. Basic fibroblast growth factor stimulates endothelial regrowth in denuded arteries in vivo. *J Clin Invest* 1990;85:2004–2008.

23. Lindner V, Lappi DA, Baird A, et al. Role of basic fibroblast growth factor in vascular lesion formation. *Circ Res* 1991;68:106–113.

24. Weiser MCM, Majack RA, Tucker A, et al. Static tension is associated with increased smooth muscle cell DNA synthesis in rat pulmonary arteries. *Am J Physiol* 1995;268:H1133-H1138.

25. Hedin U, Bottger BA, Forsberg E, et al. Diverse effects of fibronectin and laminin on phenotypic modulation of cultured arterial smooth muscle cells. *J Cell Biol* 1988;107:307–319.
26. Fritze LM, Reilly CF, Rosenberg RD. An antiproliferative heparan sulfate species produced by postconfluent smooth muscle cells. *J Cell Biol* 1985; 100(4):1041–1049.
27. Thyberg J, Hultgardh-Nilsson A. Fibronectin and the basement membrane components laminin and collagen type IV influence the phenotypic properties of subcultured rat aortic smooth muscle cells differently. *Cell Tissue Res* 1994;276(2):263–271.
28. Clowes AW, Karnovsky MJ. Suppression by heparin of smooth muscle cell proliferation in injured arteries. *Nature* 1977;265:625–626.
29. Castellot JJ, Addonizio ML, Rosenberg RD, et al. Cultured endothelial cells produce a heparinlike inhibitor of smooth muscle cell growth. *J Cell Biol* 1981;90:372–379.
30. Benitz WE, Kelley RT, Anderson CM, et al. Endothelial heparan sulfate proteoglycan. I. Inhibitory effects on smooth muscle cell proliferation. *Am J Respir Cell Mol Biol* 1990;2:13–24.
31. Li X, Tsai P, Weider ED, et al. Vascular smooth muscle cells grown on Matrigel: A model of the contractile phenotype with decreased activation of mitogen-activated protein kinase. *J Biol Chem* 1994;269:19653–19658.
32. Pauly RR, Passanti A, Crow M, et al. Experimental models that mimic the differentiation and dedifferentiation of vascular cells. *Circulation* 1992;86 (suppl III):68–73.
33. Adams JC, Watt FM. Regulation of development and differentiation by the extracellular matrix. *Development* 1993;117:1183–1198.
34. Lin CQ, Bissell MJ. Multi-faceted regulation of cell differentiation by extracellular matrix. *FASEB J* 1993;7:737–743.
35. Weiser MCM, Grieshaber NA, Schwartz PE, et al. Perlecan regulates Oct-1 gene expression in vascular smooth muscle cells. *Mol Biol Cell* 1997;8: 999–1011.
36. Weiser MCM, Belknap JK, Grieshaber SS, et al. Developmental regulation of perlecan gene expression in aortic smooth muscle cells. *Matrix Biol* 1996;15:331–340.
37. Weiser MCM, Quinn BE, Stiebellhner L, et al. Hypoxia exposure interrupts the expression of the SMC growth inhibitor, perlecan, by PA SMC. *Am J Resp Crit Care Med* 1998;157(3):A268.
38. Pukac LA, Castellot JJ Jr, Wright TC Jr, et al. Heparin inhibits c-fos and c-myc mRNA expression in vascular smooth muscle cells. *Cardiovasc Res* 1993;27(12):2238–2247.
39. Clowes AW, Clowes MM, Kirkman TR, et al. Heparin inhibits the expression of tissue-type plasminogen activator by smooth muscle cells in injured rat carotid artery. *Circ Res* 1992;70(6):1128–1136.
40. Au YP, Montgomery KF, Clowes AW. Heparin inhibits collagenase gene expression mediated by phorbol ester-responsive element in primate arterial smooth muscle cells. *Circ Res* 1992;70:1062–1069.
41. Pukac LA, Ottlinger ME, Karnovsky MJ. Heparin suppresses specific second messenger pathways for protooncogene expression in rat vascular smooth muscle cells. *J Biol Chem* 1992;267(6):3707–3711.
42. Ottlinger ME, Pukac LA, Karnovsky MJ. Heparin inhibits mitogen-activated protein kinase activation in intact rat vascular smooth muscle cells. *J Biol Chem* 1993;268(26):19173–19176.
43. Reilly CF. Rat vascular smooth muscle cells immortalized with SV40 large

T antigen possess defined smooth muscle cell characteristics including growth inhibition by heparin. *J Cell Physiol* 1990;142(2):342–351.

44. Kenagy RD, Nikkari ST, Welgus HG, et al. Heparin inhibits the induction of three matrix metalloproteinases (stromelysin, 92-kD gelatinase, and collagenase) in primate arterial smooth muscle cells. *J Clin Invest* 1994; 93(5):1987–1993.

45. Lindner V, Olson NE, Clowes AW, et al. Inhibition of smooth muscle cell proliferation in injured rat arteries: Interaction of heparin with basic fibroblast growth factor. *J Clin Invest* 1992;90(5):2044–2049.

46. Majack RA, Cook SC, Bornstein P. Regulation of smooth muscle cell growth by components of the extracellular matrix: An autocrine role for thrombospondin. *Proc Natl Acad Sci USA* 1986;83:9050–9054.

47. Grainger DJ, Witchell CM, Watson JV, et al. Heparin decreases the rate of proliferation of rat vascular smooth muscle cells by releasing transforming growth factor beta-like activity from serum. *Cardiovasc Res* 1993; 27(12):2238–2247.

48. Majack RA, Clowes AW. Inhibition of vascular smooth muscle cell migration by heparin-like glycosaminoglycans. *J Cell Physiol* 1984 118:253–256.

49. Campbell JH, Rennick RE, Kalevitch SG, et al. Heparan sulfate-degrading enzymes induce modulation of smooth muscle phenotype. *Exp Cell Res* 1992;200(1):156–167.

50. Couchman JR. Heterogenous distribution of a basement membrane heparan sulfate proteoglycan in rat tissues. *J Cell Biol* 1987;105:1901–1916.

51. Iozzo RV, Cohen IR, Grassel S, et al. The biology of perlecan: The multifaceted heparan sulfate proteoglycan of basement membrane and pericellular matrices. *Biochem J* 1994;302:625–639.

52. Danielson KG, Martinez-Hernandez A, Hassell JR, et al. Establishment of a cell line from the EHS tumor: Biosynthesis of basement membrane constituents and characterization of a hybrid proteoglycan containing heparan and chondroitin sulfate chains. *Matrix* 1992;11:22–35.

53. Hayashi K, Madri JA, Yurchenco PD. Endothelial cells interact with the core protein of basement membrane perlecan through beta 1 and beta 3 integrins: An adhesion modulated by glycosaminoglycan. *J Cell Biol* 1992; 119:945–959.

54. Chakravarti S, Horchar T, Jefferson B, et al. Recombinant domain III of perlecan promotes cell attachment through its RGDS sequence. *J Biol Chem* 1995;270:404–409.

55. Lankes W, Griesmacher A, Grunwald J, et al. A heparin-binding protein involved in inhibition of smooth muscle cell proliferation. *Biochem J* 1988; 251:831–842.

56. Damsky CH, Werb Z. Signal transduction by integrin receptors for extracellular matrix: Cooperative processing of extracellular information. *Curr Opin Cell Biol* 1992;4:772–781.

57. Clark EA, Brugge JS. Integrins and signal transduction pathways: The road taken. *Science* 1995;268:233–239.

58. Yurochko A, Liu D, Eierman D, Haskill S. Integrins as a primary signal transduction molecule regulating monocyte immediate-early gene induction. *Proc Natl Acad Sci USA* 1992;89:9034–9038.

59. Schaller M, Parsons JT. Focal adhesion kinase and associated proteins. *Curr Opin Cell Biol* 1994;6:705–710.

60. Juliano RL, Haskill S. Signal transduction from the extracellular matrix. *J Cell Biol* 1993;120:577–585.

61. Schwartz MA, Ingber DE. Integrating with integrins. *Mol Biol Cell* 1994; 5:389–393.
62. Divecha N, Irvine RF. Phospholipid signaling. *Cell* 1995;80:269–278.
63. Battaglia C, Aumailley M, Mann K, et al. Structural basis of beta-1 integrin-mediated cell adhesion to a large heparan sulfate proteoglycan from basement membranes. *Eur J Cell Biol* 1993;61:92–99.
64. Coombe DR, Watt SM, Parish CR. Mac-1 (CD11b/CD18) and CD45 mediate the adhesion of hematopoietic progenitor cells to stromal cell elements via recognition of stromal heparan sulfate. *Blood* 1994;84:739–752.
65. Hynes RO. Integrins: Versatility, modulation and signaling in cell adhesion. *Cell* 1992;69:11–25.
66. Schwartz MA, Schaller MD, Ginsberg MH. Integrins: Emerging paradigms of signal transuction. *Ann Rev Cell Biol* 1995;11:549–599.
67. Assoian RK, Marcantonio EE. The extracellular matrix as a cell cycle control element in atherosclerosis and restenosis. *J Clin Invest* 1996;98(11): 2436–2439.
68. Nikkari ST, Jarvelainen HT, Wight TN, et al. Smooth muscle cell expression of extracellular matrix genes after arterial injury. *Am J Pathol* 1994; 144:1348–1355.
69. Skinner MP, Raines EW, Ross R. Dynamic expression of $\alpha 1\beta 1$ and $\alpha 2\beta 1$ integrin receptor by human vascular smooth muscle cells. *Am J Pathol* 1994;145:1070–1081.
70. Ruoslahti E, Engvall E. Integrins and vascular extracellular matrix assembly. *J Clin Invest* 1997;99(6):1149–1152.

Chapter 12

B-Myb Represses Collagen Gene Expression in Bovine Vascular Smooth Muscle Cells

Kyriakos E. Kypreos, PhD,
Darius J. Marhamati, MD, PhD,
Matthew A. Nugent, PhD, and
Gail E. Sonenshein, PhD

Introduction

Work from several laboratories, including our own, has shown that fibrillar collagen messenger RNA (mRNA) expression varies inversely with the growth state of vascular smooth muscle cells (VSMCs). The levels of collagen mRNA are low in subconfluent cultures of exponentially growing smooth muscle cells (SMCs) and increase dramatically as the cells reach confluence.[1–5] Similarly, growth arrest of subconfluent cultures of VSMCs by serum deprivation or isoleucine deprivation results in a significant induction in fibrillar collagen mRNA levels.[6,7] On the other hand, agents that stimulate growth often inhibit collagen gene expression. For example, basic fibroblast growth factor (bFGF) is a potent mitogen for VSMCs in culture and in the vessel wall.[8–11] Kennedy and coworkers showed that treatment of human VSMCs with bFGF results in a decrease in type I collagen mRNA and protein levels, with a concomitant induction in the expression of interstitial collagenase gene.[12] Recently, work by our laboratory has implicated B-Myb as a negative regulator of collagen gene transcription and as a major intracellular link between growth and matrix gene expression.

This work was supported by National Institutes of Health Grants HL13262 and HL57326.

B-*myb*, a member of the *myb* gene family, was originally isolated based on high sequence homology (approximately 90%) with c-*myb* in the DNA-binding domain.[13] Cell synchronization studies have demonstrated that in 3T3 fibroblasts and hematopoietic cells, B-*myb* displays a late G1-specific gene expression pattern, similar to that of c-*myb*.[14-16] Work in our laboratory showed that SMCs express B-*myb* mRNA in a similar cell-cycle-dependent fashion.[17] Levels of B-*myb* mRNA were low in SMCs rendered quiescent by serum deprivation for 72 hours, and began to increase between 8 and 14 hours following serum stimulation. B-*myb* mRNA levels peaked at 24 hours. Addition of 20 ng/mL epidermal growth factor (EGF) to serum-deprived quiescent cultures also resulted in the induction in B-*myb* mRNA levels, which was detectable at 12 hours, consistent with the late G1-pattern of B-*myb* expression.[17] Furthermore, an increase in B-*myb* mRNA levels was noted following addition of insulin-like growth factor (IGF-I) to serum-deprived quiescent SMCs that had been rendered competent to proliferate by treatment with 12-O-tetradecanoylphorbol-13-acetate (TPA). This induction coincided with the G1 to S-phase transition.[17]

Detailed analysis of the functional domains of B-*myb* showed that the DNA-binding domain is located close near the amino-terminal end of the protein and is composed of three imperfect repeats of 51–52 amino acids.[18] B-Myb protein is capable of binding to the consensus c-Myb binding site (MBS) [YGRC(A/C/G)GTT(G/A)],[19] although R is preferably T/C for c-Myb and A/C for B-Myb. B-Myb was found to regulate several reporter constructs that were c-Myb regulated, including the c-*myc* gene.[20] In addition, B-Myb has also been reported to recognize a second specific consensus sequence [PuPuAAANYG].[21] Thus, B-Myb is perhaps able to regulate a second subset of genes in addition to those in common with c-Myb.

B-*myb* lacks the acidic transactivation domain conserved between c-*myb* and A-*myb*, another member of the *myb* family. B-Myb does, however, have an acidic region (amino acids 207–273) that has been shown to have the ability to impart transactivation properties on the B-Myb protein.[18] In contrast, several groups have demonstrated that B-*myb* can repress transcription, such as in the case of c-*myb*-mediated transactivation.[22,23] Tashiro et al[24] have reported the effects of B-*myb* on transcription may be cell type-specific. B-*myb* was shown to be a positive transactivator in several cell lines, including HeLa cells, whereas it was a transcriptional repressor of c-Myb-mediated transactivation in fibroblast and macrophage cell lines. These workers postulated that the C-terminal conserved region is responsible for binding to another protein, and it is this heterodimer that functions as a positive transactivator.[24] Work from our laboratory showed that B-*myb* is a negative regulator of gene expression in SMCs.[17] Specifically, B-*myb* decreased reporter activity of a multimerized MBS-element-driven promoter construct. Furthermore, the promoters of the c-*myc* and c-*myb* genes, which have been found to be stimulated by c-Myb and B-Myb in some cells,[20,25] were not induced by B-Myb in SMCs.

Indirect mechanisms of action have also been demonstrated for B-Myb. For example, without interacting with DNA, B-Myb increased the activity of the promoters of DNA polymerase α[23] and the human *hsp70* genes.[26] In the latter case, the transcriptional effects of B-Myb were found to be mediated through heat shock elements. Furthermore, v-Myb and c-Myb can interact via their transactivation domains directly with the transcriptional coactivator protein CBP (CREB [cAMP responsive element]-binding protein).[27,28]

Given our findings that B-Myb was a negative regulator of transcription in actively proliferating SMCs, we tested its effects on transcription of collagen genes, which displays an inverse pattern of expression. Our results indicate that B-Myb is a major regulator of fibrillar collagen gene expression in VSMCs. In the following sections, we will describe the findings of three separate studies, which show that B-Myb: (1) represses transcription of the promoters of type I collagen; (2) mediates the bFGF-induced signals leading to the drop in type I collagen gene expression; and (3) represses transcription of the alpha 2 type V collagen promoter in an indirect fashion via inhibiting activation by a positive regulator. We will focus predominantly on the latter two studies, since the findings of the first one were published several years ago, setting the stage for the more recent work.

B-*myb* Represses Type I Collagen Promoter Activity

The effects of B-Myb expression on the activities of the promoters of genes encoding the two chains of type I collagen were examined. An $\alpha 2(I)$ collagen promoter pMS-3.5/CAT construct, which contains 3.5 kb of sequence upstream of the promoter and 58 bp of exon 1 driving the chloramphenicol acetyltransferase (CAT) reporter gene,[29] was used for transient cotransfection analysis in bovine SMCs. The activity of the pMS-3.5/CAT vector displayed an average decrease in three experiments of $82 \pm 10.8\%$ upon cotransfection with a bovine B-*myb* vector, and similar downregulation was seen with a human B-*myb* expression vector.[17] To assess the effects of B-Myb expression on activity of the $\alpha 1(I)$ promoter, the pOB3.6, which contains 3.6 kb of the $\alpha 1(I)$ collagen promoter plus all of exon 1 and intron 1 upstream of the CAT reporter gene, was used. Upon cotransfection with bovine or human B-*myb* expression vectors, the activity of pOB3.6 was downregulated approximately 92% and 79%, respectively.[17] Therefore B-Myb expression leads to the downregulation of activity of the promoters of the genes encoding both chains of type I collagen.

bFGF-Induced Decrease in Type I Collagen Gene Transcription is Mediated by B-Myb

During the development of atherosclerotic lesions, SMCs are exposed to a variety of cytokines and growth factors, including bFGF. A member of the fibroblast growth factor family, bFGF was originally identified as an activity in pituitary extracts that stimulated growth of Swiss hamster 3T3 fibroblasts.[30] It is known for a multiplicity of biological activities both in vivo and in vitro.[31–33] Antibodies to bFGF[9] or a bFGF/toxin conjugate[10] inhibit the proliferation of VSMCs in vivo after balloon injury. Furthermore, direct administration of bFGF to the blood vessel wall stimulates in vivo SMC proliferation.[11] Together, these studies and others have indicated that bFGF plays an important role in a number of proliferative vascular disorders, including the accelerated arteriopathies that follow angioplasty and vascular bypass surgery.[31] With respect to collagen gene expression, Kennedy and coworkers showed that bFGF treatment of SMCs decreases type I collagen mRNA and protein levels.[12] Thus, we sought to determine the potential role of B-*myb* in mediating signals triggered by bFGF that result in decreased expression of the $\alpha1(I)$ collagen gene.

Treatment of Aortic SMCs with bFGF Increases B-*myb* mRNA Levels in a Dose-Dependent Fashion

We first monitored the effects of bFGF treatment on B-*myb* mRNA expression in VSMCs. Cultures of bovine aortic SMCs were plated at 1 $\times$ 10[6] cells per P-150 tissue culture plate in complete medium (10% FBS-DMEM) and treated with 0.5, 1, 2, and 5 ng/mL bFGF dissolved in carrier solution (carrier solution: 50 mmol/L Tris-HCl; pH 7.5, 0.3 M NaCl, 1 mmol/L dithiothreitol, 0.05% gelatin) or 5 μL/mL carrier solution alone (0 ng/mL bFGF) for 24 hours. RNA was isolated and analyzed by Northern blotting for B-*myb* expression (Figure 1). Equal RNA loading was verified by ethidium bromide staining of the gel. An approximate 2-fold increase (2.0 ± 0.1) in the levels of B-*myb* mRNA was observed with a concentration of bFGF as low as 0.5 ng/mL. Treatment with concentrations up to 2 ng/mL bFGF resulted in a further increase in B-*myb* mRNA (2.3 ± 0.1-fold). Interestingly, treatment with 5 ng/mL bFGF resulted in decreased induction in B-*myb* mRNA levels, as compared to 2

0   0.5   1   2   5   : ng/mL bFGF

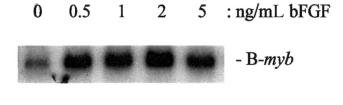

- B-*myb*

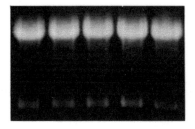

Figure 1. Dose-dependent effects of bFGF on B-*myb* mRNA expression. Sub-confluent cultures of SMCs were maintained under serum-deprivation conditions for 24 hours and then treated with carrier solution (0) or the indicated concentration of bFGF for an additional 24-hour period. Total RNA was isolated and samples (15 μg) were subjected to Northern blot analysis for the B-*myb* gene. Ethidium bromide-stained gel, confirming RNA quality and equal loading, is shown.

ng/mL bFGF. This biphasic response profile is similar to that which has been observed for bFGF-stimulated mitogenesis, where response is observed to peak and then decrease as bFGF concentration is increased.[34,35] Thus, treatment of bovine aortic SMCs with bFGF increases the B-*myb* mRNA levels. Since a concentration of 2 ng/mL bFGF had the greatest effect, it was used for the remaining studies.

Treatment of VSMCs with bFGF Decreases Type I Collagen Gene Transcription

To investigate whether the previously reported decrease in the levels of α1(I) collagen mRNA can be related to an increased rate of mRNA turnover, the effects of bFGF on the stability of α1(I) collagen mRNA were measured using 5,6-dichlorobenzimidazole riboside (DRB), a selective inhibitor of RNA polymerase II (Figure 2A). The half-life for this mRNA in control cultures was approximately 33 hours (Figure 2B). No increase in the rate of mRNA decay was seen in bFGF-treated versus control cultures (Figure 2B). Actually, the half-life of α1(I) mRNA ap-

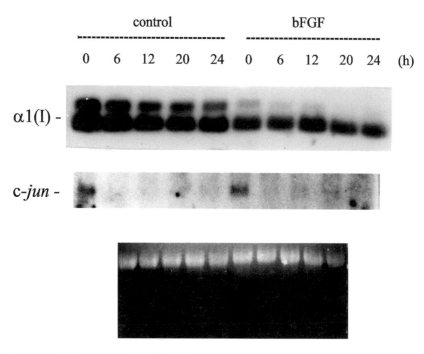

Figure 2A. Treatment with bFGF does not decrease the rate of decay of colla-gen α1(I) mRNA. Subconfluent cultures were maintained under serum-depri-vation conditions for 24 hours and then treated with carrier solution or 2 ng/mL bFGF for an additional 24-hour period. Following replacement with fresh 0.5% FBS-DMEM containing bFGF or carrier solution, 5,6-dichlorobenzimidazole ri-boside (DRB) was added to 30 µg/mL and total RNA was isolated after 0, 6, 12, 20, or 24 hours. RNA samples (10 µg) were subjected to Northern blot analysis for either α1(I) collagen or c-*jun* expression. Ethidium bromide-stained gel is shown. *(continued)*

peared to increase in the presence of bFGF, and a value of approximately 44 hours was measured. Therefore, mechanisms other than decreased mRNA stability are involved in the drop in the steady-state levels of this procollagen.

Nuclear run-off analysis was performed next to determine whether transcriptional control mechanisms play a role in the decrease in steady-state α1(I) collagen mRNA levels. Nuclei were isolated from subconfluent cultures treated with bFGF or equivalent volume of car-rier solution for 24 hours under serum-deprivation conditions. Radio-labeled run-off transcripts were isolated and used as probes. Hy-bridization to an α1(I) collagen probe was seen to decrease significantly upon bFGF treatment (Figure 3). In this and two separate experiments, an average 3.4 ± 1.5-fold drop was seen in bFGF-treated versus control cultures. Essentially equal hybridization was seen with

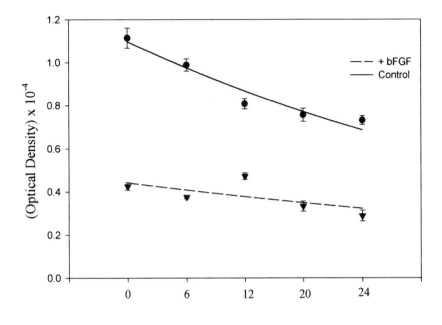

Time after DRB addition (in hours)

Figure 2B. Multiple exposures of resulting autoradiograms in Figure 2A were quantitated by scanning densitometry, and the resulting relative optical density values plotted as a function of time (in hours).

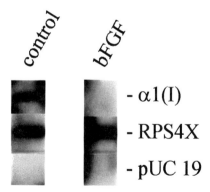

$- \alpha 1(I)$

$- RPS4X$

$- pUC\ 19$

Figure 3. bFGF decreases the rate of $\alpha 1(I)$ collagen gene transcription. Subconfluent cultures were maintained under serum-deprivation conditions for 24 hours and then treated with 2 ng/mL bFGF or carrier solution for an additional 24-hour period. Nuclei were isolated and the resulting radiolabeled RNAs (run-off transcripts) were hybridized to the indicated cDNA probes or pUC 19 vector DNA (10 μg/slot) immobilized on GeneScreen-Plus (Dupont NEN Research Products, Boston, MA) membrane. Probes included DNA for $\alpha 1(I)$ collagen, the small ribosomal subunit protein S4X, HUMRPS4X (RPS4X), and pUC 19 DNA.

the HUMRPS4X probe for the small ribosomal subunit protein S4X, confirming equal loading of the radiolabeled transcripts (Figure 3). No significant hybridization to the control pUC19 plasmid was detected. Thus, treatment with bFGF results in a drop in the rate of transcription of $\alpha1(I)$ procollagen gene that can account for the observed changes in mRNA levels.

Ectopic Expression of B-Myb Decreases Endogenous $\alpha1(I)$ Collagen mRNA Levels

To assess the effects of B-Myb on the endogenous $\alpha1(I)$ collagen gene, various transfection procedures and conditions were tested. Optimal effects were observed with lipofection; using a β-gal reporter construct and X-gal staining, a transfection efficiency of approximately 65% was estimated. Using this procedure, subconfluent SMC cultures were transfected with either a bovine B-*myb* expression vector (pB14)[17] or pBluescript KS+ plasmid, as control. Cultures were allowed to recover for 24 hours, and then incubated in complete medium or under serum-deprivation conditions for an additional 48 hours. Total RNA was isolated and subjected to Northern blot analysis for B-*myb* and $\alpha1(I)$ collagen mRNA expression. The product of the endogenous and the transfected B-*myb* genes can be distinguished based on size (3.4–4.2 kb, respectively) (Figure 4). High levels of the ectopically expressed B-*myb* were observed only in the RNA samples from cells transfected with the B-*myb* expression vector, as expected. Furthermore, the level of the endogenous B-*myb* mRNA decreased under serum-deprivation conditions, in agreement with the previously seen growth-related pattern of expression of this gene.[17]

In cultures maintained in 10% FBS-DMEM, ectopic expression of B-*myb* resulted in a modest (approximately 20%) decrease in the steady-state mRNA levels of the $\alpha1(I)$ collagen chain. The small reduction in $\alpha1(I)$ collagen mRNA is not unexpected when one considers the long half-life of this mRNA (see Figure 2). As discussed above, we previously found that $\alpha1(I)$ collagen gene expression increases significantly upon serum deprivation of subconfluent SMC cultures while B-*myb* mRNA levels drop.[6,17] If the drop in B-*myb* allowed for derepression of collagen expression, then ectopic B-*myb* expression should reduce the induction normally seen upon shifting cells from 10% FBS-DMEM to 0.5% FBS-DMEM. Serum deprivation of control cultures resulted in a 2.6 ± 0.2-fold increase in $\alpha1(I)$ collagen mRNA levels (Figure 4), as seen previously.[6] Ectopic expression of B-*myb* sig-

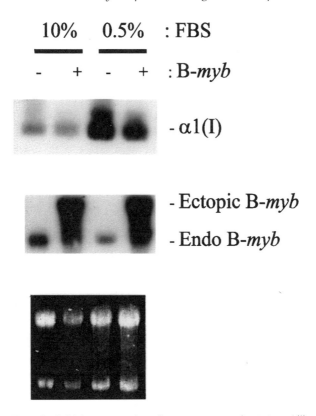

10%   0.5% : FBS

-   +   -   + : B-*myb*

- α1(I)

- Ectopic B-*myb*
- Endo B-*myb*

Figure 4. Ectopic B-Myb expression decreases steady-state α1(I) collagen mRNA levels. Subconfluent SMC cultures (5 × 10⁵ cells/P-100 tissue culture dish) were transfected with either 10 μg pB14 (bovine B-*myb* expression vector) (+) or pBluescript KS+ as control (−), using lipofectamine. Cultures were washed and allowed to recover for 24 hours in tissue culture media containing 20% FBS, and then switched to 10% FBS-DMEM or 0.5% FBS-DMEM for an additional 48 hours. RNA was isolated and samples (10 μg) subjected to Northern blot analysis for α1(I) collagen and B-*myb* expression. The positions of the RNA products of the ectopic and endogenous B-*myb* genes are indicated (ectopic and endo B-*myb*, respectively). Ethidium bromide-stained gel is shown, confirming equal loading and RNA integrity.

nificantly inhibited the induction of α1(I) collagen mRNA levels seen upon serum deprivation. Only a modest increase (1.4 ± 0.1-fold) in the level of α1(I) collagen mRNA was seen in the presence of ectopic B-*myb* expression. Thus, ectopic expression of B-*myb* decreases endogenous α1(I) collagen mRNA levels, which is seen most significantly upon conditions of serum deprivation.

B-*myb* Antisense Oligonucleotide Prevents the Drop in the Levels of α1(I) Collagen mRNA Upon bFGF Treatment

We next sought to test whether the increase in B-*myb* mRNA plays a role in the observed decrease in α1(I) collagen mRNA levels caused by bFGF. To determine this, the ability of an antisense B-*myb* oligonucleotide (5'-TGCAGCTCATCCAGCTCCTCA-3') to prevent the decrease in α1(I) collagen expression upon bFGF treatment was measured. A random oligonucleotide matched in G+C content was used (5'-GATC-CAAGTCCGAGTTTTCGC-3') as the control. We presumed that the ability of the antisense oligonucleotide to inhibit B-Myb activity would be more effective at higher cell density because of the lower endogenous levels of B-*myb* mRNA present under these conditions (see Figure 1).

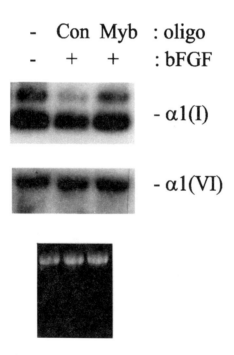

Figure 5A. B-*myb* mediates the bFGF-induced drop in α1(I) collagen mRNA levels. Confluent cultures, maintained in 10% FBS-DMEM, were treated with 2 ng/mL bFGF (+, bFGF) in the presence of 15 μmol/L control (Con) or B-*myb* antisense oligonucleotide (Myb). Alternatively, cultures were treated with 2 μL/mL carrier solution as an additional control (−, bFGF). Total RNA was extracted, and samples (15 μg) were subjected to Northern blot analysis for the indicated genes. Ethidium bromide-stained gel is shown, confirming equal RNA loading. *(continued)*

Thus, the experiments with the antisense oligonucleotide were performed in confluent cultures. Cells were incubated in the presence of 15 μmol/L of antisense B-*myb* or control oligonucleotide for 24 hours in 0.5% FBS-DMEM, to assure better uptake and stability of the oligonucleotide. Cultures were returned to complete medium (containing heat-inactivated serum) in the presence of bFGF or carrier solution and the appropriate oligonucleotide. Following a 24-hour incubation period, some cultures were used for isolation of total cellular RNA, whereas nuclear extracts were prepared from the rest of the cultures. RNA was subjected to Northern blot analysis for α1(I) and α1(VI) collagen chains (Figure 5A). Treatment with bFGF, in the presence of the control oligonucleotide, resulted in the expected decrease in the level of α1(I) collagen mRNA. However, the presence of B-*myb* antisense oligonucleotide almost completely blocked the bFGF-mediated drop in levels of message for this collagen chain. As expected, bFGF treatment had essentially no effect on the levels of α1(VI) collagen mRNA (Figure 5A).

To confirm the inhibitory effect of B-*myb* antisense oligonucleotide on B-Myb protein expression, 100 μg of the nuclear extracts, were subjected to immunoblot analysis using a B-Myb-specific antibody (C-20, Santa Cruz Biotechnology, Santa Cruz, CA) (Figure 5B). As expected, the basal levels of B-Myb protein were low in confluent cultures treated with carrier solution, and increased upon treatment with bFGF in the presence of the control oligonucleotide. However, the presence of the B-*myb* antisense oligonucleotide completely ablated the bFGF-mediated induction, confirming that treatment of SMCs with the B-*myb* antisense oligonucleotide results in inhibition of B-Myb protein synthesis (Figure 5B). As an additional control, the effect of the two oligonucleotides on the basal α1(I) collagen mRNA levels was also determined. Parallel confluent cultures of SMCs were treated with the B-*myb* anti-

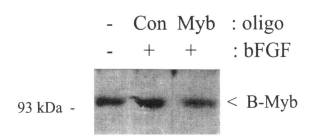

- Con Myb : oligo
- + + : bFGF

93 kDa -   < B-Myb

Figure 5B. Confluent cultures of SMCs were treated as in Figure 5A and nuclear extracts were isolated essentially by the method of Dignam-Roeder.[54] Nuclear extracts were analyzed by immunoblot analysis for the expression of B-Myb protein, using a B-Myb-specific antibody (C-20, Santa Cruz Biotechnology). Molecular weights were determined based on the migration of Benchmark protein markers (Gibco/BRL, Gaithersburg, MD). *(continued)*

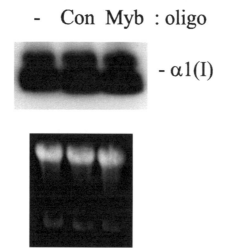

Figure 5C. Confluent cultures of SMCs maintained in 10% FBS-DMEM were treated either with 15 μmol/L of B-*myb* antisense (Myb) or control oligonucleotide (Con) for 48 hours. Alternatively, some cultures were treated with the equivalent volume of ddH2O, as an additional control (−, oligo). Total RNA was extracted, and samples (15 μg) were subjected to Northern blot analysis for the α1(I) gene. Ethidium bromide-stained gel is shown, confirming equal RNA loading.

sense or the control oligonucleotide in the absence of bFGF. RNA was isolated and analyzed for α1(I) mRNA expression (Figure 5C). Addition of the B-*myb* antisense oligonucleotide had no measurable effect on the basal α1(I) collagen mRNA levels, consistent with the low levels of basal B-*myb* mRNA levels present, and the very long half-life of α1(I) collagen mRNA. Similarly, the presence of the control oligonucleotide had no detectable effect on basal α1(I) collagen mRNA levels. Thus, the changes in α1(I) collagen mRNA expression seen upon treatment with bFGF are not due to nonspecific effects of the two oligonucleotides. Therefore, B-Myb mediates part of the negative effects of bFGF on α1(I) collagen mRNA levels.

Discussion

Here we provide evidence that B-Myb mediates signals leading to downregulation of type I collagen gene expression by bFGF. Treatment with bFGF resulted in an increase in B-*myb* expression and a decrease in the rate of α1(I) collagen transcription. Ectopic expression of B-*myb* decreased the steady-state mRNA levels of the endogenous α1(I) collagen gene, preventing the induction that would normally occur upon serum deprivation. Of note, treatment with a B-*myb* antisense oligonucleotide specifically ablated the bFGF decrease in α1(I) collagen mRNA levels. Thus, our results identify the transcription factor B-Myb as an important mediator of signals controlling expression of α1(I) collagen by bFGF.

In most cells examined, B-*myb* is cell-cycle expressed, with high mRNA levels detected in exponentially growing cells, and barely detectable levels in serum-deprived quiescent cultures.[36] While B-*myb* has been implicated in control of cell-cycle progression in fibroblasts,[37] it does not appear to be involved in promoting cell-cycle entry in bovine VSMCs. Contrary to results in fibroblasts, in SMCs, B-Myb does not stimulate transcription of genes known to promote growth of cells, including c-*myc* and c-*myb*.[17] Furthermore, co-microinjection of SMCs with vectors expressing both B-*myb* and the competence factor c-*myc*[38,39] did not promote entry of these cells into the S phase, whereas c-*myc* and either c-*myb* and A-*myb* effectively induced S-phase entry in 75%-80% of the cells.[40] Thus, the decrease in α1(I) collagen gene expression, caused by B-*myb*, is not likely due to a nonspecific, cell-cycle effect.

The mechanism of the repression of type I collagen gene expression by B-Myb remains to be elucidated. The α1(I) collagen promoter contains several putative Myb-binding sites, raising the possibility of a direct interaction of B-Myb with this promoter. However, indirect mechanisms have also been demonstrated. For example, B-Myb increases the activity of the DNA polymerase α promoter, without directly interacting with the DNA.[23] Furthermore, the transcriptional effects of c-*myb* have also been found to be mediated through heat shock elements, such as in the case of the human *hsp70* gene, without direct interaction of c-Myb with the DNA.[41] An additional possibility is that the effects of B-Myb on α1(I) collagen gene expression are mediated through protein-protein interactions with other nuclear factors. Recently, it has been reported that v-Myb and c-Myb can interact directly with the transcriptional coactivator CBP via their transactivation domains.[27,28] In addition, v-Myb and c-Myb associate directly with members of the C/EBP family of transcription factors, and this association is required for the Myb-induced transactivation of many genes, including neutrophil elastase,[42,43] *mim*-1,[44,45] and *tom*-1.[46] Thus, B-Myb could repress collagen gene expression via inhibiting a coactivator protein that would normally lead to gene activation. As discussed in the following section, the effects of B-Myb on the promoter of the α2 chain of type V collagen appear to be through such an indirect mechanism, although not involving CREB elements. Work is in progress to elucidate the mechanism of the inhibition of type I collagen gene transcription by B-Myb in VSMCs.

Our data constitute the first report to directly implicate the growth-regulated gene B-*myb* as a specific mediator of the effects of bFGF in

VSMCs. Binding of bFGF to cell-surface receptors triggers signals that result in an induced expression of B-*myb*, which in turn inhibits type I collagen gene expression. Identification of B-*myb* in the bFGF-induced inhibition of collagen gene expression provides important information about the potential mechanism of action of this growth factor during tissue remodeling at the sites of vascular injury. Understanding the role of this gene in extracellular matrix gene expression during the development of atherosclerosis may lead the way to important clinical applications for the prevention and treatment of the disease.

B-Myb Inhibits Transactivation of the α2 Type V Collagen Promoter Through Novel Elements Within the First Exon

We next sought to determine whether B-*myb* has a similar inhibitory effect on transcription of another matrix gene whose expression varies inversely with growth, the fibrillar type V collagen.

Ectopic Expression of B-Myb Decreases α2(V) Collagen Gene Expression

To begin to test the effects of B-*myb* on the promoter of the α2 chain of type V collagen gene, transient cotransfection analysis was performed. The pST2.5 α2(V) collagen promoter CAT reporter construct, containing 2,350 bp of promoter and upstream sequences and 150 bp of exon 1,[47] was cotransfected into bovine aortic SMCs with increasing doses of the bovine B-*myb* expression vector pB14 (Figure 6A). A significant downregulation was observed; at doses as low as 2.5 mg of B-*myb* vector, an average decrease of 3.7-fold was seen. In three separate experiments, an average decrease in α2(V) promoter activity of 3.6 ± 1.0-fold was measured upon cotransfection of the pB14 vector. Thus, B-*myb* expression downmodulates the activity of the α2 type V collagen promoter.

To assess the effects of B-Myb on the endogenous α2(V) collagen gene, lipofection was again used in transfection analysis, as outlined above. Subconfluent SMC cultures were transfected with either the bovine B-*myb* expression vector pB14 or pBluescript KS+ plasmid, as control. Cultures were allowed to recover for 24 hours, and then incubated in complete media or under serum-deprivation conditions for an additional 48 hours. Total RNA was isolated and subjected to Northern blot analysis for B-*myb* and α2(V) collagen mRNA expression. Ectopically expressed B-*myb* mRNA (4.2 kb) was observed only in the RNA samples from cells transfected with the B-*myb* expression vector, as

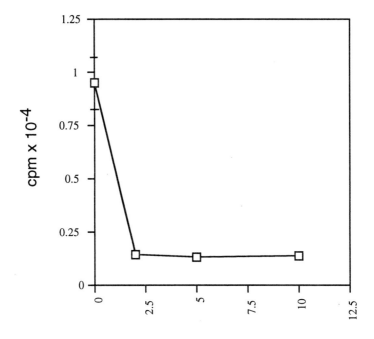

Cotransfected B-*myb* Expression Vector (Total μg of DNA)

Figure 6A. B-*myb* decreases α2(V) collagen expression. Promoter activity. Bovine aortic SMCs, plated at a density of 5 × 10[5] cells/P-100 in 10% FBS-DMEM, were allowed to grow for 1 day (subconfluent cultures). Using the calcium phosphate precipitation method, these cultures were transfected in duplicate with 25 μg pST2.5 collagen α2(V) promoter-reporter construct[47] in the presence of the indicated amounts of B-*myb* expression vector and pBluescript KS+ plasmid DNA to make up a total of 50 μg DNA/P-100 dish. Extracts containing equal amounts of protein were assayed for CAT activity. *(continued)*

expected (Figure 6B). Again, the level of the endogenous B-*myb* mRNA (3.4 kb) decreased under serum-deprivation conditions. In cultures maintained in complete medium (10% FBS-DMEM) ectopic expression of B-*myb* resulted in a small but significant (approximately 1.6-fold) decrease in the steady-state mRNA levels of the α2(V) collagen chain, consistent with the long half-life of this mRNA.[17]

As with type I collagen, α2(V) collagen gene expression was found to increase significantly upon serum deprivation of subconfluent SMC cultures,[48] correlating with the drop in B-*myb* mRNA levels. Thus, we next assessed whether ectopic B-*myb* expression would reduce the increase normally seen upon shifting cells from 10% FBS-DMEM to 0.5%

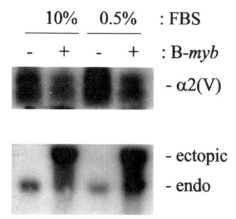

Figure 6B. Endogenous α2(V) collagen mRNA levels. Subconfluent SMC cultures were transfected using lipofectamine with either 10 μg pB14 bovine B-*myb* expression vector (+), or pBluescript KS+ as control (−). Cultures were allowed to recover for 24 hours in 20% FBS-DMEM, and then switched to 10% FBS-DMEM or 0.5% FBS-DMEM for an additional 48 hours. RNA was isolated and samples (10 μg) were subjected to Northern blot analysis for α2(V) collagen (upper panel) and B-*myb* expression (lower panel). The positions of the RNA products of the ectopic and endogenous B-*myb* genes are indicated (ectopic and endo, respectively).

FBS-DMEM (Figure 6B). Serum deprivation of control cultures was shown to result in a significant, 2-fold increase in α2(V) collagen mRNA levels.[48] Ectopic expression of B-*myb* completely prevented the induction in α2(V) collagen mRNA levels upon serum deprivation, and resulted in levels lower than those seen in exponentially growing control cultures. Thus, ectopic expression of B-*myb* decreases endogenous α2(V) collagen mRNA levels, and prevents the induction seen under serum-deprivation conditions.

The B-Myb-Responsive Region of the α2(V) Collagen Gene Maps to a 250-bp Fragment

To map the responsive elements, we compared the effects of B-*myb* on the pST2.5 vector with a series of nested deletion α2(V) collagen promoter constructs. These reporter constructs contained approximately 150 bp of exon 1 sequences, and upstream sequences ranging from 1050 bp (termed pST1.2) to 150 bp (termed pST0.3).[47] B-*myb* cotransfection caused a significant decrease in activity of all of the α2(V) promoter-CAT constructs, but not of the parental (pBLCAT3) vector (Figure 7A). Furthermore, a smaller α2(V) collagen promoter CAT construct, pST0.25

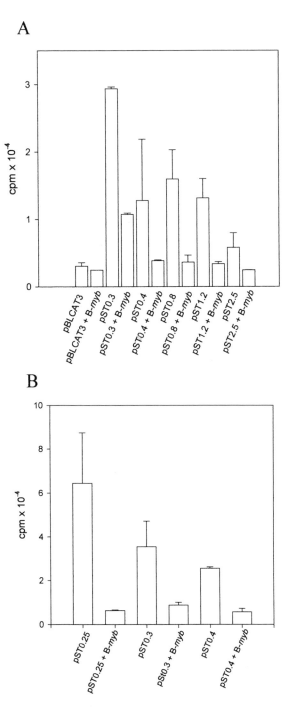

Figure 7. Effects of B-*myb* localize to a 250-bp region of the α2(V) collagen gene. A series of α2(V) collagen promoter nested deletion CAT reporter constructs (pST0.25 to pST2.5) were employed. **A and B:** Subconfluent cultures of SMCs were transfected with reporter constructs in the absence or presence of 3 μg of B-*myb* expression vector, using the calcium phosphate precipitation method, as described in the legend for Figure 6A. Extracts containing equal amounts of protein were assayed for CAT activity.

containing a 250-bp insert (100 bp of promoter and 150 bp of exon 1 sequences) was similarly downregulated (Figure 7B). Thus, the region-mediating negative regulation of this promoter maps to an approximately 250-bp fragment.

Mutation of Two CRE-Like Elements Ablates Negative Regulation by B-Myb

Previous work has shown that c-Myb can interact directly with the transcriptional activator CBP.[27,28] In turn, CBP interacts with a phosphorylated form of CREB that binds DNA directly through CRE (cAMP responsive elements) and activates expression of cAMP-inducible genes.[49] Computer analysis revealed the presence of two CRE-like elements in exon 1 of the α2(V) collagen gene fragment present in all of the responsive constructs. These CRE-like elements were located 11 bp apart from each other at +84 and +103 bp, respectively. To determine whether protein factors found in nuclear extracts from bovine aortic SMCs can bind to these two elements, electrophoretic mobility shift analysis (EMSA) was performed using a double stranded oligonucleotide (wt MRF-V: 5'-ACAGC**TGACTTCA**TGGTGCTACAAT**AACCTCA**GAATC-3') that contained the two CRE-like putative matrix regulatory factor (MRF)-binding elements (in bold). Nuclear extracts were prepared from subcon-

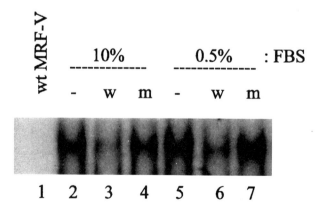

Figure 8. Protein binding to a 35-bp region in exon 1 that contains two CRE-like elements. Subconfluent cultures of bovine aortic SMCs (5 × 10⁵ cells/P-150) were maintained in 10% FBS-DMEM or switched to 0.5% FBS-DMEM for 48 hours. Nuclear extracts were isolated as described previously[54] and used in EMSA with the double stranded wt MRF-V oligonucleotide (−). Competition analysis was performed with a 250X molar excess of unlabeled wild type (w) or the mutant MRF-V (m), where indicated. Lane 1 corresponds to the free probe.

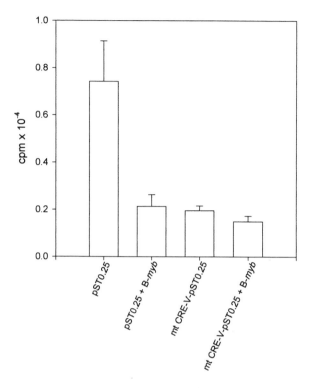

Figure 9. Introduction of mutations into the two CRE-like elements in exon 1 ablates negative regulation by B-Myb. Bovine aortic SMCs were plated at a density of 5×10^5 cells/P-100 plate in 10% FBS-DMEM. Using the calcium phosphate precipitation method, these subconfluent cultures were transfected with 25 μg pST0.25 or mt MRF-V-pST0.25 plasmid in the absence or presence of 5 μg pact-B-*myb* expression vector. Extracts containing equal amounts of protein were assayed for CAT activity.

fluent cultures maintained in normal tissue culture medium, or following 48 hours of serum deprivation when type V collagen expression increases.[48] EMSA performed with either extract resulted in the appearance of one slowly migrating protein/DNA complex. Furthermore, a higher level of binding was observed with the extracts from the serum-deprived cells (Figure 8). Competition assays performed using excess unlabeled oligonucleotide confirmed the specificity of this complex. A mutated version of MRF-V oligonucleotide (mt MRF-V: 5'-CAGC*TTCTAGAA*TGGT-GCTACAAA*AGATCTAGAA*T-3'), containing 6 point-mutations (underlined and italicized) in each of the two CRE-like elements, was similarly used in competition EMSA; this oligonucleotide competed much less effectively for binding to the probe (Figure 8). These data indicate that protein factors present in nuclear extracts of bovine aortic SMCs

bind to these two elements. Furthermore, serum deprivation results in enhanced formation of this complex, which correlates with the induction in
$\alpha 2(V)$ collagen gene expression.

To determine whether the effects of B-Myb on $\alpha 2(V)$ collagen transcription are mediated through its two elements, site-directed mutage-
nesis was performed. The same two sets of six mutations in the mt
MRF-V probe that ablated binding were introduced into the pST0.25
vector; the new vector was termed mt MRF-V-pST0.25. Subconfluent
cultures of SMCs were cotransfected with either the wt pST0.25 or mt
MRF-V-pST0.25 reporter construct in the absence or presence of the B-
myb expression vector (pact-B-Myb). Introduction of the mutation severely reduced $\alpha 2(V)$ collagen basal promoter activity. In three separate experiments, an average 3.3 ± 0.2-fold decrease in activity was
observed (Figure 9). Expression of B-*myb* had little effect on the activity of the mt MRF-V-pST0.25 reporter construct (Figure 9). As expected,
cotransfection of pact-B-*myb* resulted in a 3.3 ± 0.6-fold drop in the activity of the wt pST0.25 vector, essentially to that of the basal activity of
the mutant $\alpha 2(V)$ promoter construct. Thus, these two elements play a
significant role in the downregulation of the $\alpha 2(V)$ collagen promoter
activity by B-Myb. Furthermore, factors that interact with these two elements appear to positively regulate this promoter.

Binding of SMC Nuclear Extracts to MRF-V is Not Mediated by CREB Factors

To directly assess the binding of CREB to the MRF-V sequence, we
performed EMSA using an oligonucleotide containing the classical
CRE element within the somatostatin gene promoter (SOMCRE) as
competitor[50] (5'-CTTGGCTGACGTCAGAGAGA-3'). Nuclear extracts
were prepared from SMCs in complete medium or following serum
deprivation for 48 hours, as above. The expected increase in binding to
the MRF-V probe was seen with nuclear extracts from serum-deprived
cultures (Figure 10). Competition with 500X molar excess of unlabeled
SOMCRE oligonucleotide had only a minor effect on binding, whereas,
successful competition with unlabeled wt MRF-V confirmed the binding specificity (Figure 10). Thus, formation of the slowly migrating
complex appears mediated through proteins distinct from CREB.

B-Myb Decreases Complex Formation

Since the absence of B-Myb in nuclear extracts from cells incubated
under serum-deprivation conditions correlated with enhanced binding
to the two elements within MRF-V, we next sought to determine whether

10%   0.5%   :FBS

- V C - V C

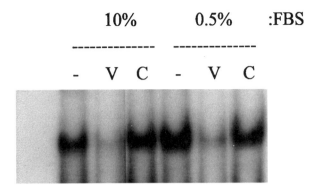

Figure 10. CREB factors are not present in the MRF-V protein binding complex. Nuclear extracts, prepared as described in the legend for Figure 8, were used in EMSA with the wt MRF-V oligonucleotide as probe. Competition analysis was performed by addition of 500X molar excess of unlabeled wt MRF-V (V), or SOMCRE (C).

B-Myb ablated the formation of the slowly migrating complex. To assess this, a purified fusion protein that contains the N-terminal end (345 amino acids) of murine B-Myb fused to the glutathione-S-transferase (GST) moiety (NB-Myb-GST) was added to the binding reactions. Purified GST protein was used as control. Significant binding was seen with nuclear extracts from 48-hour serum-deprived SMC cultures, where the levels of the endogenous B-Myb expression are very low. Addition of 200 ng of purified NB-Myb-GST to the binding reaction resulted in slightly

200 ng   400 ng

- + - + - : GST

- - + - + : NB-Myb-GST

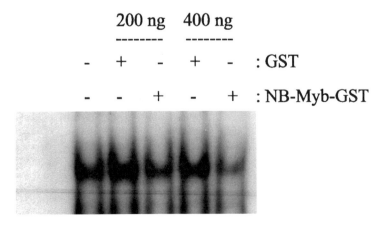

Figure 11. B-Myb decreases complex formation. Subconfluent cultures of bovine aortic SMCs (5×10^5 cells/P-150 dish) were switched to 0.5% FBS-DMEM for 48 hours. Nuclear extracts were isolated and used in EMSA with the wt MRF-V oligonucleotide as probe. To assay for the effects of B-Myb on complex formation, 200 ng or 400 ng of purified NB-Myb-GST or GST protein were added to the binding reaction.

reduced formation of the complex (Figure 11). Addition of 400 ng of NB-Myb-GST dramatically decreased complex formation (Figure 11). No similar decrease in binding was seen upon addition of either 200 ng or 400 ng of purified GST protein alone to the binding reaction. In fact, a slight increase in formation of the complex was noted (Figure 11). The decrease in binding caused by NB-Myb-GST did not appear to be due to direct competition for DNA binding since purified NB-Myb-GST protein did not yield any shifted complexes with wt MRF-V probe in EMSA. These data suggest that B-Myb decreases the complex formation through protein-protein interactions that result in decreased affinity to the elements in the MRF-V sequence. Furthermore, the N-terminal end of B-Myb appears to mediate this inhibitory effect.

DNA-Binding and Carboxyl-Terminal Conserved Domains of B-Myb Are Required for Inhibition

To further identify regions of B-Myb required for the inhibition of α2(V) collagen expression, a series of mutant B-*myb* expression vectors were used. The mutant B-*myb* vectors contained deletions in either the DNA-binding domain (pact-B-*myb*-1), in the acidic region (pact-B-*myb*-2), or in the carboxyl-terminal conserved region (pact-B-*myb*-3) of B-Myb.[18] The effects of these mutations on the ability of B-Myb to inhibit the activity of the pST0.25 α2(V) collagen promoter construct were determined in cotransfection assays using subconfluent SMCs in 10% FBS-DMEM. Cotransfection of wt B-*myb* expression vector resulted in the expected decrease in the α2(V) collagen promoter activity (Figure 12). Deletion of the amino-terminal end of B-Myb completely ablated this inhibition. In fact, a slight induction in pST0.25 activity (1.8 ± 0.5-fold) was seen (Figure 12). This finding is consistent with the EMSA showing involvement of the region in protein-protein interactions. In contrast, deletion of the acidic region had little effect; the pact-B-*myb*-2 expression vector reduced pST0.25 promoter activity to the same extent as the wild-type vector. Cotransfection of pST0.25 with carboxyl-terminal deleted pact-B-*myb*-3 resulted in a 2.8 ± 0.6-fold induction in the activity of this collagen promoter (Figure 12). Thus, both the DNA binding and the carboxyl-terminal conserved domains of B-Myb are required for inhibition of α2(V) collagen promoter activity.

Discussion

We have shown that B-Myb downregulated the promoter activity of the α2 chain of type V collagen indirectly through inhibition of posi-

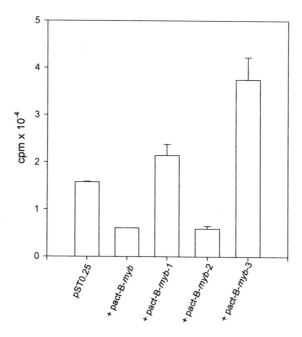

Figure 12. Effects of various B-Myb deletion mutants on inhibition of α2(V) collagen promoter activity. Bovine aortic SMCs were plated at a density of 5×10^5 cells/P-100 tissue culture plate in 10% FBS-DMEM, and allowed to grow for 1 day. Using the calcium phosphate precipitation method, these subconfluent cultures were transfected in triplicate with 25 μg α2(V) collagen reporter construct pST0.25 in the absence or presence of 5 μg wild-type (pact-B-*myb*) or mutant B-*myb* expression vector. The mutant B-*myb* expression vectors used were: pact-B-*myb*-1, deletion in the DNA-binding domain; pact-B-*myb*-2, deletion in the conserved acidic domain; and pact-B-*myb*-3, deletion in the carboxyl-terminal conserved region of B-*myb*. Extracts containing equal amounts of protein were assayed for CAT activity.

tive-acting factors interacting with two elements of the MRF-V sequence located within exon 1. EMSA and supershift analysis indicated that binding of a protein complex to the two elements correlated directly with the level of α2(V) collagen gene expression, ie, binding was elevated with serum deprivation when type V collagen levels are high. Mutation of the elements decreased basal promoter activity to the level seen upon coexpression of B-Myb, and furthermore ablated the inhibitory effect of B-Myb. Last, a protein(s) within the complex appeared to interact directly with B-Myb. Interestingly, Tashiro and coworkers postulated the C-terminal conserved region of B-Myb is responsible for binding to another protein,[24] and we observed that the carboxyl-terminal conserved region of B-Myb was required for the negative regulation of the α2(V) collagen promoter. Thus, these data support the model, illustrated in Figure 13, that the downregulation of α2(V) collagen gene expression by B-Myb involves inhibition of positive transactivation signals mediated via the two elements located within the MRF-V region of exon 1. Furthermore, they suggest that B-Myb is a major intracellular mediator of growth-related signals leading to this inverse relationship between matrix gene expression and the proliferative state of the VSMC.[2,4,5,48,51]

Our initial attempts have failed to identify the nature of the protein components binding to the elements within MRF-V sequence. Although these binding elements share high homology with a CRE consensus sequence, competition EMSA ruled out involvement of CREB; furthermore, based on a lower level of homology with an AP-1 element, competition EMSA was performed that similarly ruled out products of the c-*fos*/c-*jun* family. Interestingly, Greenspan et al[52] observed that genes encoding the α2(V) and α1 chain of type III collagen, which also responds inversely to growth state,[2,6] have a high level of homology in the MRF-V region of exon 1, consistent with a potentially important role for this region in regulation of collagen gene expression. A more detailed understanding of the mechanism of regulation of collagen promoter activity by B-Myb, therefore, awaits identification and cloning of this putative B-Myb interacting factor.

Deletion in the DNA-binding domain of B-*myb* (pact-B-*myb*-1) resulted in a modest level of transactivation of the α2(V) collagen promoter rather than the downregulation normally seen. These findings suggest that an intact DNA-binding domain is required for the inhibition. This appears, at least in part, due to the involvement of this region in protein-protein interaction with proteins binding to MRF-V. Purified amino-terminal NB-Myb-GST protein was found to significantly decrease the formation of the slowly migrating complex, although it does not bind directly to the wt MRF-V probe. This observation is in agreement with the work of Ying et al,[53] who found that the DNA-binding domain of A-Myb binds to a 110-kD nuclear protein. These workers speculated that this interaction was responsible for the B-cell-specific transactivation of the c-*myc* promoter by A-Myb. However, the nature and exact function of the 110-kD nuclear protein remains to be characterized.

One intriguing possibility is that B-Myb binding to the α2(V) collagen promoter facilitates its interaction with the protein complexes binding to the MRF-V sequence. Interestingly, the smallest pST0.25 α2(V) collagen promoter fragment contains several putative B-Myb-binding sites with homology with the AGAAANYG sequence of Mizuguchi et al.[21] Preliminary EMSA performed using purified N-terminal B-Myb-GST fusion protein (NB-Myb-GST) has confirmed binding to a 60-bp region (−20 to +40 bp relative to the start site of transcription). We are in the process of preparing site-directed mutations within this region to test the functional role of this binding. This analysis, however, may be

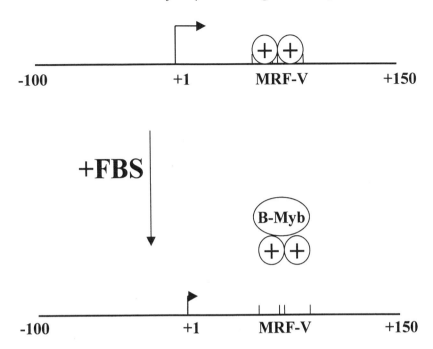

Figure 13. Model of the mechanism of B-Myb inhibition of α2(V) promoter activity in VSMCs. The data presented support a model in which positive transactivation signals are mediated by factor binding to two elements termed Matrix Regulatory Factor of type V collagen (MRF-V), which are located within exon 1 of the α2(V) collagen gene. The downregulation of α2(V) promoter activity by B-Myb, which follows its induction upon addition of fetal bovine serum (FBS), is mediated via direct B-Myb-MRF-V factor interaction. This interaction ablates MRF-V-factor binding and thus transactivation of the α2(V) collagen promoter.

complex in light of the findings of Cogswell et al,[25] who noted that mutation of all five MBS elements within the c-*myc* promoter were needed to ablate transactivation by c-Myb.

As mentioned above, deletion of the carboxyl-terminal end of B-Myb (pact-B-*myb*-3) ablated the ability of B-Myb to inhibit type V collagen expression, suggesting involvement of this region in inhibition. This finding is in agreement with the work of Tashiro et al,[24] who further found that the effects of B-Myb were cell type specific. This led these investigators to postulate that B-*myb* effects on transcriptional regulation require cell type-specific binding of a cofactor to the carboxyl-terminal conserved region. Of note, we also found that the effect of B-*myb* on the α2(V) collagen promoter is cell type-specific; no repression of the activity of this collagen promoter by B-*myb* was observed in NIH3T3 fibroblasts, although a significant inhibition was detected in IMR 90 human lung fibroblasts, and in neonatal rat VSMCs. The exact nature of the protein that mediates these effects is currently under investigation.

Conclusion

Collagen gene expression is strongly linked to the proliferative state of the cell in VSMCs. Agents that promote cell growth decrease collagen production, suggesting that a growth-related gene(s) mediates signals involved in the formation and remodeling of the extracellular matrix. We have provided evidence that B-*myb*, a member of the *myb* gene family, is an important intracellular mediator of signals relating SMC growth state to the level of matrix gene expression. In VSMCs, B-*myb* is activated by growth-promoting signals mediated via bFGF, serum, IGF-1, EGF, and cell density. B-Myb inhibits transcription of genes encoding both types I and V collagen. These observations implicate B-Myb in driving the downregulation of matrix gene expression seen in proliferating SMCs in culture. Experiments are in progress using transgenic mouse models to test whether B-Myb plays a similar role within the vessel wall in vivo. If transgenic animals display greatly reduced levels of matrix proteins when high levels of B-Myb are achieved, such downregulation would suggest that B-Myb functions as an antifibrotic gene in VSMCs. As a potent inhibitor of collagen expression, B-*myb* would represent a specific candidate gene for future gene therapy experiments aimed at the control and treatment of diseases involving excess matrix deposition by the VSMC, particularly the major diseases of atherosclerosis and restenosis. Lastly, since B-*myb* is widely expressed in many cell types, the possibility that it similarly affects connective tissue expression in other cell types deserves additional investigation.

Acknowledgments   We thank J. Foster for use of the densitometer, and F. Ramirez, R. Moreland, R. Watson, and S. Ishii for providing cDNA clones.

References

1. Jones PA, Scott-Burden T, Gevers W. Glycoprotein, elastin, and collagen secretion by rat smooth muscle cells. *Proc Natl Acad Sci USA* 1979;76:353–357.
2. Beldekas J, Gerstenfeld L, Sonenshein GE, et al. Cell density and estradiol modulation of procollagen type III in cultured calf smooth muscle cells. *J Biol Chem* 1982;257:12252–12256.
3. Stepp MA, Kindy MS, Franzblau C, et al. Complex regulation of collagen gene expression in cultured bovine aortic smooth muscle cells. *J Biol Chem* 1986;261:6542–6547.

4. Liau G, Chan LM. Regulation of extracellular matrix RNA levels in cultured smooth muscle cells: Relationship to cellular quiescence. *J Biol Chem* 1989;264:10315–10320.

5. Ang AH, Tachas G, Campbell JH, et al. Collagen synthesis by cultured rabbit aortic smooth-muscle cells. Alteration with phenotype. *Biochem J* 1990;265:461–469.

6. Kindy MS, Chang C-J, Sonenshein GE. Serum deprivation of vascular smooth muscle cells enhances collagen gene expression. *J Biol Chem* 1988; 263:11426–11430.

7. Chang C-J, Sonenshein GE. Increased collagen gene expression in vascular smooth muscle cells cultured in serum or isoleucine deprived medium. *Matrix* 1991;11:242–251.

8. Winkles JA, Friesel R, Burgess WH, et al. Human vascular smooth muscle cells both express and respond to heparin-binding growth factor I (endothelial cell growth factor). *Proc Natl Acad Sci USA* 1989;84:7124–7128.

9. Lindner V, Reidy MA. Proliferation of smooth muscle cells after vascular injury is inhibited by an antibody against basic fibroblast growth factor. *Proc Natl Acad Sci USA* 1991;88:3739–3743.

10. Casscells W, Lappi DA, Olwin BB, et al. Elimination of smooth muscle cells in experimental restenosis: Targeting of fibroblast growth factor receptors. *Proc Natl Acad Sci USA* 1992;89:7159–7163.

11. Edelman ER, Nugent MA, Smith LT, et al. Basic fibroblast growth factor enhances the coupling of intimal hyperplasia and proliferation of vasa vasorum in injured rat arteries. *J Clin Invest* 1992;89:465–473.

12. Kennedy SH, Qin H, Lin L, et al. Basic fibroblast growth factor regulates type I collagen and collagenase gene expression in human smooth muscle cells. *Am J Pathol* 1995;146:764–771.

13. Nomura N, Takahashi M, Matsui M, et al. Isolation of human cDNA clones of myb-related genes, A-myb and B-myb. *Nucl Acids Res* 1988;16: 11075–11083.

14. Lam EW, Robinson C, Watson RJ. Characterization and cell cycle-regulated expression of mouse B-myb. *Oncogene* 1992;7:1885–1890.

15. Golay J, Capucci A, Arsura M, et al. Expression of c-myb and B-myb, but not A-myb, correlates with proliferation in human hematopoietic cells. *Blood* 1991;77:149–158.

16. Reiss K, Travali S, Calabretta B, et al. Growth regulated expression of B-myb in fibroblasts and hematopoietic cells. *J Cell Physiol* 1991;148:338–348.

17. Marhamati DJ, Sonenshein GE. B-Myb expression in vascular smooth muscle cells occurs in a cell cycle-dependent fashion and down-regulates promoter activity of type I collagen genes. *J Biol Chem* 1996;271:3359–3365.

18. Nakagoshi H, Takemoto Y, Ishii S. Functional domains of the human B-myb gene product. *J Biol Chem* 1993;268:14161–14167.

19. Howe KM, Watson RJ. Nucleotide preferences in sequence-specific recognition of DNA by c-myb protein. *Nucl Acids Res* 1991;19:3913–3919.

20. Nakagoshi H, Kanei-Ishii C, Sawazaki T, et al. Transcriptional regulation of the c-myc gene by the c-*myb* and B-*myb* gene products. *Oncogene* 1992;7:1233–1239.

21. Mizuguchi G, Nakagoshi H, Nagase T, et al. DNA binding activity and transcriptional activator function of the human B-Myb protein compared with c-Myb. *J Biol Chem* 1990;265:9280–9284.

22. Foos G, Grimm S, Klempnauer KH. Functional antagonism between mem-

bers of the myb family: B-myb inhibits v-myb-induced gene activation. *EMBO J* 1992;11:4619–4629.

23. Watson R, Robinson C, Lam E. Transcription regulation by murine B-myb is distinct from that by c-myb. *Nucl Acids Res* 1993;21:267–272.

24. Tashiro S, Takemoto Y, Handa H, et al. Cell type-specific trans-activation by the B-myb gene product: Requirement of the putative cofactor binding to the C-terminal conserved domain. *Oncogene* 1995;10:1699–1707.

25. Cogswell J, Cogswell WM, Kuehl WM, et al. Mechanism of c-myc regulation by c-*myb* in different cell lineages. *Mol Cell Biol* 1993;13:2858–2869.

26. Kamano H, Klempnauer KH. B-Myb and cyclin-D1 mediate heat shock element dependent activation of the human HSP70 promoter. *Oncogene* 1997;14:1223–1229.

27. Oelgeschlager M, Janknecht R, Krieg J, et al. Interaction of the co-activator CBP with Myb proteins: Effects on Myb-specific transactivation and on the cooperativity with NF-M. *EMBO J* 1996;15:2771–2780.

28. Dai P, Akimaru H, Tanaka Y, et al. CBP as a transcriptional coactivator of c-Myb. *Genes Dev* 1996;10:528–540.

29. Boast S, Su M-W, Ramirez F, et al. Functional analysis of cis-acting DNA sequences controlling transcription of the human type I collagen genes. *J Biol Chem* 1990;265:13351–13356.

30. Gospodarowicz D, Cheng J, Lui G, et al. Isolation of brain fibroblast growth factor by heparin-Sepharose affinity chromatography: Identity with pituitary fibroblast growth factor. *Proc Natl Acad Sci USA* 1984;81:6963–6967.

31. Klagsbrun M, Edelman ER. Biological and biochemical properties of fibroblast growth factors: Implications for the pathogenesis of atherosclerosis. *Atherosclerosis* 1989;9:269–278.

32. Burgess WH, Maciag T. The heparin-binding (fibroblast) growth factor family of proteins. *Annu Rev Biochem* 1989;58:575–606.

33. Rifkin DB, Moscatelli D. Recent developments in the cell biology of basic fibroblast growth factor. *J Cell Biol* 1989;109:1–6.

34. Fannon M, Nugent MA. Basic fibroblast growth factor binds its receptors, is internalized, and stimulates DNA synthesis in Balb/c3T3 cells in the absence of heparan sulfate. *J Biol Chem* 1996;271:17949–17956.

35. Bikfalvi A, Klein S, Pintucci G, et al. Biological roles of fibroblast growth factor-2. *Endocr Rev* 1997;18:26–45.

36. Lyon J, Robinson C, Watson R. The role of Myb proteins in normal and neoplastic cell proliferation. *Crit Rev Oncog* 1994;5:373–388.

37. Sala A, Calabretta B. Regulation of BALB/c 3T3 fibroblast proliferation by B-myb is accompanied by selective activation of cdc2 and cyclin D1 expression. *Proc Natl Acad Sci USA* 1992;89:10415–10419.

38. Campisi J, Gray H, Pardee AB, et al. Cell-cycle control of c-myc but not c-ras expression is lost following chemical transformation. *Cell* 1984;36:241–247.

39. Kelly K, Cochrant C, Stiles C, et al. The regulation of c-myc by growth signals. *Cell* 1983;35:603–610.

40. Marhamati DJ, Bellas RE, Arsura M, et al. A-myb is expressed in bovine vascular smooth muscle cells during the late G1-to-S phase transition and cooperates with c-myc to mediate progression to S phase. *Mol Cell Biol* 1997;17:2448–2457.

41. Kanei-Ishii C, Yasukawa T, Morimoto R, et al. c-Myb-induced trans-activation mediated by heat shock elements without sequence-specific DNA binding of c-Myb. *J Biol Chem* 1994;269:15768–15775.

42. Oelgeschlager M, Nuchprayoon I, Luscher B, et al. C/EBP, c-Myb, and

PU.1 cooperate to regulate the neutrophil elastase promoter. *Mol Cell Biol* 1996;16:4717–4725.

43. Nuchprayoon I, Simkevich CP, Luo M, et al. GABP cooperates with c-myb and C/EBP to activate the neutrophil elastase promoter. *Blood* 1997;89: 4546–4554.

44. Mink S, Kerber U, Klempnauer KH. Interaction of C/EBPβ and v-Myb is required for synergistic activation of the mim-1 gene. *Mol Cell Biol.* 1996; 16:1316–1325.

45. Burk O, Mink S, Ringwald M, et al. Synergistic activation of the chicken mim-1 gene by v-Myb and C/EBP transcription factors. *EMBO J* 1993;12: 2027–2038.

46. Burk O, Worpenberg S, Haenig B, et al. H. tom-1, a novel v-Myb target gene expressed in AMV- and E26-transformed myelomonocytic cells. *EMBO J* 1997;16:1371–1380.

47. Truter S, Di Liberto M, Inagaki Y, et al. Identification of an upstream regulatory region essential for cell type-specific transcription of the pro-alpha 2(V) collagen gene (COL5A2). *J Biol Chem* 1992;267:25389–25395.

48. Brown KE, Lawrence R, Sonenshein GE. Concerted modulation of $\alpha 1(\text{XI})$ and $\alpha 2(\text{V})$ collagen mRNAs in bovine vascular smooth muscle cells. *J Biol Chem* 1991;266:23268–23273.

49. Arias J, Alberts AS, Binde P, et al. Activation of cAMP and mitogen responsive genes relies on a common nuclear factor. *Nature* 1995;370:226–229.

50. Montiminy MR, Sevarino KA, Wagner JA, et al. Identification of a cyclic-AMP-responsive element within the rat somatostatin gene. *Proc Natl Acad Sci USA* 1986;83:6682–6686.

51. Kindy MS, Sonenshein GE. Regulation of oncogene expression in cultured aortic smooth muscle cells: Post-transcriptional control of c-myc mRNA. *J Biol Chem* 1986;261:12865–12868.

52. Greenspan DS, Lee ST, Lee BS, et al. Homology between alpha 2(V) and alpha 1 (III) collagen promoters and evidence for negatively acting elements in the alpha 2(V) first intron and 5 flanking sequences. *Gene Expr* 1991;1:29–39.

53. Ying G-G, Arsura M, Introna M, et al. The DNA binding domain of the A-*myb* transcription factor is responsible for its B cell-specific activity and binds to a B cell 110-kDa nuclear protein. *J Biol Chem* 1997;272:24921–24926.

54. Dignam JD, Lebovitz RM, Roeder RG. Accurate transcription initiation by RNA polymerase II in a soluable extract from isolated mammalian nuclei. *Nuc Acids Res* 1983;11:1475–1489.

Chapter 13

Mechanical Forces in Vascular Growth and Development

B. Lowell Langille, PhD

Introduction

Unlike most tissues, the vasculature must assume mature function very shortly after the first differentiation of the cells that comprise it. Furthermore, this system must continuously remodel throughout development, first as primitive vessels form and reorganize, then as the circulation accommodates changing perfusion requirements of developing peripheral tissues. This capacity of blood vessels to restructure persists throughout life; it is expressed when the adult circulation adapts to many chronic changes in cardiovascular function including those associated with exercise training, reproductive cycles and pregnancy, and it is critical to the development of vascular pathologies including hypertension, atherosclerosis, and restenosis.[1]

It is now clear that this coordination of vascular development with tissue perfusion demands is achieved in large part by a direct sensitivity of vascular tissues to the hemodynamic forces associated with blood pressure and blood flow. Thus, the tensile stresses imposed by blood pressure stimulate growth of vessel wall thickness, whereas the flow-related forces (shear forces) stimulate growth of vessel diameter. This capacity to remodel in response to hemodynamic changes is particularly important during fetal and neonatal life, when arteries assume their mature structure and when large changes in hemodynamic function occur.

Supported by the Medical Research Council of Canada and The Heart and Stroke Foundation of Ontario.

From: Weir EK, Archer SL, Reeves JT (eds). *The Fetal and Neonatal Pulmonary Circulations.* Armonk, NY: Futura Publishing Company, Inc.; ©1999./

Developmental Changes in Hemodynamic Stresses Imposed on Arteries

Blood pressure (P) imparts a circumferential tensile stress (S) on tissue arterial wall tissue that is given by the Law of LaPlace,

$$S = P \times h/R$$

where h = wall thickness and R = vessel radius. In contrast, flow imparts a frictional force, or shear stress (τ), that is proportional to fluid viscosity (μ) and the velocity gradient near the endothelial surface ($\partial v / \partial r$),

$$\tau = \mu \partial v / \partial r$$

Initial assessments of both tensile and shear stresses imposed on large arteries distant from branch sites revealed only modest variations among different anatomic sites and between species. Several investigators have inferred that these observations could be generalized, and that mechanical stresses were controlled around physiological set points by local negative feedback. However, more recent data indicates that arterial wall stresses are more variable than was originally believed, especially when different stages of development were compared. Particularly large variations in hemodynamic loads occur at parturition, with systemic arterial pressures doubling within days to weeks,[2] pulmonary arterial pressures declining by more than 50%,[3] and massive redistribution of blood flows following the closure of central cardiovascular shunts (foramen ovale, ductus arteriosus) and the dramatic changes in tissue perfusion demands that occur as the neonate adjusts to ex utero life.[4] In many tissues (brain, muscle, skin, adrenal glands), blood flow decreases abruptly at birth, presumably because the dramatic rise in arterial PaO_2 that accompanies lung ventilation[4] means that oxygen delivery demands can be met with reduced perfusion. It is important to note that these abrupt changes are not superimposed on stable prenatal or postnatal hemodynamics; both late gestation and the early postnatal period are characterized by rapidly changing tissue perfusions.[4]

Finally, although the remodeling that arteries undergo in direct response to altered hemodynamics is undoubtedly central to vascular adaptations to neonatal life, it is complemented by additional responses to nonhemodynamic stimuli. For example, systemic arterial accumulation of connective tissue (elastin and collagen) accelerates dramatically in the days preceding parturition, apparently as a preadaptation to the elevation in arterial pressure that will subsequently occur postpartum.[2,4] Available evidence indicates that this accumulation is driven by late gestational increases in circulating cortisol levels.[5]

Tensile Arterial Wall Stresses During Development

Many years ago, Wolinsky and Glagov[6] showed that tensile aortic wall stress was remarkably invariant among species whose body weight varied by more than four orders of magnitude. (These authors actually showed that tension per "lamellar unit," ie, one elastic lamella and one adjacent smooth muscle cell [SMC] layer, was relatively constant; however, a similar invariance in tensile wall stress can be inferred because the number of elastic lamellae was proportional to wall thickness.) This finding, coupled with observation that experimental increases in wall tension gave rise to wall thickening, led to the inference that wall stress was regulated to set value; however, these authors subsequently showed that aortic wall stress increased substantially with age, and we have found that thoracic aortic wall stress is 2- to 3-fold higher in adult sheep than in newborn lambs and almost 4-fold higher than in the late gestation fetus.[7] The increase in the tensile stress with age was due to both an increase in arterial pressure and a decrease in relative wall thickness (wall thickness/radius is halved between neonatal and adult life).

Arterial Shear Stresses

Time-averaged shear stresses of 10–15 dynes/cm^2 are frequently cited as characteristic of central arteries, but these values are based on limited data, generally from larger animals. Shears are higher in smaller animals; thus, values for flow rates[8–10] and diameters (unpublished data) for mouse aortas indicate time-averaged shear stress (approximately 100 dynes/cm^2) that are an order of magnitude greater than those of larger species. The reasons for these high shear stresses are associated with the relatively high blood flow requirements imposed by a large surface area:body weight ratio in smaller species.[11] Data on developing arteries are lacking, but in this case, small body size is superimposed on the additional metabolic requirements of tissue growth and development, so higher shears are expected. This is especially true for some vessels that carry high blood flow rate; shear stresses in the umbilical arteries of late gestation sheep fetuses average 30–40 dynes/cm^2 (unpublished data).

Shear Stress–Induced Arterial Remodeling

Flow-induced changes in arterial diameter return wall shear stress toward normal levels. This negative feedback involves acute vasomotor responses and then chronic wall restructuring, and both phases are driven by endothelial cell sensitivity to shear stresses.[12] Acute vasomotor responses are predominantly mediated by nitric oxide (NO) release,[13] a response that probably is amplified over time by increased expression of the endothelial nitric oxide synthase (eNOS) gene.[14]

Structural changes with long-term blood flow alterations involve both tissue growth and reorganization. Experimental decreases in flow rates in developing arteries slow accumulation of endothelial and smooth muscle cells,[6] the two cell types found in the intima/media of healthy arteries. This finding was thought to be due solely to inhibition of cell replication; however, we have shown that both apoptosis and inhibition of cell proliferation can be induced by experimental blood flow reductions in developing arteries.[15]

Arterial elastin accumulation also is influenced by blood flow alterations. Elastin is a very important matrix constituent in large arteries since it bears much of the wall tension generated by blood pressure; therefore, it is a major determinant of resting vessel diameter. We found that both spontaneous and experimental reductions in blood flow rates inhibit elastin accumulation in immature arteries.[5,16] Also, reorganization of elastin, as well as net accumulation, is important in arterial remodeling. Elastin in large arteries is laid down in concentric, fenestrated lamellae. New elastin is deposited randomly onto the surfaces of lamellae,[17] except from some targeting to fenestrae,[18] therefore pre-formed elastin must be reorganized during remodeling, probably through coordinated synthesis and degradation. An endogenous vascular elastase was identified in developing arteries and its expression during normal development suggests a role in normal remodeling. Furthermore, it appears to be important in arterial remodeling associated with pulmonary hypertension.[19]

Recently, we observed an important feature of developmental remodeling of elastic lamellae in large arteries.[20] We manipulated blood flow in postnatal rabbit carotid arteries and then used laser scanning confocal microscopy to optically section through whole mount arterial preparations that were fixed at physiological distension to preserve in situ morphology. We found that fenestrae that perforated elastic lamellae increase both in size and number during postnatal growth, such that the space occupied by the fenestrae increased more than 20-fold between 3 weeks of age and adulthood. This enlargement of fenestrae occurred while the lamellae accumulated large amounts of new elastin, and despite preferential deposition at fenestrae.[18] Thus, production and enlargement of fenestrae contributes substantially to growth of the lamellae. Importantly, experimental manipulations of blood flow dramatically altered growth of fenestrae; they enlarged much more rapidly when flow rates were increased, and they became smaller when flow rates were suppressed. Changes in other matrix constituents have not been widely studied, but total collagen contents are relatively insensitive to decreases in blood flow.[16]

Recent important observations have linked early, NO-mediated, vasomotor responses and chronic remodeling in response to altered blood flow rate. Rudic et al[21] found that mice with a null mutation of the eNOS gene failed to exhibit chronic arterial narrowing of the carotid artery in response to reduced blood flow. This finding is consistent with observations that inhibition of NO production with L-NAME suppresses flow-induced remodeling.[22]

Particularly striking examples of the effects of blood flow-related remodeling on arterial development can be seen in the perinatal period. For example, the abdominal aorta experiences a > 95% reduction in blood flow at parturition at birth,[23] due to loss of the placenta, and the diameter of this vessel becomes greatly reduced within a few days.[24] There is also an interesting and quite subtle aspect to this remodeling of the abdominal aorta that links adaptations to shear and wall tension. Before birth, when arterial pressure is low, the vessel has a very large radius but very thin wall, so tensile wall stress imposed on this vessel is substantially above that imposed on other systemic arteries (see Equation 1). Immediately after birth, the radius is reduced and, because wall mass is conserved, the wall thickens. As a result, wall tension is reduced and becomes comparable with that experienced by other systemic vessels.[24] Thus, the abdominal aorta appears programmed to assume wall tensions typical of other arteries in early postnatal life, when arterial pressure and wall tensions start to rise dramatically.

Remodeling Due to Increased Blood Pressure and Wall Tension

Increased blood pressure and tensile stress induce adaptive wall thickening throughout life. During development, tension-induced wall thickening partially offsets increasing arterial pressure and decreasing h/R, although tensile stress still increases by several fold between fetal and adult life.[7] In adults, hypertension induces arterial wall thickening comprised of cellular hyperplasia and/or hypertrophy[25] and accumulation of matrix.[26,27] Originally, Folkow[28] implicated this remodeling in the progression of hypertension, arguing that any persistent physiological increase in blood pressure would cause wall thickening that encroached on the lumen of small resistance vessels, thereby increasing flow resistance and further elevating pressure, a phenomenon now referred to as the "vascular amplifier." This positive feedback loop might be entered in different ways: developmental abnormalities might produce abnormally thick-walled resistance vessels, or the wall thickness might be enhanced by the growth-promoting actions of some hypertensive agonists (eg, angiotensin II[29-31]). Increased flow resistance still would drive positive feedback, albeit from a different start point. More recent data indicate that the narrowed lumen of hypertensive vessels is not entirely due to increased wall mass[32]; however, the vascular amplifier model remains a focus of hypertension research.

Although increased wall tissue mass is a hallmark of hypertension, it is noteworthy that hypertension also induces apoptotic cell death.[33,34] Cell death in the setting of net cell accumulation probably reflects the subtle reorganization of wall tissues that occurs as remodeling vessels take on a new geometry.

Although perinatal development involves increases in systemic arterial pressure and in wall tension, pulmonary arterial pressures decrease dramatically after birth by more than 50%. Wall tension undoubtedly decreases also, before again starting to rise,[35] but the effects of decreased wall tension on arterial development are not well understood. We recently off-loaded circumferential tension in rabbit carotid arteries by excising the contralateral carotid artery, opening it longitudinally and sewing it as a cuff around the test vessel. The cuff limited distension under pressure of the native vessel and therefore reduced the wall tension that it bears. The cuffing vessel remained viable, but profound alterations to the cuffed artery occurred by 3 weeks that were manifested by medial thinning, cell loss through apoptosis, and matrix degradation (unpublished data). These findings suggest that decreases in wall tension induce active atrophy of arterial tissue.

Integration of Pressure–Induced and Flow–Induced Remodeling

The capacity of arteries to selectively increase arterial diameter in response to a flow stimulus, but to increase wall thickness in response to increased pressure, raises intriguing questions concerning how such selective remodeling is achieved. How do SMCs preferentially deliver newly synthesized tissue in the circumferential versus the radial direction in response to these two stimuli? Our observations on the reshaping of fenestrae in elastic lamellae when blood flow is altered[20] provide insights into radial versus circumferential growth. Thus, formation and enlargement of fenestrae when flow is increased should contribute to increased vessel circumference (and length) but not to wall thickness. In contrast, the increases in lamellar thickness that occur with increased arterial pressure[36] may simply reflect accretion of newly synthesized elastin onto inner and outer lamellar surfaces. The large proportion of wall tension borne by elastin at resting blood pressure may indicate that stress-selective remodeling of elastin imposes such changes in vessel geometry on other wall constituents.

Mechanotransduction by Vascular Cells

Much important, but poorly understood, data has been collected concerning how many cell types respond to mechanical loads.[37,38] Typically, individual cells respond to a single force via multiple mechanosensors that activate multiple signal transduction cascades. While the links between sensor and transduction pathway are frequently known, there is rarely an understanding of how this signaling is integrated to produce cellular responses such as growth and remodeling. In arteries, flow (shear stress) is sensed by endothelium and there is evidence that some responses to circumferential stretch are also endothelium-dependent[39]; however, most evidence points toward mechanotransduction of circumferential stretch by smooth muscle. It appears, however, that some similar mechanotransduction mechanisms are employed by both cell types.

Transduction of shear stress by endothelium

Recent work has focused on shear sensing at focal adhesion plaques.[38,40] Shear stress exerted on the apical surface of endothelial cells is ultimately transmitted to the basal surface of the cell where forces may be concentrated at adhesion plaques. At these sites, the extracellular domains of integrins bind extracellular matrix constituents and their cytoplasmic domains are coupled by a complex of proteins to stress fibers and to signal transduction pathways.[41] Thus, shear induces tyrosine phosphorylation (activation) of focal adhesion kinase (FAK),[40,42] association of FAK with the Grb-2/mSos (Ras activating) signaling pathway[40] and Ras activation.[43] Activation of mitogen-activated protein (MAP) kinase appears to be downstream from these events because dominant negative mutations of both FAK and mSos attenuate shear-induced MAP kinase activation.[40]

G-protein coupled receptors also may sense shear since the intracellular signals that they produce (inositol triphosphate and diacylglyerol, activation of the phospholipase C/PKC pathway) are also produced by shear stress.[44] In addition, the G-protein inhibitor, GDPβS, blocks shear-induced NO and cGMP production.[45] Signaling may converge with FAK-mediated responses at the MAP kinase pathway, since shear-induced activation of the MAP kinase pathway is suppressed by inhibition of G_{i2}.[46] Finally, putative shear sensors in endothelium include mechanosensitive ion channels.[44] Most attention has focused on inwardly rectifying K^+ channels, which appear to be important to some physiological responses to shear stress, eg, shear-induced NO release[47] and transforming growth factor-β1 (TGF-β1) expression.[48]

Transduction of tension by smooth muscle

Less work has been done on force transduction by smooth muscle and much of it has focused on acute myogenic responses rather than remodeling. Vascular SMCs express stretch-activated cation channels[49] and integrin-related signaling is also a strong candidate for mechanotransduction, especially since stretch-induced phosphorylation of FAK and paxillin has been demonstrated in nonvascular smooth muscle.[50] Several intracellular signals that are responsive to stretch of smooth muscle mirror those seen in shear stressed endothelium, including phospholipase $C/IP_3/DAG/$protein kinase $C,$[37] NF-κB,[51] and, more recently, the Erk 1/Erk 2[52] and Jnk/SAPK pathways[53]; however, the downstream events that they regulate are not well defined. One downstream event that is important to stretch-induced remodeling is production of angiotensin II, which may be important to both matrix and cell accumulation in hypertension. In one scenario, angiotensin II drives cell proliferation through platlet-derived growth factor (PDGF) production,[54] and collagen synthesis through release of TGF-β.[55]

Recently, we showed that expression of the primary gap junctional protein found in vascular smooth muscle, connexin 43, was dramatically upregulated by stretching SMCs.[56] Nuclear run-on assays indicated transcriptional control, although CAT reporter constructs failed to reveal a regulatory region within 2 kb of the transcriptional start site. The functional significance of this finding is still under investigation, but we suspect a role in coordination of remodeling, given our recent finding that null mutation of the gene in mice led to aberrant developmental remodeling of the heart.[57]

Conclusion

Developmental growth and remodeling of the arterial system are regulated by a direct sensitivity of vascular tissues to the mechanical loads that are imposed on them. Pressure-related tensile stresses regulate growth of vessel wall thicknesses and flow-related shear stresses control growth of arterial diameter. The growth modulation and remodeling that is driven by this sensitivity to mechanical loads involves cell proliferation and cell death, as well as synthesis, degradation, and remodeling of extracellular matrix. Recent studies have provided important insights into how these remodeling processes are integrated during arterial development, but more work is needed in this area. Similarly, critically important progress has been made in elucidating how vascular cells sense mechanical inputs and transduce these inputs into biochemical signaling cascades; however, very little is known concerning how this signal transduction drives and integrates cellular responses that are important in vascular remodeling. The perinatal development imposes acute and severe challenges on this regulation because of the profound changes in blood pressures and blood flow distribution that occur at birth.

References

1. Langille BL. Blood flow-induced remodeling of the artery wall. In: Bevan JA, Kaley G, Rubanyi G, eds: *Flow-Dependent Regulation of Vascular Function.* New York: Oxford; 1995:277–299.
2. Heymann MA, Iwamoto HS, Rudolph AM. Factors affecting changes in the neonatal systemic circulation. *Ann Rev Physiol* 1981;43:371–383.
3. Davidson D. Pulmonary hemodynamics at birth: Effect of acute cyclooxygenase inhibition in lambs. *J Appl Physiol* 1988;64:1676–1682.
4. Bendeck MP, Langille BL. Changes in blood flow distribution in the perinatal period in fetal sheep and lambs. *Can J Physiol Pharmacol* 1992;70: 1576–1582.
5. Bendeck MP, Keeley FW, Langille BL. Perinatal accumulation of arterial wall constituents: Relation to hemodynamic changes at birth. *Am J Physiol* 1994;267:H2268-H2279.
6. Wolinsky H, Glagov S. A lamellar unit of aortic medial structure and function in mammals. *Circ Res* 1967;XX:99–111.
7. Wells SM, Langille BL, Adamson SL. In vivo and in vitro mechanical properties of the sheep thoracic aorta in the perinatal period and adulthood. *Am J Physiol (Heart Circ Physiol)* 1998;274:H1749-H1760.
8. Sarin SK, Sabba C, Groszmann RJ. Splanchnic and systemic hemodynamics in mice using a radioactive microsphere technique. *Am J Physiol* 1990; 258:G365-G369.
9. Wang P, Ba ZF, Burkhardt J, et al. Trauma-hemorrhage and resuscitation in the mouse: Effects on cardiac output and organ blood flow. *Am J Physiol* 1993;264:H1166-H1173.
10. Barbee RW, Perry BD, Ré RN, et al. Microsphere and dilution techniques for the determination of blood flows and volumes in conscious mice. *Am J Physiol* 1992;263:R728-R733.
11. Langille BL, Gotlieb AI, Kim DW. Vascular tissue response to experimentally altered local blood flow conditions. In: Westerhof N, Gross DR, eds: *Vascular Dynamics.* New York: Plenum; 1989:229–235.
12. Langille BL. Chronic effects of blood flow on the artery wall. In: Frangos JA, ed: *Physical Forces and the Mammalian Cell.* San Diego: Academic Press; 1993:249–274.
13. Kanai AJ, Strauss HC, Truskey GA, et al. Shear stress induces ATP-independent transient nitric oxide release from vascular endothelial cells, measured directly with a porphyrinic microsensor. *Circ Res* 1995;77:284–293.
14. Ranjan V, Xiao Z, Diamond SL. Constitutive NOS expression in cultured endothelial cells is elevated by fluid shear stress. *Am J Physiol* 1995;269:H550-H555.
15. Cho A, Mitchell L, Koopmans D, et al. Effects of changes in blood flow rate on cell death and cell proliferation in carotid arteries of immature rabbits. *Circ Res* 1997;81:328–337.

16. Langille BL, Bendeck MP, Keeley FW. Adaptations of carotid arteries of young and mature rabbits to reduced carotid blood flow. *Am J Physiol* 1989;256:H931-H939.

17. Davis EC. Immunolocalization of microfibril and microfibril-associated proteins in the subendothelial matrix of the developing mouse aorta. *J Cell Sci* 1994;107:727–736.

18. Davis EC. Elastic lamina growth in the developing mouse aorta. *J Histochem Cytochem* 1995;43:1115–1123.

19. Zhu L, Wigle D, Hinek A, et al. The endogenous vascular elastase that governs development and progression of monocrotaline-induced pulmonary hypertension in rats is a novel enzyme related to the serine proteinase adipsin. *J Clin Invest* 1994;94:1163–1171.

20. Wong LCY, Langille BL. Developmental remodeling of the internal elastic lamina of rabbit arteries: Effect of blood flow. *Circ Res* 1996;78:799–805.

21. Rudic RD, Shesely EG, Maeda N, et al. Direct evidence for the importance of endothelium-derived nitric oxide in vascular remodeling. *J Clin Invest* 1998;101:731–736.

22. Tronc F, Wassef M, Esposito B, et al. Role of NO in flow-induced remodeling of the rabbit common carotid artery. *Arterioscler Thromb Vasc Biol* 1996;16:1256–1262.

23. Bendeck MP, Keeley FW, Langille BL. Arterial elastin, collagen and DNA accumulation: Relation to hemodynamic changes at birth. *Am J Physiol* 1994;267:H2268-H2279.

24. Langille BL, Brownlee RD, Adamson SL. Perinatal aortic growth in lambs: Relation to blood flow changes at birth. *Am J Physiol* 1990;259:H1247-H1253.

25. Owens GK. Control of hypertrophic versus hyperplastic growth of vascular smooth muscle cells. *Am J Physiol* 1989;257:H1755-H1765.

26. Keeley FW, Johnson DJ. The effect of developing hypertension on the synthesis and accumulation of elastin in the aorta of the rat. *Biochem Cell Biol* 1986;64:38–43.

27. Keeley FW, Alatawi A. Response of aortic elastin synthesis and accumulation to developing hypertension and the inhibitory effect of colchicine on this response. *Lab Invest* 1991;64:499–507.

28. Folkow B. Physiological aspects of primary hypertension. *Physiol Rev* 1982;62(2):347–497.

29. Stouffer GA, Owens GK. Angiotensin II-induced mitogenesis of spontaneously hypertensive rat-derived cultured smooth muscle cells is dependent on autocrine production of transforming growth factor-β. *Circ Res* 1992;70:820–828.

30. Gibbons GH, Pratt RE, Dzau VJ. Vascular smooth muscle cell hypertrophy vs. hyperplasia: Autocrine transforming growth factor-$\beta 1$ expression determines growth response to angiotensin II. *J Clin Invest* 1992;90:456–461.

31. Kato H, Suzuki H, Tajima S, et al. Angiotensin II stimulates collagen synthesis in cultured vascular smooth muscle cells. *J Hypertens* 1991;9:17–22.

32. Heagerty AM, Aalkjaer C, Bund SJ, et al. Small artery structure in hypertension: Dual processes of remodeling and growth. *Hypertension* 1993;21:391–397.

33. Hamet P, DeBlois D, Dam T-V, et al. Apoptosis and vascular wall remodeling in hypertension. *Can J Physiol Pharmacol* 1996;74:850–861.

34. Sharifi AM, Schiffrin EL. Apoptosis in aorta of deoxycorticosterone ac-

etate-salt hypertensive rats: Effect of endothelin receptor antagonism. *J Hypertens* 1997;15:1441–1448.

35. Leung DYM, Glagov S, Mathews MB. Elastin and collagen accumulation in rabbit ascending aorta and pulmonary trunk during postnatal growth: Correlation of cellular synthetic response with medial tension. *Circ Res* 1977;41:316–323.

36. Berry CL, Greenwald SE. Effects of hypertension on the static mechanical properties and chemical composition of the rat aorta. *Cardiovas Res* 1976; 10:437–451.

37. Osol G. Mechanotransduction by vascular smooth muscle. *J Vasc Res* 1995;32:275–292.

38. Shyy JY-J, Chien S. Role of integrins in cellular responses to mechanical stress and adhesion. *Curr Opin Cell Biol* 1997;9:707–713.

39. Katusic ZS, Shepherd JT, Vanhoutte PM. Endothelium-dependent contraction to stretch in canine basilar arteries. *Am J Physiol* 1987;252:H671.

40. Li S, Kim M, Hu Y-L, et al. Fluid shear stress activation of focal adhesion kinase: Linking to mitogen-activated protein kinases. *J Biol Chem* 1997; 272:30455–30462.

41. Clark EA, Brugge JS. Integrins and signal transduction pathways: The road taken. *Science* 1995;268:233–239.

42. Ishida T, Peterson TE, Kovach NL, et al. MAP kinase activation by flow in endothelial cells: Role of β_1 integrins and tyrosine kinases. *Circ Res* 1996; 79:310–316.

43. Li YS, Shyy JYJ, Li S, et al. The Ras-JNK pathway is involved in shear-induced gene expression. *Mol Cell Biol* 1996;16:5947–5954.

44. Davies PF. Flow-mediated endothelial mechanotransduction. *Physiol Rev* 1995;75:519–560.

45. Kuchan MJ, Jo H, Frangos JA. Role of G proteins in shear stress-mediated nitric oxide production by endothelial cells. *Am J Physiol (Cell Physiol)* 1994;267:C753-C758.

46. Jo H, Sipos K, Go Y-M, et al. Differential effect of shear stress on extracellular signal-regulated kinase and N-terminal Jun kinase in endothelial cells G_{i2}- and G[beta]/[gamma]-dependent signaling pathways. *J Biol Chem* 1997;272(2):1395–1401.

47. Cooke JP, Rossitch E Jr, Andon NA, et al. Flow activates an endothelial potassium channel to release an endogenous nitrovasodilator. *J Clin Invest* 1991;88:1663–1671.

48. Ohno M, Cooke JP, Dzau VJ, et al. Fluid shear stress induces endothelial transforming growth factor beta-1 transcription and production: Modulation by potassium channel blockade. *J Clin Invest* 1995;95:1363–1369.

49. Ohya Y, Adachi N, Nakamura Y, et al. Stretch-activated channels in arterial smooth muscle of genetic hypertensive rats. *Hypertension* 1998;31:254–258.

50. Smith PG, Garcia R, Kogerman L. Mechanical strain increases protein tyrosine phosphorylation in airway smooth muscle cells. *Exp Cell Res* 1998; 239:353–360.

51. Hishikawa K, Oemar BS, Yang Z, et al. Pulsatile stretch stimulates superoxide production and activates nuclear factor-κB in human coronary smooth muscle. *Circ Res* 1997;81:797–803.

52. Franklin MT, Wang CLA, Adam LP. Stretch-dependent activation and desensitization of mitogen-activated protein kinase in carotid arteries. *Am J Physiol (Cell Physiol)* 1997;273:C1819-C1827.

53. Hamada K, Takuwa N, Yokoyama K, et al. Stretch activates Jun N-termi-

nal kinase/stress-activated protein kinase in vascular smooth muscle cells through mechanisms involving autocrine ATP stimulation of purinoceptors. *J Biol Chem* 1998;273:6334–6340.

54. Li Q, Muragaki Y, Ueno H, et al. Stretch-induced proliferation of cultured vascular smooth muscle cells and a possible involvement of local renin-angiotensin system and platelet-derived growth factor (PDGF). *Hypertens Res* 1998;20:217–223.

55. Li Q, Muragaki Y, Hatamura I, et al. Stretch-induced collagen synthesis in cultured smooth muscle cells from rabbit aortic media and a possible involvement of angiotensin II and transforming growth factor-β. *J Vasc Res* 1998;35:93–103.

56. Cowan DB, Lye SJ, Langille BL. Regulation of vascular connexin43 gene expression by mechanical loads. *Circ Res* 1998;82:786–793.

57. Reaume A, de Sousa PA, Kulkarni S, et al. Cardiac malformation in neonatal mice lacking connexin 43. *Science* 1995;267:1831–1834.

Section III

Mechanisms of Hemodynamic Control in the Neonate

Chapter 14

Lung Arteriolar Endothelial Cell Proliferation at Birth:
Possible Roles of Stretch and Hypoxia

John T. Reeves, MD

Introduction

When the lung arteries fail to dilate at birth, health or even life itself is threatened. In the instant of birth, mammals are ejected from the womb's protective environment into an independent existence in a harsh and dangerous world. The environment is transformed from aquatic to atmospheric, from iso- to poikilothermic, from an absence to the presence of gravity, while simultaneously the lifeline for gas exchange is severed. Physiologically, the newborn is suddenly on its own, where the first priorities are to acquire oxygen and eliminate carbon dioxide, immediately, and for the rest of its life. Air must be brought to the alveoli where the respiratory gases can be exchanged in the flowing blood. If the process fails or is flawed, death or disability results.

For its part, the lung circulation must quickly initiate and then maintain the transition from a high to a low resistance circuit. Much research has examined the preparation of the lung circulation for birth and the chemically mediated vasodilation that accompanies it.[1–11] The focus of this chapter is on how, with the onset of ventilation, mechanical forces might affect *endothelial cells* and thereby contribute to the lowering of vascular resistance following birth. Other than the reports from Haworth's laboratory,[12,13] the mechanical forces acting on endothelial cells at birth have received little attention.

At birth, lung inflation suddenly lengthens and dilates the pul-

This work was supported in part by National Institutes of Health Grants HL-14985 and HL-SCOR 56481.

From: Weir EK, Archer SL, Reeves JT (eds). *The Fetal and Neonatal Pulmonary Circulations.* Armonk, NY: Futura Publishing Company, Inc.; ©1999.

monary arterioles, which mechanically stretches the endothelial cells,[13] possibly impeding their function of covering completely the basement membrane of the arteriolar wall. Smooth muscle cells would also be stretched.[12] Here, we speculate that endothelial cells will replicate, primarily to diminish the stress, and in addition, to participate in subsequent postnatal vascular growth. When transition to a low resistance circuit is prevented, both stretch[14] and vascular growth[10] are affected, and endothelial cell replication rates may be altered. The following discussion will review (with emphasis on the mechanics of vasodilation) some of the salient features of the history of our understanding of the transition of the pulmonary circulation at birth, and focus on the mitotic activity of endothelial cells in the pulmonary arterial walls: (1) in calves, in the days following normoxic birth when the normal transition occurs; and (2) in other calves, when the normal transition is prevented by postnatal hypoxia. The concepts emerging from these animal experiments are that the very high replication rates of endothelial cells in lung arterioles shortly after birth accompany mechanical stresses on the endothelium, and that the replication rates are substantially altered when hypoxia interferes with the normal transition. The possibility is considered that even temporary abnormalities in the transition may have lasting residual impact.

Historical Background

. . . in the embryo . . . the two ventricles . . . are nearly equal in all respects. . . . It is only when the lungs are used . . . that the difference . . . of strength . . . between the two ventricles begins to be apparent.[15]

William Harvey

Anatomy and Early Physiology

In medicine, the understanding of what goes wrong begins with an analysis of how things go right. So briefly, how did we come to our current understanding of the normal circulatory transition from the fetal to the air breathing lung? In 1628, William Harvey[15] left a clue, as noted above, that the lung circulation of the fetus was very different from that following the onset of breathing. According to Ardran et al,[16] the matter rested there until, in 1871, Schultz reported that the systemic arterial pressure fell at birth, while Cohnstein and Zuntz reported the opposite in 1884 and 1888. In 1937, Hamilton et al[17] inserted needles directly through the chest walls of dog and rabbit fetuses and found similar pressures in the two ventricles, but that, with the onset of breathing in the rabbit, *"inspiration lowered the right ventricular pressure more than the left."* They correctly attributed this to a reduced pulmonary vascular resistance. Unfortunately, the rabbit's fetal ventricular systolic pressures were only approximately 20 mm Hg; the right ventricular systolic pressures after birth were not clearly different from the fetal values, and thus the authors' contemporaries[18,19] were not convinced by the findings.

About the same time, Barclay et al[19] obtained excellent radiographs at rates of up to 200 frames per minute showing patterns of blood flow through the heart and great vessels of exteriorized sheep fetuses. In a report of little more than two pages, which reviewed prior angiograms in 13 fetuses of varying gestational age, they did not comment on respiration, but they concluded *"that closure of the ductus was followed by a reduction in the average pulmonary circulation time. . . ."* They spoke of *" . . . halving of the pulmonary circulation time through closure of the ductus . . ."* as though ductal closure caused the increased lung blood flow. Ten years later, Ardran et al reviewed the films and found that Barclay's lambs had been breathing spontaneously when the ductus was closed; they concluded that the observed increased pulmonary blood flow was not necessarily due to ductal closure.[16]

> *"But inspection of their original data, which are still available, shows that this reduction in pulmonary circulation time could equally well be ascribed to the onset of breathing, and that the change is of a progressive character as aeration of the lungs proceeds."[16]*

Even though Barclay et al may not have correctly interpreted their own experiments,[19] in retrospect, their data were the first to indicate that lung blood flow increases following birth.

In the late 1940s, Jesse Edwards, the noted pathologist at the Mayo Clinic in Rochester, Minnesota, began studying the pulmonary vascular changes at birth, as a result of the burgeoning interest in congenital heart disease.[20] The newly developed technique of cardiac catheterization was being introduced in children with congenital heart disease, surgeons were developing new corrective operations, and pathologists were finding remarkably thickened lung arterioles in the children who died.[20] Edwards and colleagues soon realized that: *"Study of the structure of the pulmonary vascular tree in certain congenital cardiac malformations and in other conditions makes it imperative that anatomic base lines be established."[21]* His laboratory conducted in humans the first examination of age-related changes in normal pulmonary arteries from fetus to adult. Civin and Edwards,[21] drawing on their own observations and those of Hamilton et al,[17] suggested that: *" . . . shortly after birth, when the lungs are expanding, [muscular arteries] become dilated [and] this may be the anatomic expression of progressive relative fall in . . . resistance to pulmonary blood flow after birth."* Although these were remarkably accurate conclusions for the time, these anatomic studies could not show the rate, magnitude, or mechanisms of the changes in the lung circulation at birth.

Dawes' Emphasis on Mechanical Dilation of the Lung Circulation at Birth

The whole picture suddenly changed with the remarkable experiments conducted in 1951, and published in 1952, from Dawes's laboratory.[16] The authors utilized the exteriorized sheep fetus which had been developed by Barclay, but they made direct measurements of vascular pressures (Figure 1). With the onset of ventilation, pressures fell immediately in both pulmonary and systemic circulations. Then, within moments and following occlusion of the umbilical cord, pressure rose in the aorta, but continued to fall in the pulmonary artery. Because the work was done in Oxford's Nuffield Institute, where Barclay had pioneered cardiopulmonary cineradiography in fetal lambs, radio opaque contrast injections could be used to estimate the effect of breathing on changes in

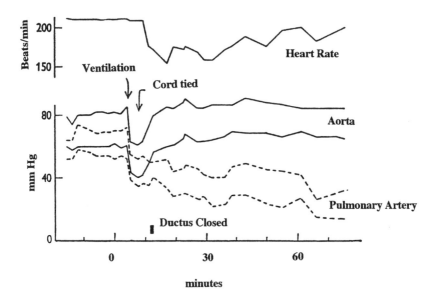

Figure 1. First demonstration of the decrease over time in pulmonary arterial pressure with onset of ventilation of the fetal lung. Shown from above and downward are heart rate, systolic and diastolic pressures in the aorta, and (as broken lines) systolic and diastolic pressures in the pulmonary artery. Onset of artificial ventilation and the tying of the umbilical cord are indicted by arrows. Angiographic demonstration of closure of the ductus is indicated by the vertical bar. (Modified from Reference 16.)

lung blood flow and on the patency of the ductus arteriosus. The radiographs indicated a clear and immediate shortening of pulmonary circulation time of the contrast material, which implied that the lung blood flow increased markedly with onset of breathing, not with ductal closure. Further, as had been noted before,[19] ductal behavior was variable with regard to both when, and how completely, closure occurred.

> *It is important to note that the fall in pulmonary arterial pressure, which is communicated to the systemic arterial system because the ductus arteriosus is still open, occurs immediately on beginning artificial ventilation and before the closure of the ductus arteriosus. Our impression from these observations is that the changes in pulmonary arterial pressure and circulation time are primarily due to aeration of the lungs. Whether these changes are in any way responsible for the closure of the ductus arteriosus remains to be seen.[16]*

Not only did the pulmonary vascular resistance fall with the onset of breathing, but the fall was sudden and large. Dawes and his group[11] and subsequent investigators[3–8,22–25] using more sophisticated preparations would confirm the basic findings, but the foundations to our understanding were laid by the observations made in 1951.

What was going on? Air contains both oxygen and nitrogen, and the 'aeration' mentioned by Ardran et al[16] was not necessarily identical to oxygenation, as Dawes et al soon observed. Because *"a single sudden inflation even with nitrogen has on occasion caused a four fold increase in [pulmonary blood] flow"[24]* (Figure 2), Dawes felt that simply inflating the lungs reduced the resistance to blood flow, and the composition of the gas did not matter significantly. The morphologist, Reynolds, who worked with Dawes in 1951, promptly used guinea pigs to search for an anatomic mechanism that explained the fall in vascular resistance with the first inflation of fetal lungs. He concluded[26] that *"in the fetus, resistance to blood flow in the lung is high owing to the presence of coiled and erythrocyte-packed arterial capillaries . . . On aeration of the lungs, the extension of the arterial capillaries in the lung lowers the resistance to blood flow . . . "* Although his suggestion that coiled fetal precapillary lung arteries straighten with lung inflation has not been confirmed, his work was an early attempt to understand mechanical factors that might dilate lung vessels at birth. A few years later, Riley,[27] Permutt, and coworkers (see review in Reference 28) proposed that inflation of alveoli places radial traction on the small lung arteries, thereby increasing their diameters. Though this mechanism could nicely account for much of the sudden and large vasodilation with the first breath, to the knowledge of this author, the hypothesis has not been directly tested for the fetal-newborn transition.

Dawes's mechanical view of the sudden fall in lung vascular resistance at birth was vigorously challenged by Leonard Strang at a London meeting of perinatologists (Cassin S, personal communication). Strang,

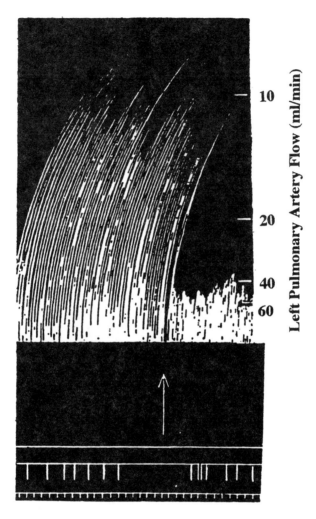

Figure 2. Increase in pulmonary blood flow in a fetal lung with inflation by a single breath of nitrogen (at the arrow). Note that smaller deflections indicate larger flows. (Modified from Reference 49.)

while visiting Harvard, had worked in Cook's laboratory studying the role of CO_2 in the control of the lung circulation in the fetal and newborn lamb.[1] Apart from the vasodilating effect of oxygen on the lung circulation at birth, the work at Harvard had led him to think that an important effect of ventilation, either with air or with N_2, was to lower CO_2, which then relieved vasoconstriction in the fetal lung and thereby reduced resistance to lung blood flow. To resolve the controversy, Dawes and Strang collaborated[11,22] in further research, which showed that each one

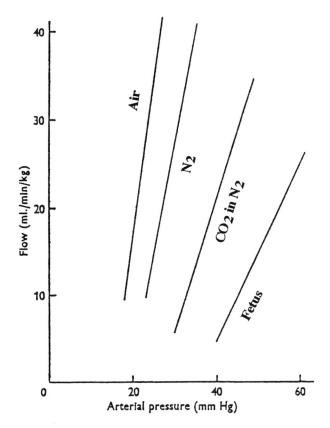

Figure 3. Pulmonary flow pressure curves in near-term fetal lambs when the lungs were ventilated with different gas mixtures. Some vasodilation (a shift of the line to the left) occurred with a mixture of carbon dioxide in nitrogen (CO_2 in N_2, to keep the fetal P_{CO_2} and pH unchanged during ventilation). Progressively greater vasodilation occurred with N_2 alone and with air. (Modified from Reference 22.)

was partly right. Dawes was partly in the right in that ventilation with N_2 lowered resistance, even when fetal P_{CO_2} was maintained (Figure 3). Strang was partly right in that acutely lowering P_{CO_2} per se, had an important effect in reducing lung vascular resistance at birth (Figure 3). Not under contention, but confirmed by these experiments, was that there was an additional vasodilating role of O_2 in the acute changes at birth (Figure 3). Dawes and Strang et al not only provided an excellent example of collaboration in a relaxed atmosphere to resolve opposing views, but their work also indicated that the changes that occur at birth were more complicated than expected, and that simplistic explanations would no longer suffice. Key mechanisms ensuring survival of the species are often defended by multiple, complimentary, and interacting strategies.

The Endothelium at Birth: Both Chemical and Mechanical Influences

In recent years, the endothelial cell has received increased focus as a mediator of some of the pulmonary vascular changes following birth. Endothelial production of prostacyclin (PGI_2) may play a smaller role than originally thought,[2] but increasing evidence supports an important role for the endothelial production of nitric oxide (NO). For example in the fetal lamb, inhibiting the formation of NO blocks approximately half of the fall in resistance following the onset of ventilation[8] (Figure 4). Endothelin, initially considered a pulmonary vasoconstrictor, could, following birth, play an important vasodilating role in the mediation of the NO response.[6,9] Inspection of Figure 4 suggests that the other half of the large ventilation-related fall in pulmonary vascular resistance was not accounted for by the NO mechanism. Mechanical forces are probably at work, although they may not involve the uncoiling of arterioles as postulated by Dawes[24] and Reynolds.[26] With lung inflation, the mechanically induced longitudinal and (as noted above) radial traction on the arterioles causes the endothelial cells to flatten, thereby helping to open the lumena[13] (Figure 5). Mechanical forces can powerfully stimulate mi-

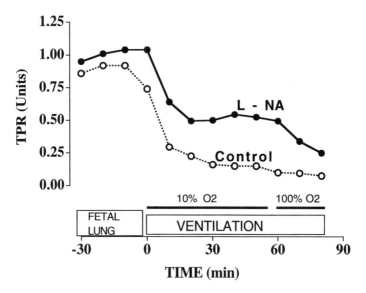

Figure 4. Total pulmonary resistance (TPR) in near-term fetal lambs when the lung is ventilated with hypoxic or hyperoxic mixtures, either with or without inhibition by nitro-L-arginine (L-NA) of nitric oxide synthase. (Redrawn from Reference 8.)

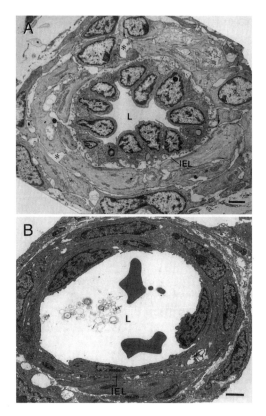

Figure 5. Electron micrographs of transverse sections through small muscular arteries from **A**: a stillborn pig, and **B**: a newborn pig within 5 minutes after birth. The bar indicates 2 μm. IFL = internal elastic lamina; L = lumen.(Reproduced with permission from Reference 50.)

tosis especially in endothelial cells, but also in smooth muscle cells,[29] with consequences that have implications for vascular function, remodeling, and growth. The replication of arterial cells, particularly in the endothelium, during the transition is the focus of this chapter.

Postnatal Arterial Endothelial Replication in Normoxia

Hypotheses

We reasoned that if the endothelial cells are stretched at birth as proposed from Haworth's laboratory,[12,13] and if stretch stimulates endothelial replication,[29,30] then there should be high endothelial replication following birth. A parallel line of reasoning is that if flow increases in the small lung arteries after birth, and if increasing shear increases endothelial replication,[29,31] then increased arteriolar flow also would be a stimulus for endothelial replication after birth. High endothelial replication rates after birth could: (a) maintain the integrity of the lining layer by providing more cells to cover the basement membrane of the arterial lumen; (b) allow each cell to be more firmly anchored to the basement membrane by having a larger number of cells; and (c) promote long-term maintenance of low tone and vascular resistance via a larger population of lung endothelial cells available to supply endothelial-dependent relaxing factor.

The main pulmonary artery (MPA), in contrast to the arterioles, would not be stretched by lung inflation and would not have increased flow, or dilate at birth. Further, shear forces are less in the larger than the smaller arteries, and endothelial flattening was not observed in the MPA after birth.[13] We expected less endothelial replication after birth in the large pulmonary arteries than in the small, and thus endothelial cell replication in an arterial segment would likely vary according to the hemodynamic stresses within that segment.

Approach

We approached the question of pulmonary arterial endothelial cell replication rates after birth in vivo using newborn calves which, like human babies, show rapid decreases in pulmonary arterial pressures

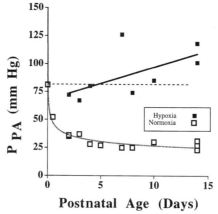

Postnatal Age (Days)

Figure 6. Mean pulmonary arterial pressure (P PA) versus postnatal age in normoxic calves, and those placed shortly after birth in a hypoxic chamber to give a fetal-like arterial PO_2 of 20–30 mm Hg. (Data are compiled from References 32–36.) The broken line indicates values measured in near-term fetal calves.[37]

(Figure 6) and resistances after birth.[32–34] In calves of postnatal age of approximately 2–14 days, we labeled, over 24 hours, the endothelial cells in the S phase of replication, using the thymidine analog, bromodeoxyuridine (BrdU).[35,36] After sacrificing the calves, we then examined endothelial replication rates with postnatal age in large and small pulmonary arteries by comparing the percentage of labeled to total nuclei. We thus measured how endothelial cell replication varied with postnatal age and with arterial segment.

Endothelial Replication in Large and Small Pulmonary Arteries in Normoxia

We were surprised by the high rate of endothelial replication in the smaller arteries in the youngest calves (aged 1–2 days), where more than 25% of lung arterioles were labeled with BrdU[36] (Figure 7A). Replication rates rapidly fell with increasing postnatal age, and by day 14, only approximately 1% of the endothelial cells appeared to be replicating. Perhaps this should not have been a surprise, because on reviewing the data (from piglets) of Hall[13] and Haworth[14] (Figure 7B), one sees the very rapid change during the first day of postnatal life in endothelial cell shape (as measured by a ratio of volume to surface area) in arterioles of approximately the same size as those we measured. If endothelial cell

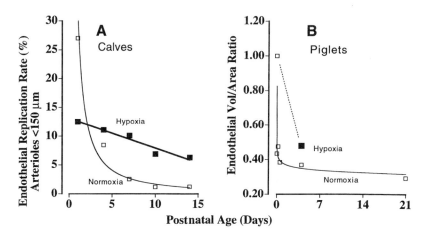

Figure 7. A: Endothelial replication rates, as measured with bromodeoxyuridine (BrdU), in calves of different postnatal ages reared in normoxic or hypoxic environments.[36] B: Shape change in arteriolar endothelial cells in piglets of different postnatal ages reared in normoxic or hypoxic environments.[13,14] Note that shape change shown here as the ratio of cell volume to surface area is the inverse of that which was originally reported.[13,14]

volume is little changed, but surface area is increasing rapidly, then one may assume that the cells are being stretched, which would then stimulate replication. Although the increase in endothelial cell surface area occurred quickly after birth, the rate of change was short lived, such that after the first postnatal day, there was little further increase in surface area (Figure 7B). Of interest in the calves, the high rate of endothelial cell replication was also short lived, such that after day 4, replication rates remained low (Figure 7A). If mechanical stresses on endothelium in calves resembled those in piglets, then the possibility exists that in the calves, following a fall in mechanical stress on the endothelial cell, replication rates fell. Also, the possibility exists that following a stabilization of mechanical stress, there would be stabilization at a low level of endothelial cell replication. An association between mechanical stress on endothelial cells and replication rate does not indicate cause and effect, particularly when the association is in different experiments and different species. However, the possibility deserves further examination.

With the available data, what can be said about how much circumferential stretch occurred in the different vascular segments in the transition from the fetus to postnatal day 1 or 2? How does this compare with the endothelial replication rates in the segments? Complicating the issue is that we did not have replication rates in the fetus, and further, we depended on previously reported measurements of fetal arterial pressure.[37] However, taking the fetal systemic and pulmonary arterial pressure in the term calf as 81 mm Hg,[37] given the circulatory changes known to occur at birth, and using the measurements made shortly after birth in these calves, then one can make assumptions about the hemodynamic and blood gas changes that likely occurred from fetal life to early neonatal life (Table 1).

For the pulmonary arterioles on postnatal day 1 or 2, compared to the fetus, pulmonary arterial pressure was markedly lower, but flow could have increased, even by an order of magnitude. Because pressure was much less than in the fetus and flow was much higher, the luminal diameters of the lung arterioles must have increased substantially during the first 2 days of postnatal life (Table 1), and the increased diameters would be expected to stretch the endothelium lining the arteriolar wall and to promote endothelial replication.

In the MPA, the situation would be expected to be much different. Because the MPA flow was likely high in fetal life (two-thirds of combined output from both ventricles), flow might not be much increased in the first day or two after birth. This, combined with the fall in pulmonary arterial pressure, would suggest little or no increase in arterial diameter of the MPA on days 1 and 2 compared to the fetus (Table 1). The percentages of replicating endothelial cells were much lower than in the arterioles and did not change with postnatal age[36] (Figure 8).

Table 1

Hemodynamic and Blood Gas Factors Possibly Affecting Endothelial Cell Replication in Arteries Soon After Birth

Estimated Changes From Fetus to Newborn

Locus	Aterial Pressure	Flow	Arterial Diameter	PO$_2$	Endothelial Replication on Days 1–2
Pulmonary/					
Arteriole	Decreased	+++	+++	+++	27.0%
MPA	Decreased	+	±	±	3.6%
Aorta	Increased	+	++	+++	12.3%

MPA = main pulmonary artery.

For the aorta, the pressures measured on days 1–2 (113 mm Hg) were approximately 30 mm Hg higher than reported fetal values, and the diameter in the aorta (and stretch of the endothelial cells) would be expected to increase following birth (Table 1). Endothelial replication rates were rather high in the aorta on days 1–2, and they fell with increasing postnatal age (Table 1). One could postulate that those arterial segments (lung arterioles and aorta) which probably increased in diameter at birth (causing endothelial stretch) would show more endothelial

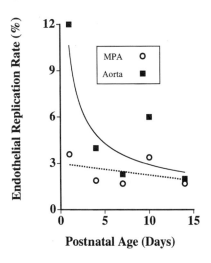

Figure 8. Endothelial replication rates from the main pulmonary artery (MPA) and aorta in normoxic calves of different postnatal ages.

replication on the first postnatal days than segments (MPA) which did not increase in diameter.

While our analysis has focused on endothelial stretch from an increased arterial diameter as a likely cause of the high replication rates

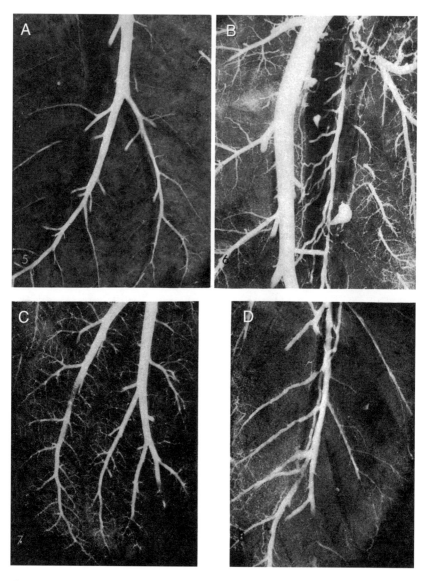

Figure 9. Radiographs of 1-cm thick lung slices from young calves having postmortem pulmonary arterial injections of a fine suspension of barium sulphate.[33] A: Normoxic calf, aged 6 hours. B: Normoxic calf, aged 1 week. C: Normoxic calf, aged 4 months. D: Hypoxic calf, aged 4 months.

in the arteriole and aorta, there are many other contributing factors, including increased flow and oxygenation following birth (Table 1).

Replication in Lung Arterial Media and Adventitia Following Normoxic Birth

While the pulmonary arterial circulation is rapidly dilating after birth, it is also rapidly growing, as is the bronchial circulation (Figure 9, A and B), and such growth should contribute to replication within the endothelium and the other layers of the arteriolar walls. Thus, it is of considerable interest to compare for the lung arterioles, the magnitude and the time course of the changes in endothelial replication with those in the media and adventitia of these same calves.[35] The media and adventitia (Figure 10) have higher replication rates on days 1 and 4 than on day 14, so in both of these layers, as with endothelium, replication rates fell with increasing age.[35,36] However, on day 1, endothelial replication was greater than in the other two layers. This finding is compatible with greater stimulation of replication in the endothelial layer. Whether, on day 1, a greater replication-related stimulation for endothelium than for

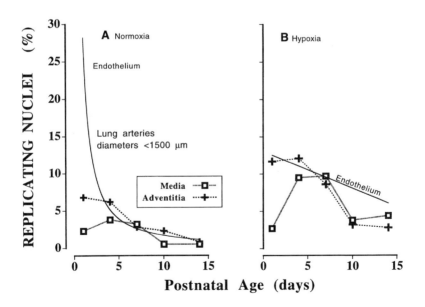

Figure 10. Endothelial replication rates (percent replicating nuclei) for endothelium (unbroken line), media (squares), and adventitia (crosses) for calves of different postnatal ages reared in either normoxic (**A**), or hypoxic (**B**) environments.[35,36]

media or adventitia is due to mechanical stretch, angiogenesis, and/or other factors, requires future research.

Postnatal Arterial Endothelial Replication in Hypoxia

Hypotheses

In the calf, neonatal hypoxia prevents the transition of the lung circulation to a low resistance circuit (Figure 6), but systemic arterial pressure rises above the fetal levels, much as in normoxia. Arteriolar vasodilation and normal angiogenesis of the lung arterioles could be retarded[33] (Figure 9, C and D), which might inhibit endothelial replication. However, with the onset of breathing, longitudinal stretch of arterioles should occur, and with prolonged hypoxic pulmonary hypertension, the arteriolar walls become markedly thickened,[34] both of which might stimulate endothelial replication. We therefore expected that neonatal hypoxia would alter the time course, magnitude, and mechanisms of endothelial replication, but we could not predict what these alterations would be.

Approach

Our approach[35,36] was identical to that in the normoxic calves, except that we interrupted the normal neonatal transition of the pulmonary circulation by placing the newborn calves at age 12–24 hours in an hypobaric chamber at a simulated altitude of 4,570 m ($P_B = 430$ mm Hg), and maintaining them there, where they had arterial PO_2 values of 20 to 32 mm Hg, ie, PO_2 values similar to those in the term fetus.[37]

Endothelial Replication in Small Pulmonary Arteries in Hypoxia

When there was severe neonatal hypoxia, pulmonary arterial pressures[34,36] did not show the normal postnatal decrease, and instead, were little different from those in fetal life[37] (Figure 6). Normal pulmonary arteriolar vasodilation did not occur and, in the early postnatal period, mechanical forces on endothelial cells were probably altered by the hypoxia. Indeed, endothelial replication rates, for arterioles less than 150 μm, were different in hypoxic versus normoxic calves[36] (Figure 7A). At age 1–2 days, replication rates in hypoxia (12.5%) were approximately half of those in normoxia (27%). One could postulate that while on the one hand, there had been longitudinal stretch as normally occurs with lung inflation, that on the other hand, hypoxia would have maintained high arteriolar tone, and this high tone would oppose the mechanical vasodilation mediated by inflation of alveoli. Thus, normal circumferential stretch might not occur. Consistent with this concept is the report of Allen and Haworth[14] that in newborn piglets made hypoxic for the first 4 days of life, flattening of the arteriolar endothelial cells was much less than normal (Figure 7B). Thus, less than normal postnatal endothelial stretch probably contributed to reducing endothelial cell replication rates in the first day or two of life in hypoxia. Future research will need to consider the interaction of stretch, shear, hypoxia per se, and other factors on the altered endothelial replication rates when hypoxia is imposed from birth.

In hypoxic calves older than 1–2 days, the endothelial replication rates were actually higher than in the normoxic calves (Figure 7A). The mechanisms are not clear for the persistence of high arteriolar endothelial replication rates during the first 2 postnatal weeks in hypoxic calves. Mechanical stretch of the arteriolar wall seems unlikely, because the effects of lung inflation should have been completed and the arterioles have remained constricted. Thus, by 1–2 weeks postnatally, neither longitudinal nor circumferential stretch would likely be stimulating mitosis of endothelial cells, and one looks for other factors, eg, the metabolic activity of other cells in the arteriolar wall.

Replication in Lung Arteriolar Adventitia and Media Following Birth in Hypoxia

In the adventitia of the small arterioles and with hypoxia, replication rates were 2- to 3-fold higher than in normoxia, for each of the time points observed[35] (Figures 10A vs. 10B). These higher rates in hypoxia (approximately 12% of nuclei were labeled with BrdU) were apparent at the first measurement on days 1–2, and they were sustained through day 4; during this interval they were similar to rates in the endothelium in hypoxia. The comparison of replication in the adventitia with that in the endothelium in these early postnatal days was of interest, because hypoxic exposure appeared to reduce replication rates in the endothelium, but to increase rates in the adventitia.

In the media, hypoxic exposure elicited a complex response (Figures 10A and 10B). Compared to normoxia, hypoxic exposure had no effect on replication on days 1–2. However, hypoxic exposure of 4–7 days was associated with rates that were nearly 3-fold higher (Figure 10B), after which the rates were decreased, but not to normoxic levels. One notes in Figure 10B that a high replication rate in the adventitia *preceded* that in the media. The findings are reminiscent of those with hypoxia in the adult rat, where the earliest and largest increases in thymidine incorporation occurred in the adventitia of the lung arteries.[38] These findings both in the newborn calf and in the adult rat raise the possibility that the early mitotic activity in the adventitia, possibly mediated by the sensing of hypoxia per se, affected replication in the media and even in the endothelium. Adventitial fibroblasts are known to possess autocrine and paracrine mitotic activity and to promote the production of matrix in both the adventitia and medial cells.[39-41]

Because each of the layers of the arteriolar wall has a unique function, it is not surprising that each has a unique proliferative behavior. The different proliferative behaviors are perhaps best illustrated by the responses to hypoxic exposure during the first day or two of postnatal life. Thus with hypoxic exposure, replication appeared to be enhanced in the adventitia, depressed in the endothelium, and unchanged in the media. Clarification of these different in vivo behaviors requires further research, but is critical to our understanding of vascular function in the lung.

Short-Term Consequences of Hypoxia-Related Mitogenesis in Lung Arterioles

The possible consequences of this hypoxia-related increased mitotic activity in the arteriolar wall are considered next. Clearly, in the wall itself, the adventitia and the media become greatly thickened, and this thickening contributes directly to narrowing of the arteriolar lumen and a failure of transition to a low resistance lung circulation. Not only is the media thickened, but the contractile elements within the smooth muscle cells increase,[14] as does their capacity to secrete matrix.[41] For the endothelium, the morphological consequences of a persisting high replication rate during the first 2 weeks of life are not so clear, because the endothelium is not obviously thickened in the calves, though morphometric analysis has not been done. What is likely, however, is that endothelial function is altered. For example, in pulmonary hypertensive neonatal lambs, endothelin (ET-1) protein is increased approximately 3-fold, while the endothelin A (ET_A, vasoconstrictive[9]) receptors are greatly increased and the endothelin B (ET_B, vasodilator[9]) receptors are greatly decreased[6]—all of which is likely to tilt endothelial function toward vasoconstriction rather than vasodilation. These changes in endothelin metabolism will also promote mitogenic activity for smooth muscle and possibly for fibroblasts. But whether or not the mitogenic activity in the lung arterioles in hypoxic pulmonary hypertension contributes to vascular tone remains to be seen. What is clear relative to the short-term consequences of neonatal hypoxia, however, is that newborn calves maintained under these severely hypoxic conditions often develop, within 2–3 weeks, heart failure that may be fatal. Marked thickening of the arteriolar wall is present, compatible with the increased mitotic activity in the media and adventitia, and with increased production of matrix proteins.

Long-Term Consequences of Early Neonatal Hypoxia

There is increasing recognition of the potential in the systemic circulation for fetal and infant origins of adult disease.[42] For example, adults who were small at birth are more likely to have severe systemic hypertension than adults with normal birth weight. Apparently, by mechanisms that we do not understand, even transient adverse health events in early life can have adverse health consequences much later in life.[42] Whether such a concept holds true for the pulmonary circulation remains to be seen. The first report (of which the author is aware) that raises the possibility that early hypoxic pulmonary hypertension may have lasting effects is that of a 15-year-old girl who was born and lived in Leadville, Colorado, at 10,150 feet (3,100 m).[43] She was asymptomatic and an outstanding high school athlete. On routine examination she was found to have clinical and electrocardiographic evidence of pulmonary hypertension. During cardiac catheterization, mean pulmonary arterial pressure was 44 mm Hg at rest and 109 mm Hg on mild exercise. She was moved to a residence at sea level, where 11 months later her resting (17 mm Hg) and exercise (38 mm Hg) pressures were normal. After an absence of 18 months, she returned to Leadville, and 6 months later repeat cardiac catheterization showed that her pulmonary hypertension had returned to the previous level. It is thus probable that this young woman has a pulmonary circulation that is hyperreactive to hypoxia. However, whether or not her lung circulation became entirely normal during her 18 months at sea level, it retained mechanisms that rapidly reestablished chronic pulmonary hypertension on reexposure to hypoxia.

What are the effects of neonatal hypoxia that has lasted only for days or weeks, rather than years? In two articles published independently in 1990, transient neonatal hypoxia in rats was followed by an increased pulmonary pressor response to hypoxia some weeks or months later, when the rats were adult.[45,46] There are similar findings from a recent report from Sartori et al[47] in normal human subjects. Ten healthy 21-year-old adults who were known to have had transitory hypoxic pulmonary hypertension during their first week of life were taken to high altitude on Monta Rosa, in Northern Italy (4,559 m). Over 2 days they developed higher systolic pulmonary artery pressures (62 mm Hg) than did ten normal controls without such history (50 mm Hg). Remarkably, it seems possible from studies in both humans and in experimental animals that a period of perinatal hypoxia of relatively brief duration may alter the lung circulation at some time, even years, later.

Also, prenatal stimuli affecting the lung circulation may be retained after birth. In 1971, Goldberg et al[44] suggested that maternal hypoxia in rats caused thickened pulmonary arterioles in the newborn, and the thickening persisted for up to 25 days of postnatal life. Chronic narrowing of the ductus arteriosus in the near-term sheep fetus, a maneuver known to elevate fetal pulmonary arterial pressure, caused severe pulmonary hypertension after birth of the lambs.[25] Recent preliminary evidence in the fawn-hooded rat, which spontaneously develops pulmonary hypertension and abnormal pulmonary parenchymal structure at Denver's altitude,[48] indicates that the pressure elevation (as measured by right heart hypertrophy) and abnormalities in lung parenchyma can be ameliorated by a period of pre- and/or postnatal hyperbaria to simulate sea level PO_2 (Le Cras TD, Abman SH, personal communication). Studies are needed which confirm or deny that stimuli affecting the lung circulation in the perinatal period have recognizable effects later in life.

Conclusion

William Harvey's remarkable statement of 1628, "*It is only when the lungs are used . . . that the difference . . . of strength . . . between the two ventricles begins to be apparent,*"[15] implies that with ventilation of the lungs at birth, the right ventricle *begins* to beat with less force. He did not indicate how long after the lungs were 'used' that the process begins. Perhaps he suspected, as shown by Dawes more than three centuries later, that the process begins, and dramatically so, with the first breath. This first breath both stretches and dilates the small resistance arteries, thus lowering vascular resistance. Part of the lowered resistance develops because the arteriolar endothelial cells are stretched and thereby flattened, which in turn increases luminal diameter at crucial loci in the small arteries. At this time, during the first 2 days of life, the endothelial cells of the arterioles have very high replication rates. We speculate that the two events, endothelial stretch and marked replication, are linked, and we have postulated that endothelial stretch may be an important causative factor in this high replication rate (Figure 11). It is also interesting to speculate whether the early postnatal mitotic activity of the endothelium helps maintain a stable and normal low lung vascular resistance.

Even if our concepts are only partially correct, they raise other questions, some of which are listed here. What is the role of shear stress and increasing PO_2 on endothelial replication at birth? Is the endothelium communicating with other cells in the vascular wall and promoting neovascularization and/or angiogenesis? If metabolic activity of the en-

HYPOTHETICAL SCHEMA

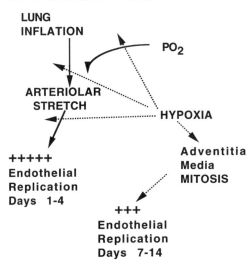

Figure 11. Hypothetical schema that might account for high endothelial replication rates in very young (aged 1–4 days) normoxic neonatal calves (unbroken lines). The possible effects of a hypoxic environment, which could blunt
replication rates during days 1–4 but might account for persistence of high
replication rates on days 7–14, are shown as broken lines.

dothelial cell is directed at replication, then how can the cell effectively
perform its endothelial-dependent vasodilating function, which seems
to be so essential for neonatal health?

When hypoxia interferes with the normal fetal-to-neonatal transition of the lung circulation, high arteriolar tone inhibits the normal dilation of the arterioles and partially inhibits endothelial stretch. Early
postnatal endothelial replication also seems to be partially inhibited,
possibly because there is less mechanical stress on the endothelial cell
(Figure 11). But what are the roles of a low postnatal PO_2 and of altered
shear forces? Also, we do not understand the mechanisms for the persistence of high endothelial replication for at least 2 weeks in the hypoxic
environment. Abnormal signaling between the cell layers of the arteriolar wall are likely occurring (Figure 11), but what are these signals, and
what is controlling them? If abnormal signals between cells are occurring, do they account for the abnormal lung vascular growth patterns in
the hypoxic neonate? Finally, is it true that neonatal pulmonary hypertension results in an altered lung circulation later in life, and if so, how
do the lung vessels "remember" their abnormal neonatal experiences?
We have come a long way since Harvey, but much of the journey remains ahead.

Dedication

It is my great pleasure to dedicate this chapter to Estelle Grover. She was for my colleague, Dr. Robert F. Grover, a constant companion in life and research and she was for many of us a model of dedication and practical wisdom. In addition, she was a collaborator in what were the defining studies in my own career, namely, our studies with the Colorado State University veterinarians, Arch Alexander and Don Will, in chronic pulmonary hypertension at high altitude. The 1958 studies in cattle continued into the winter in the coldest barn I have ever known, at 10,000 feet in Fairplay, Colorado. The intravenous fluids froze, and my fingers and toes nearly suffered the same fate. Estelle never faltered, setting the example for us all. In 1960, she participated in every phase of our study at 12,700 feet on Mount Evans, from setting up the corral and moving in the cattle and sheep, to performing blood gas analyses using the laborious Riley bubble technique while being frequently exposed to lightening strikes above tree line, and finally, analyzing the data.

References

1. Cook CD, Drinker PA, Jacobson HN, et al. Control of pulmonary blood flow in the foetal and newly born lamb. *J Physiol* 1963;169:10–29.
2. Davidson D. Pulmonary hemodynamics at birth: Effect of acute cyclooxygenase inhibition in lambs. *J Appl Physiol* 1988;64:1676–1682.
3. Rudolph AM. Fetal and neonatal pulmonary circulation. *Annu Rev Physiol* 1979;41:383–395.
4. Rudolph AM. Circulatory changes at birth. *J Perinat Med* 1988;16(suppl 1):9–21.
5. Teitel DF, Iwamoto HS, Rudolph AM. Changes in the pulmonary circulation during birth-related events. *Pediatr Res* 1990;27:372–378.
6. Ivy DD, Le Cras TD, Horan MP, et al. Increased lung preproET-1 and decreased ETB-receptor gene expression in fetal pulmonary hypertension. *Am J Physiol* 1998;274:L535–L541.
7. Steinhorn RH, Morin FC, Fineman JR. Models of persistent pulmonary hypertension of the newborn (PPHN) and the role of cyclic guanosine monophosphate (GMP) in pulmonary vasorelaxation. *Semin Perinatol* 1997;21:393–408.
8. Cornfield DN, Chatfield BA, McQueston JA, et al. Effects of birth-related stimuli on L-arginine-dependent pulmonary vasodilation in ovine fetus. *Am J Physiol* 1992;262:H1474–H1481.
9. Perreault T, Baribeau J. Characterization of endothelin receptors in newborn piglet lung. *Am J Physiol* 1995;268:L607–L614.
10. Stenmark KR, Durmowicz AG, Dempsey EC. Modulation of vascular wall phenotype in pulmonary hypertension. In: Bishop JE, Reeves JT, Laurent GJ, eds: *Pulmonary Vascular Remodelling*. London: Portland Press; 1995:171–212.
11. Dawes GS. *Foetal and Neonatal Physiology*. Chicago: Year Book Publishers; 1968:79–90.
12. Haworth SG. Development of the normal and abnormal pulmonary circulation. *Exp Physiol* 1995;80:843–853.

13. Hall SM, Haworth SG. Normal adaptation of pulmonary arterial intima to extrauterine life in the pig: Ultrastructural studies. *J Pathol* 1986;149:55–66.
14. Allen KM, Haworth SG. Impaired adaptation of pulmonary circulation to extrauterine life in newborn pigs exposed to hypoxia: An ultrastructural study. *J Pathol* 1986;149:205–212.
15. Harvey W. *On the Motion of the Heart and Blood in Animals.* [Willis's translation, revised and edited by Bowie A.] London: George Bell & Sons; 1889:82.
16. Ardran GM, Dawes GS, Prichard MML, et al. The effect of ventilation of the foetal lungs upon the pulmonary circulation. *J Physiol* 1952;118:12–22.
17. Hamilton WF, Woodbury RA, Woods EB. The relation between systemic and pulmonary pressures in the fetus. *Am J Physiol* 1937;119:206–212.
18. Abel S, Windle WF. Relation of the volume of pulmonary circulation to respiration. *Anat Rec* 1939;75:451–463.
19. Barclay AE, Franklin KJ, Pritchard MML. Pulmonary circulation times before and after functional closure of the ductus arteriosus. *J Physiol* 1942; 101:375–377.
20. Edwards JE, Douglas JM, Burchell HB, et al. Pathology of the intrapulmonary arteries and arterioles in coarctation of the aorta associated with patent ductus arteriosus. *Am Heart J* 1949;38:205–233.
21. Civin WH, Edwards JE. The postnatal structural changes in intrapulmonary arteries and arterioles. *Arch Pathol* 1951;51:192–200.
22. Cassin S, Dawes GS, Mott JC, et al. The vascular resistance of the foetal and newly ventilated lung of the lamb. *J Physiol* 1964;171:61–79.
23. Cassin S, Dawes GS, Ross BB. Pulmonary blood flow and vascular resistance in immature fetal lambs. *J Physiol* 1964;171:80–89.
24. Dawes GS. The pulmonary circulation after birth. In: Adams W, Veith I, eds: *Pulmonary Circulation.* New York: Grune & Stratton; 1959:199–203.
25. Levin DL, Hyman AI, Heymann MA, et al. Fetal hypertension and the development of increased pulmonary vascular smooth muscle: A possible mechanism for persistent pulmonary hypertension of the newborn. *J Pediatr* 1978;92:265–269.
26. Reynolds SRM. The fetal and neonatal pulmonary vasculature in the guinea pig in relation to hemodynamic changes at birth. *Am J Anat* 1956;98:97–121.
27. Riley RL. Effects of lung inflation on the pulmonary vascular bed. In: Adams W, Veith I, eds: *Pulmonary Circulation.* New York: Grune & Stratton; 1959:147–159.
28. Permutt S. Pulmonary mechanics and the pulmonary blood vessels. In: Wagner WW, Weir EK, eds: *The Pulmonary Circulation and Gas Exchange.* Armonk, New York: Futura Publishing Co; 1994:147–165.
29. Bishop JE, Butt RP, Low RB. The effect of mechanical forces on cell function: Implications for pulmonary vascular remodelling due to hypertension. In: Bishop JE, Reeves JT, Laurent GJ, eds: *Pulmonary Vascular Remodelling.* London: Portland Press; 1995:213–240.
30. Dawes KE, Bishop JE, Peacock AJ, et al. The role of endothelium in vascular remodelling. In: Bishop JE, Reeves JT, Laurent GJ, eds: *Pulmonary Vascular Remodelling.* London: Portland Press; 1995:241–270.
31. Langille LB. Remodeling of developing and mature arteries: Endothelium, smooth muscle and matrix. *J Cardiovasc Pharmacol* 1993;21(suppl 1):S11–S17.
32. Reeves JT, Leathers JE. Circulatory changes following birth of the calf and the effect of hypoxia. *Circ Res* 1964;15:343–354.

33. Reeves JT, Leathers JE. Post-natal development of pulmonary and bronchial arterial circulations in the calf and the effect of hypoxia. *Anat Rec* 1967;157:641–655.

34. Stenmark KR, Fasules J, Hyde DM, et al. Severe pulmonary hypertension and adventitial changes in newborn calves at 4300 m. *J Appl Physiol* 1987;62:821–830.

35. Belknap JK, Orten EC, Ensley B, et al. Hypoxia increases bromodeoxyuridine labeling indices in bovine neonatal pulmonary arteries. *Am J Cell Mol Biol* 1997;16:366–371.

36. Stiebellehner L, Belknap JK, Ensley B, et al. Lung endothelial cell proliferation in normal and pulmonary hypertensive neonatal calves. *Am J Physiol* 1998;275 *(Lung Cell Mol 19)*: L593–L600.

37. Reeves JT, Daoud FA, Gentry M. Growth of the fetal calf and its arterial pressure, blood gases and hematological data. *J Appl Physiol* 1972;32:240–244.

38. Meyrick B, Reid L. Hypoxia and incorporation of 3H-thymidine by cells of the rat pulmonary arteries and alveolar wall. *Am J Pathol* 1979;96:51–70.

39. Stenmark KR, Mecham RP. Cellular and molecular mechanisms of pulmonary vascular remodeling. *Annu Rev Physiol* 1997;59:89–144.

40. Keeley FW, Rabinovitch M. Vascular matrix in hypertension. In: Bishop JE, Reeves JT, Laurent GJ, eds: *Pulmonary Vascular Remodelling*. London: Portland Press; 1995:149–169.

41. Stenmark KR, Durmowicz AG, Roby JD, et al. Persistence of the fetal pattern of tropoelastin gene expression in severe neonatal bovine pulmonary hypertension. *J Clin Invest* 1994;93:1234–1242.

42. Barker DJP. *Fetal and Infant Origins of Adult Disease*. London: British Medical Journal; 1992.

43. Grover RF, Vogel JHK, Voigt GC, et al. Reversal of high altitude pulmonary hypertension. *Am J Cardiol* 1966;18:928–932.

44. Goldberg SJ, Levy RA, Siassi B, et al. The effects of maternal hypoxia and hyperoxia upon the neonatal pulmonary vasculature. *Pediatrics* 1971;48: 528–533.

45. Hakim TS, Mortola JP. Pulmonary vascular resistance in adult rats exposed to hypoxia in the newborn period. *Can J Physiol Pharmacol* 1990;68: 419–424.

46. Hampl V, Herget J. Perinatal hypoxia increases hypoxic pulmonary vasoconstriction in adult rats recovering from chronic exposure to hypoxia. *Am Rev Respir Dis* 1990;142:619–624.

47. Sartori C, Trueb L, Alleman Y, et al. Transitory perinatal hypoxic pulmonary hypertension predisposes to exaggerated pulmonary vasoconstriction in young adults exposed to high altitude. *FASEB J* 1997;11:A135.

48. Kim DH, Le Cras TD, Horan MP, et al. Impaired expression of lung endothelial nitric oxide synthase and abnormal alveolarization in the fawnhooded rat: Implications for the risk of developing pulmonary hypertension. *Pediatr Res* 1998;43:288A.

49. Dawes GS, JC Mott, Widdicombe JG, et al. Changes in the lungs of the newborn lamb. *J Physiol* 1953;121:141–162.

50. Haworth SG, Hall SM, Chew M, et al. Thinning of fetal pulmonary arterial wall and post natal remodelling: Ultrastructural studies on the respiratory unit arteries of the pig. *Virchows Arch* 1987;411:161–171.

Chapter 15

Physiologic Roles of Nitric Oxide in the Perinatal Pulmonary Circulation

*Steven H. Abman, MD, John P. Kinsella, MD,
Thomas A. Parker, MD, Laurent Storme, MD,
and Timothy D. Le Cras, PhD*

Introduction

At birth, pulmonary vascular resistance (PVR) rapidly falls from high fetal levels, allowing pulmonary blood flow to increase nearly 10-fold and enabling the lung to assume its postnatal role in gas exchange. Mechanisms that contribute to the normal decrease in PVR at birth include increased oxygen tension, rhythmic distension of the lung, shear stress, and enhanced production of vasodilator substances, including nitric oxide (NO). Failure of the pulmonary circulation to successfully achieve or sustain this decrease in PVR causes severe hypoxemia in several neonatal cardiopulmonary disorders that constitute the syndrome known as persistent pulmonary hypertension of the newborn (PPHN). PPHN is a major clinical problem, contributing substantially to morbidity and mortality in both full-term and premature neonates. Diseases such as idiopathic PPHN, meconium aspiration, sepsis, asphyxia, acute respiratory distress syndrome (RDS), lung hypoplasia, and others, are often included within the PPHN syndrome. This syndrome is characterized by high PVR, right-to-left extrapulmonary shunting of blood across the ductus arteriosus (DA) or foramen ovale, and marked hypoxemia. Mechanisms that cause severe pulmonary hypertension after birth are incompletely understood, but can include

From: Weir EK, Archer SL, Reeves JT (eds). *The Fetal and Neonatal Pulmonary Circulations*.
Armonk, NY: Futura Publishing Company, Inc.; ©1999.

altered pulmonary vascular tone, growth, and structure. Understanding basic mechanisms of normal functional and structural development of the pulmonary circulation in utero, and mechanisms that contribute to sustained pulmonary vasodilation at birth, may provide insights into the syndrome of PPHN and its treatment.

The endothelial cell is now recognized as playing a critical role in modulating vascular tone, growth, and structure in many experimental and clinical settings. The vascular endothelium produces several vasoactive products that regulate the perinatal lung circulation, including NO. NO has potent effects on vascular tone and reactivity, and can modulate endothelial and smooth muscle cell (SMC) growth and vessel structure. Its effects are also dependent upon other enzymes, such as soluble guanylate cyclase (sGC), cyclic guanosine monophosphate (cGMP)-specific phosphodiesterases, cGMP kinase, and other proteins, which comprise the "NO-cGMP cascade." This chapter will provide a review of the physiologic roles of the NO-cGMP cascade in regulation of the pulmonary circulation during fetal life, and the contribution of NO to pulmonary vasodilation at birth. We will further discuss how changes in the NO-cGMP cascade may contribute to the pathophysiology of neonatal pulmonary hypertension and briefly consider implications for the treatment of PPHN.

Physiology of the Developing Lung Circulation

Due to high PVR in the normal fetus, the pulmonary circulation receives less than 10% of combined ventricular output, with most of the right ventricular output crossing the widely patent DA to the aorta.[1–3] Although fetal pulmonary blood flow is low, it is essential for providing substrates, hormones, and oxygen to allow for normal lung growth, as evidenced by lung hypoplasia after occlusion of the left pulmonary artery during late gestation.[4] The pulmonary circulation undergoes changes in both vascular structure and function throughout fetal life. With advancing fetal age, pulmonary blood flow increases with lung growth and increased vessel number. However, PVR increases with gestational age when calculated on the basis of fetal lung or body weight. Thus, pulmonary vascular tone appears to increase during late gestation, especially prior to birth. Mechanisms that contribute to high fetal PVR include the lack of a gas-liquid interface, low oxygen tension, low basal production of vasodilator products (ie, PGI_2 and NO), increased production of vasoconstrictors (including endothelin-1 [ET-1]), and altered SMC reactivity (ie, enhanced myogenic tone).

The acute pulmonary vasodilator response to several stimuli, such as acetylcholine and increased oxygen tension, and the vasoconstrictor response to acute hypoxia increase with advancing gestation in the ovine fetus.[5,6] In addition to high basal tone, the fetal lung circulation is further characterized by its capability to oppose vasodilation during prolonged exposure to vasodilator stimuli. Several vasodilators (ie, increased O_2, acetylcholine, histamine, bradykinin, and prostaglandins) increase pulmonary blood flow, but this response is often transient, as blood flow returns toward baseline values despite continued treatment.[7,8] This response can also be observed during mechanical increases in pulmonary blood flow caused by partial compression of the DA (Figure 1).[9] Mechanisms underlying time-dependent increases in PVR despite prolonged exposure to dilator stimuli are uncertain, but suggest that the fetal lung circulation may have the capacity for autoregulation, which serves to maintain high PVR in utero. Interestingly, agents that directly stimulate smooth muscle relaxation independent of endothelial release of vasodilators, such as cGMP, atrial natriuretic peptide, and K^+-channel agonists, cause more sustained pulmonary vasodilation than endothelium-dependent stimuli.[7,10] We have hypothesized that this capacity for time-dependent autoregulation may be partially due to increased myogenic responses in the fetal lung, which may be masked by NO release (as discussed below).

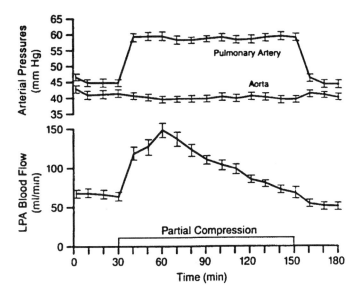

Figure 1. Time-dependent response of pulmonary blood flow during partial compression of the ductus arteriosus. As shown, ductus compression increases pulmonary artery pressure (PAP) and blood flow, but despite constant PAP, blood flow returns to basal levels over time. LPA = left pulmonary artery. (Reproduced with permission from Reference 9.)

The NO-cGMP Cascade in the Fetal Pulmonary Circulation

Maturational changes in endothelial function, especially with regard to the NO-cGMP cascade, may account for changes in pulmonary vasoregulation during fetal life. NO is produced during conversion of L-arginine to L-citrulline by the enzyme, NO synthase (NOS).[11,12] This step requires a unique five-electron oxidation of a terminal guanidinium nitrogen on L-arginine. NOS activity is dependent on the availability of other substrates and cofactors, including oxygen, tetrahydrobiopterin, nicotinamide adenine dinucleotide phosphate (NADPH), flavin adenine dinucleotide (FAD), flavin mononucleotide (FMN), and calmodulin. NOS functions as a homodimer, with each monomer consisting of reductase and oxygenase domains. A binding site for calmodulin bridges these domains, and following activation by calcium, permits the transfer of electrons from NADPH via the flavins to the heme catalytic site. Once produced, NO rapidly diffuses to underlying SMCs and causes vasodilation by stimulating soluable guanylate cyclase, and increasing cGMP production. Elevated cGMP stimulates cGMP kinase, increases calcium-activated K^+-channel activity, and causes membrane hyperpolarization.[11,13,14] This lowers intracellular calcium in the SMC by decreasing calcium entry through L-type channels, and causes vasodilation. In some settings, NO has been shown to directly stimulate K^+ channels or voltage-gated Ca^{2+} channels independent of increased cGMP.[15,16] Hemodynamic (eg, shear stress), hormonal, paracrine, and pharmacological stimuli can regulate vascular NOS expression. NOS activity is affected by multiple factors, including substrate and cofactor availability, superoxide production (which inactivates NO and forms peroxynitrite), superoxide dismutase activity, and other factors (as discussed below).

Three NOS isoforms have been identified: two are considered as constitutive (type I, neuronal [nNOS]; and type III, endothelial [eNOS]). Activity of the constitutive NOS isoforms is dependent upon changes in intracellular calcium after stimulation by physiologic, biochemical, and pharmacological stimuli. The third NOS isoform (type II, iNOS) is the so-called "inducible" isoform, and is largely regulated by transcriptional mechanisms. Since calmodulin is tightly bound to type II NOS, its activity is largely calcium-independent, and it is capable of generating large amounts of NO. Although originally characterized by cell-specific expression in neurons (type I), endothelium (type III), and macrophages (type II), further work has now demonstrated that diverse cells can express each isoform, and that each of these isoforms has been identified within the fetal lung. Endothelial NOS (type III) activity is also dependent upon its subcellular localization within the endothelial cell.[17] Of the three NOS isoforms, eNOS is uniquely associated with cell membranes, which is due to myristoylation and palmitoylation of the protein. Acylation of these sites targets eNOS to plasmalemmel microdomains, or caveolae, which may allow for eNOS to be more effectively located for interactions with blood-borne substances, other enzyme or receptor systems contained within caveolae, and the endothelial cytoskeleton.[17]

Lung eNOS mRNA and protein are present in the early fetus and increase with advancing gestation in utero and during the early postnatal period in rats.[18] In sheep, lung eNOS mRNA, protein, and activity increase markedly at 113–118 days (term = 147 days). The timing of this increase in lung eNOS content immediately precedes an increased capacity to respond to endothelium-dependent vasodilators.[3,5,6] Although most studies of the perinatal lung have focused on the role of eNOS in vasoregulation, the other NOS isoforms, including neuronal (type I) NOS and inducible (type II) NOS, have been identified by immunostaining in the rat and human fetal lungs.[19] Lung nNOS mRNA and protein increase during development in the fetal rat,[18] but data is limited regarding its site of expression within the fetal lung. Inducible (type II) NOS has also been detected by immunostaining in the ovine fetal lung, and is predominantly expressed in airway epithelium and vascular smooth muscle, but not vascular endothelium. This is in striking contrast with past observations that lung eNOS expression is predominantly localized within endothelial cells (Figure 2).

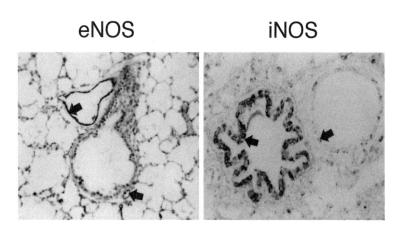

eNOS   **iNOS**

Figure 2. Immunohistochemistry comparing the preferential distribution of endothelial (type III; eNOS) and "inducible" (type II; iNOS) NO synthase in the late gestation fetal lung. As shown, eNOS is most striking in vascular endothelium throughout the lung, whereas iNOS expression is especially strong in airway epithelium, with light staining of vascular smooth muscle. Arrows point to positive staining.

Whether the "nonendothelial" (types I and II) isoforms contribute to the physiologic responses of NO-dependent modulation of fetal pulmonary vascular tone has been uncertain. Treatment of pregnant rats with an iNOS (type II)-selective antagonist caused constriction of the great vessels (main pulmonary artery and thoracic aorta) and DA in fetal rats.[20] It is unclear, however, whether these changes were due to the direct effects of iNOS blockade in the fetus or secondary to alterations in placental perfusion and fetal oxygenation. To determine the potential role of iNOS as a source of NO in the fetal lung, we measured the pulmonary vascular effects of selective iNOS antagonists in chronically prepared fetal lambs.[21] We found that selective iNOS antagonists (including aminoguanidine and ethylisothiourea) increase fetal PVR at doses that do not inhibit acetylcholine-induced pulmonary vasodilation.[21] In contrast, the nonselective NOS antagonist, nitro-L-arginine (L-NA), elevated PVR but completely blocked acetylcholine-induced vasodilation. These findings support the speculation that iNOS may also modulate pulmonary vascular tone in utero, but further work is needed to clarify the relative roles of the different NOS isoforms in NO production in the fetal lung. Differences in sites of expression may have physiologic implications in nonvascular tissue. For example, we speculate that high iNOS expression in airway epithelium may imply roles in regulation of airway bronchomotor tone, epithelial fluid production, or other functions.

Vascular responsiveness to NO is also dependent upon several SMC enzymes, including sGC, cGMP-specific (type V) phosphodiesterase (PDE5), and cGMP kinase. Several studies have shown that sGC, which produces cGMP in response to NO activation, is active at least as early as 0.7 of term gestation in the ovine fetal lung.[22,23] Similarly, PDE5, which limits cGMP-mediated vasodilation by hydrolysis and inactivation of cGMP, is also active in utero.[24] Infusions of selective PDE5 antagonists, including zaprinast, dipyridamole, E4021, and DMPPO, cause potent and sustained fetal pulmonary vasodilation.[24] In the fetal lung, PDE5 expression has been localized to vascular smooth muscle, and PDE5 activity is high in comparison with the postnatal lung.[25,26] Thus, PDE5 activity appears to play a critical role in pulmonary vasoregulation during the perinatal period, and must be accounted for in assessing responsiveness to endogenous NO and related vasodilator stimuli.

Physiologic Roles for NO in the Normal Fetal Lung

Various studies have demonstrated several physiologic roles for the NO-cGMP cascade in pulmonary vasoregulation in the perinatal period. In vivo studies of the pulmonary hemodynamic effects of NOS antagonists demonstrate that basal NO release modulates pulmonary vascular tone during late gestation.[27] Since NOS blockade increases PVR at least as early as 0.75 gestation (112 days) in the fetal lamb, endogenous NOS activity appears to contribute to vasoregulation throughout late gestation.[23] In addition, NOS inhibition selectively attenuates pulmonary vasodilation to such stimuli as acetylcholine,[27] oxygen,[28] and increased flow or shear stress[29] in the normal fetus, without altering the vasodilator response to endothelium-independent agonists (including inhaled NO, atrial natriuretic peptide, and lemakalim). These findings demonstrate the important role of basal and stimulated NO release in fetal pulmonary vasoregulation. Since acetylcholine and oxygen cause pulmonary vasodilation by stimulating NO release,[27–29] maturational changes in the NO-cGMP cascade are likely to account for past observations of increasing pulmonary vasodilation to these agents with advancing fetal age. In vitro studies suggest that pharmacological agents which cause vasodilation by stimulating NO release are less potent in fetal than neonatal or adult pulmonary arteries.[22] In contrast, pulmonary artery relaxation due to direct stimulation of smooth muscle with sodium nitroprusside (which releases NO) is not different between fetal, newborn, and adult vessels.[22] Thus, basal NOS activity modulates PVR during late gestation in the ovine fetus, and maturational changes in endothelial cell function may contribute to developmental changes in pulmonary vascular tone and reactivity. Parallel in vivo studies of fetal pulmonary vasoreactivity support these in vitro observations; exogenous NO or agents that directly increase smooth muscle cGMP content cause more sustained fetal pulmonary vasodilation than many endothelium-dependent agonists.[30]

Past studies have shown that endogenous NO activity lowers PVR in utero and mediates vasodilation to various stimuli. Recent observations from our laboratory suggest that NO may play an additional role in modulating the high myogenic responsiveness of the fetal lung. The *myogenic response* is commonly defined by increased vasoconstriction caused by acute elevation of intravascular pressure, or "stretch stress."[31] Past in vitro studies have demonstrated the presence of a myogenic response in pulmonary arteries from adult cats,[32] and also that fetal pulmonary arteries have greater myogenic activity than neonatal or adult arteries.[33] To determine whether the myogenic response is operative and contributes to lung vasoregulation in vivo, we performed a series of experiments in chronically prepared fetal lambs during acute compression of the DA with an inflatable occluder. Partial DA compression elevates mean pulmonary artery pressure (PAP) and increases pulmonary blood flow, causing a progressive fall in PVR during the initial 30 minutes of compression. The immediate response within the first few minutes, however, is characterized by a brief rise in PVR, followed by pulmonary vasodilation.[33a] The net effect on tone is likely related to a balance between responses to at least two interactive forces: shear stress, which causes NO-dependent vasodilation, and stretch stress, which may provoke vasoconstriction through a myogenic response. NOS inhibition not only blocks pulmonary vasodilation, but it actually causes a marked rise in PVR (Figure 3). In addition, stepwise incremental increases in PAP by progressive compression of the DA did not increase flow but elevated PVR, demonstrating that increased intravascular pressure induced vasoconstriction. Thus, these findings support our hypothesis that NOS inhibition unmasks a potent myogenic response, which maintains high PVR in the normal fetus. We speculate that downregulation of NO, such as observed in experimental pulmonary hypertension, may further increase myogenic activity, increasing the risk for unopposed vasoconstriction in response to stretch stress at birth.

Although NO production increases cGMP content in vascular smooth muscle, NO-induced vasodilation is limited by the rapid hydrolysis or extrusion of cGMP.[11,34,35] For example, brief infusions of various PDE5 inhibitors, including dipyridamole, zaprinast, E4021, and DMPPO, cause marked and sustained increases in fetal pulmonary blood flow.[24] PDE5 blockers also augment and prolong pulmonary vasodilator responses to acetylcholine and inhaled NO in the normal fetus and in an experimental model of PPHN.[26] Maturational studies have also shown that lung PDE5 activity is highest during fetal life, rapidly decreases after birth, and remains low during adult life. Thus, physiologic and biochemical studies demonstrate that high PDE5 activity contributes to high PVR and limits responsiveness to pulmonary vasodilator stimuli in the normal fetus. PDE5 activity also contributes to experimental pulmonary hypertension caused by chronic hypoxia in adult rats[35a] and perinatal pulmonary hypertension in fetal lambs (see below).

The role of endogenous NO in the regulation of pulmonary vascular tone during late gestation is well established; however, little is known of its potential role in the pulmonary circulation during early stages of lung development. In addition to its effects on vascular tone, NO influences endothelial and SMC growth in vitro.[36,37] Since eNOS protein is present at a stage of lung development when blood flow is absent or minimal, it has been hypothesized that NO may potentially contribute to angiogenesis during early lung development.[38] Whether early eNOS expression implies a role in promoting vascular growth or is merely a marker of growing endothelial cells is unknown. Recent studies report conflicting data regarding the effects of eNOS activity in promoting new vessel formation in different experimental models of angiogenesis. Although NO can inhibit endothelial cell mitogenesis and proliferation, it has also been shown to mediate the angiogenic

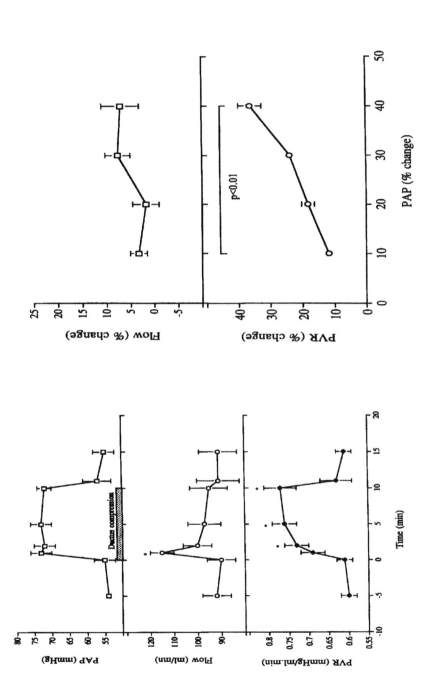

Figure 3. Inhibition of NOS activity unmasks the presence of intense myogenic responses in the fetal pulmonary circulation. Ductus compression after nitro-L-arginine (L-NA) treatment causes paradoxical increases in pulmonary vascular resistance (PVR) **(left panel)**. Serial brief incremental increases in pulmonary artery pressure (PAP) do not increase flow after L-NA treatment **(right panel)**. (Reproduced with permission from Reference 33a.)

effects of substance P and vascular endothelial growth factor in vitro.[36,37] Growing bovine aortic endothelial cells in culture express greater eNOS mRNA and protein than confluent cells, but NOS inhibition does not affect their rate of proliferation.[39] NO has also been shown to decrease smooth muscle proliferation in vitro,[40] but other studies suggest that NO has biphasic, dose-dependent effects on fetal pulmonary artery SMC growth.[41] High doses of NO donors inhibit SMC growth, but low doses cause paradoxical stimulation. Whether NO modulates SMC growth in vivo remains controversial; one study reported the failure of chronic NOS inhibition to alter pulmonary vascular structure during late gestation in the fetal lamb.[42] Thus, although multiple studies have examined the role of NO in vascular growth and remodeling, its effects vary between experimental settings and remain controversial.

Role of NO in the Fall in PVR at Birth

Within minutes after delivery, PAP falls and blood flow increases in response to birth-related stimuli. Mechanisms contributing to the fall in PVR at birth include establishment of an air-liquid interface, rhythmic lung distension, increased oxygen tension, and altered production of vasoactive substances.[1] Physical stimuli, such as increased shear stress, ventilation, and increased oxygen, cause pulmonary vasodilation in part by increasing production of vaosodilators, NO and PGI_2.[27,29,43–46] Pretreatment with the arginine analogue, L-NA, blocks NOS activity and attenuates the decline in PVR after delivery of near-term fetal lambs.[27] These findings suggest that about 50% of the rise in pulmonary blood flow at birth may be directly related to the acute release of NO. Specific mechanisms that cause NO release at birth include the marked rise in shear stress, increased oxygen, and ventilation.[27,29] Recent studies from Cornfield et al suggest that increased PaO_2 triggers NO release, which augments vasodilation through cGMP kinase-mediated stimulation of K^+ channels.[14] The important role of NO activity during the transitional circulation has been confirmed in experiments of chronic treatment of fetal lambs with a NOS antagonist.[42]

Although these studies were performed in term animals, similar mechanisms also contribute to the rapid decrease in PVR at birth in premature lambs.[23] The pulmonary vasodilator responses to ventilation with hypoxic gas mixtures (or, rhythmic distension) of the lung or increased PaO_2 are partly due to stimulation of NO release in premature lambs at least as early as 112–115 days (0.7 term).[23] Other vasodilator products, including PGI_2, also modulate changes in pulmonary vascular tone at birth.[43,46–48] Rhythmic lung distension and shear stress stimulate both PGI_2 and NO production in the late gestation fetus[9,29]; increased O_2 tension triggers NO activity but does not appear to alter PGI_2 production in vivo.[28,48]

Thus, although NO does not account for the entire decrease in PVR at birth, NOS activity appears important in achieving postnatal adaptation of the lung circulation. Transgenic eNOS knockout mice successfully make the transition at birth without evidence of PPHN.[49] This finding suggests that eNOS $-/-$ mice may have adaptive mechanisms, such as a compensatory vasodilator mechanism (ie, upregulation of other NOS isoforms or dilator prostaglandins) or less constrictor tone. Interestingly, these animals are more sensitive to the development of pulmonary hypertension at relatively mild decreases in PaO_2. We speculate that isolated eNOS deficiency alone may not be sufficient for the failure of postnatal adaptation, but that decreased ability to produce NO in the setting of a perinatal stress (ie, hypoxia or hypertension, or upregulation of vasoconstrictors) may cause PPHN (see below).

Experimental Studies of the NO-cGMP Cascade in PPHN

Some newborns fail to achieve or sustain the normal decline in PVR after birth, and constitute the clinical syndrome known as PPHN.[50] As a clinical syndrome, PPHN includes diverse cardiac and pulmonary disorders, or it can manifest as an idiopathic disorder, in the absence of significant cardiac or pulmonary disease. Although these diverse diseases have features that are distinct from each other, they are generally included within this clinical syndrome because they share a common pathophysiologic feature: high PVR leading to right-to-left shunting of blood across the DA or foramen ovale and marked hypoxemia. Despite multiple therapeutic strategies, morbidity and mortality in neonates with severe PPHN remain high. Although cardiac and lung function contribute significantly to the clinical course of neonates with PPHN, abnormalities of the pulmonary circulation are critical features of PPHN. PPHN is characterized by altered pulmonary vascular reactivity, structure, and in some cases, growth. Diseases associated with this syndrome of PPHN are often characterized as fitting into one of three categories: (1) maladaptation—vessels are presumably of normal structure but have abnormal vasoreactivity; (2) excessive muscularization—increased SMC thickness and increased distal extension of muscle to vessels that are usually nonmuscular; and (3) underdevelopment—lung hypoplasia associated with decreased pulmonary artery number.[51] Clinically, many conditions combine mixtures of alterations in structure and function; for example, congenital diaphragmatic hernia incorporates elements from each of these categories. It is likely that not all newborns with PPHN have structural lung vascular lesions; altered pulmonary vasoreactivity can be due to an acute or short-term insult (group B streptococcal sepsis, meconium aspiration, and acute asphyxia).

Several experimental models have been studied to explore the pathogenesis and pathophysiology of PPHN.[52,53] Such models have included exposure to acute or chronic hypoxia after birth, chronic hypoxia in utero, placement of meconium into the airways of neonatal animals, sepsis, and others. Although each model demonstrates interesting physiologic changes that may be especially relevant to particular clinical settings, most studies examine only brief changes in the pulmonary circulation, and mechanisms underlying altered lung vascular structure and function of PPHN remain poorly understood. Clinical observations that neonates with severe PPHN who die during the first days after birth already have pathological signs of chronic pulmonary vascular disease suggest that intrauterine events may play an important role in this syndrome. Adverse intrauterine stimuli during late gestation, such as decreased lung blood flow, changes in substrate or hormone delivery to the lung, chronic hypoxia, chronic hypertension, inflammation, or others, may potentially alter lung vascular function and structure, contributing to abnormalities of postnatal adaptation.

Several investigators have examined the effects of chronic intrauterine stresses, such as hypoxia or hypertension, in animals in order to attempt to mimic the clinical problem of PPHN. Whether chronic hypoxia alone can cause PPHN is controversial. An early report that maternal hypoxia in rats increases pulmonary vascular smooth muscle thickening in newborns has not been replicated with more extensive studies in maternal rats or guinea pigs.[54] However, animal studies suggest that hypertension, due to either renal artery ligation or partial or complete closure of the DA, can cause structural and physiologic changes that resemble features of clinical PPHN.[55]

Pulmonary hypertension induced by early closure of the DA in fetal lambs alters lung vascular reactivity and structure, causing the failure of postnatal adaptation at delivery, and providing an experimental model of PPHN.[56,57] In this model, partial closure of the DA acutely increases PAP and flow, but after 1 hour, blood flow returns toward baseline values.[9] Over days, PAP and PVR progressively increase, but flow remains low and PaO_2 is unchanged.[56] Thus, this model illustrates the effects of chronic intrauterine hypertension, but not high flow, on intrauterine lung vascular structure and function. Marked right ventricular hypertrophy and structural remodeling of small pulmonary arteries develops after 8 days of hypertension. After delivery, these lambs have persistent elevation of PVR despite mechanical ventilation with high oxygen concentrations.[56,57] Thus, physiologic and structural studies suggest that this experimental model of PPHN mimics many of the abnormalities found in severe idiopathic PPHN in the human newborn.

To determine whether changes in the NO-cGMP system contributes to pulmonary vascular abnormalities in PPHN, our laboratory and others have studied endothelial and smooth muscle cell function in this experimental model (Figure 4). That chronic hypertension can alter NO production or activity was first suggested in physiologic studies of pulmonary vasodilation of hypertensive and control lambs.[58] McQueston and coworkers[58] found that pulmonary vasodilator responses to acetylcholine and increased oxygen, which act in part by stimulating NO release, were impaired after chronic hypertension. Responsiveness to atrial natriuretic peptide, which causes vasodilation by directly increasing smooth muscle cGMP content, independent of NO release by vascular endothelium, remains relatively intact. These findings suggested that intrauterine hypertension impairs endothelial function, and that the ability to produce NO may be impaired. Subsequent molecular and biochemical studies have demonstrated that chronic pulmonary hypertension decreases lung eNOS mRNA and protein expression and

Abnormal NO-cGMP Cascade in PPHN

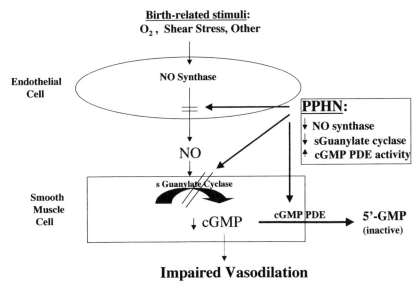

Figure 4. Schematic illustratiion of the potential role of abnormalities of the NO-cGMP (nitric oxide-cyclic guanosine monophosphate) cascade in the pathophysiology of persistent pulmonary hypertension of the newborn (PPHN). PDE = phosphodiesterase.

total NOS activity.[59] Thus, these studies support the hypothesis that vascular injury in utero can decrease vasodilator responsiveness to birth-related stimuli by reducing lung eNOS content and NO production. Whether impaired NOS activity in utero also contributes to hypertensive structural remodeling of pulmonary arteries (including smooth muscle hypertrophy or hyperplasia) is uncertain.

As described above, pulmonary vasodilation to endogenous NO is also dependent upon several other factors, including smooth muscle sGC and cGMP-specific PDE5 activities.[30] Recent studies have examined sGC and PDE5 activities after chronic DA closure in this experimental model of PPHN. Steinhorn and coworkers reported impaired sGC activity in hypertensive lambs, as reflected by decreased generation of cGMP and reduced vascular relaxation to NO stimulation in vitro.[60] In addition, Hanson and coworkers found marked elevation of lung PDE5 activity, suggesting that rapid cGMP hydrolysis may limit cGMP-dependent pulmonary vasodilation after chronic hypertension.[25,26] Thus, decreased lung eNOS protein and activity in the presence of decreased sGC and elevated PDE5 activities limits the ability to sustain smooth muscle cGMP, favoring vasoconstriction and high PVR in experimental PPHN. These observations may have clinical implications regarding potential strategies for enhancing responsiveness to vasodilator therapy of PPHN (see below).

Thus, alterations in the NO-cGMP cascade appear to play an essential role in the pathogenesis and pathophysiology of experimental PPHN. Abnormalities of NO production and responsiveness contribute to altered structure and function of the developing lung circulation, leading to failure of postnatal cardiorespiratory adaptation. Insights into mechanisms underlying altered vasoreactivity may provide new treatment strategies for clinical PPHN.

Abnormal Lung Growth and the Risk for Pulmonary Hypertension

Although abnormal pulmonary vascular function in the perinatal period has primarily been studied with regard to the immediate events at birth and the early postnatal period, it is possible that abnormalities of lung vascular development may increase the risk for the late development of pulmonary hypertension. For example, Hampl and Herget have previously reported that perinatal hypoxia can subsequently increase the risk for pulmonary vascular disease in adult rats.[61] In addition, children with lung hypoplasia, including bronchopulmonary dysplasia, congenital diaphragmatic hernia, and primary lung hypoplasia, are at risk for the development of pulmonary hypertension. Mechanisms linking the effects of perinatal events, such as transient perinatal hypoxia or abnormal lung growth, with subsequent abnormalities of the pulmonary circulation are unknown. The fawn-hooded rat (FHR) strain is characterized by platelet abnormalities and systemic hypertension, and has been used to study genetic risk factors for the development of idiopathic pulmonary hypertension.[62] Unlike other rat strains, FHRs develop progressive pulmonary hypertension when exposed to slight decreases in alveolar PO_2. We hypothesize that early maturational abnormalities in lung growth or pulmonary vasoreactivity could predispose the FHR for subsequent development of pulmonary hypertension. Since endogenous NO modulates hypoxic pulmonary vasoconstriction and may influence vessel growth, we further hypothesized that decreases in lung eNOS content may contribute to the risk of pulmonary hypertension in FHRs. We measured lung eNOS content and lung growth in FHR and control strains (Fischer and Sprague-Dawley rats [SDR]) at late fetal and postnatal ages (days 1 and 7, and weeks 3 and 10). We found that lung to body weight ratios were reduced in fetal and newborn FHR by 20% and 40% compared with control rats. In comparison with SDR, FHR lung eNOS protein was decreased to $69 \pm 8\%$, $56 \pm 8\%$, and $68 \pm 7\%$ at fetal, newborn, and day 7 ages, respectively ($p < 0.05$ at each age). Histology revealed striking changes in lung maturation and growth in FHR at all ages, including reduced alveolar number, as determined by radial

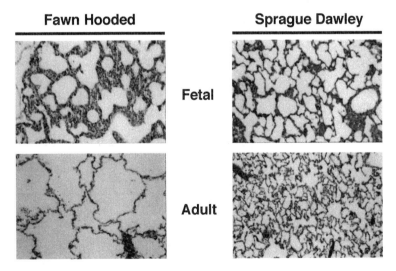

Figure 5. Abnormal alveolarization in the fawn-hooded rat, a genetic strain that develops pulmonary hypertension with mild decreases in alveolar PO_2. As shown, lung histology of fetal (upper panels) and adult (lower panels) show striking differences in lung maturation and growth between fawn-hooded and control (Sprague-Dawley) rat strains.

count (FHR 58 ± 2% of SDR at day 7, p<0.05; Figure 5). We conclude that in comparison with other rat strains, lung eNOS content is decreased in the FHR fetus and newborn, and remains low throughout adult life. In addition, the FHR has decreased alveolarization, with histological signs of delayed lung maturation. We speculate that reduced vascular surface area and decreased lung eNOS expression increase the susceptibility of the FHR for subsequent development of progressive pulmonary hypertension, and that decreased NO production may be associated with disorders of abnormal lung growth and development. The relationships between early perinatal events and late pulmonary vascular function and structure may lead to new insights into mechanisms of pulmonary hypertension in older children and adults.

Clinical Implications

Inhaled NO therapy was studied in newborns with severe PPHN after early reports demonstrated its potent and selective pulmonary vasodilator effects in adults with primary pulmonary hypertension and in perinatal animals.[30,63,64] Roberts and coworkers reported acute increases in postductal arterial saturation without systemic hypotension in six neonates during brief treatment with inhaled NO at 80 ppm.[65] Kinsella and coworkers also reported acute improvement in oxygenation and pulmonary hypertension (as directly assessed by echocardiogram) during brief treatment (up to 4 hours), but lower doses of inhaled NO (6–20 ppm) were used.[66] In addition to the acute response to inhaled NO, the latter report further demonstrated clinical recovery after continued low dose NO treatment.[66] The efficacy of this low dose NO strategy was subsequently demonstrated in consecutive patients who met clinical criteria of severe PPHN refractory to conventional therapy, including high-frequency oscillatory ventilation (HFOV), while meeting criteria for extracorporial membrane oxygenation (ECMO) therapy. As reported in the initial report, low dose NO (6 ppm) caused sustained improvement in oxygenation without evidence of tachyphylaxis or a need for higher doses. In some cases, clinical responsiveness was sustained with even lower doses of inhaled NO (1–3 ppm). During the initial studies, 13 of 15 consecutive patients with severe PPHN that met ECMO criteria were successfully treated without the need for ECMO therapy.[66,67] More recently, two multicenter randomized studies have demonstrated the success of inhaled NO therapy in improving oxygenation and decreasing the need for ECMO therapy.[68,69] Although clinical improvement during inhaled NO therapy occurs with many disorders associated with PPHN, not all neonates with acute hypoxemic respiratory failure and pulmonary hypertension respond well to inhaled NO.[70] Several mechanisms may explain the clinical variability in responsiveness to inhaled NO therapy. An inability to deliver NO to the pulmonary circulation due to poor lung inflation is the major cause of poor responsiveness. In some settings, administration of NO with HFOV has improved oxygenation more effectively than during conventional ventilation in the same patient. In addition, poor NO responsiveness may be related to myocardial dysfunction or systemic hypotension, severe pulmonary vascular structural disease, and unsuspected or missed anatomic cardiovascular lesions (such as total anomalous pulmonary venous return, coarctation of the aorta, alveolo-capillary dysplasia, and others). Another mechanism of poor responsiveness to inhaled NO may be altered SMC responsiveness. As described from animal studies, decreased sGC or increased PDE5 activities may limit the vasodilator response to NO. For example, inhibition of PDE5 activity with dipyridamole or zaprinast may augment the vasodilator response to inhaled NO in experimental studies.

Although the primary physiologic abnormality in premature neonates with RDS is surfactant deficiency or dysfunction, severe RDS is associated with pulmonary hypertension. The presence of high PVR is associated with severe lung disease and poor outcome.[71] Although pulmonary hypertension in this setting may be due to the mechanical effects of low lung volumes, pulmonary vasoconstriction contributes to high PVR in some patients. As suggested by the marked vasodilator responsiveness to inhaled NO in premature animals,[72] low dose inhaled NO therapy (5 ppm) can improve oxygenation in selected premature neonates with severe RDS.[73] In addition to lowering PVR and improving pulmonary blood flow, low dose inhaled NO may further improve oxygenation in the absence of severe pulmonary hypertension by reducing intrapulmonary shunt, as demonstrated in adult respiratory distress syndrome (ARDS). Whether inhaled NO can safely improve oxygenation and mortality without adverse sequelae, such as increased risk of chronic lung disease or intracranial hemorrhage, is under study. Although NO may prove toxic to the premature lung, recent studies suggest that inhaled NO may decrease lung inflammation in experimental RDS in premature lambs.[74]

Conclusion

Experimental studies have clearly shown the important role of the NO-cGMP cascade in the regulation of vascular tone and reactivity of the fetal and transitional pulmonary circulation, and that abnormalities in this system contribute to abnormal pulmonary vascular tone and reactivity in an experimental model of PPHN. Although inhaled NO therapy can dramatically improve oxygenation in sick neonates with severe

PPHN and premature neonates with RDS, responsiveness is poor in some patients. Further studies of the NO-cGMP cascade may provide helpful insights into novel clinical strategies for more successful treatment of neonatal pulmonary vascular disease. In addition, since studies of vascular growth suggest important functions of NO in angiogenesis, we speculate that fetal NO production may contribute to normal lung vascular development. Mechanisms linking abnormal lung growth, the risk for pulmonary hypertension, and regulation of the NO-cGMP cascade may have important therapeutic implications in the clinical setting.

References

1. Heymann MA, Soifer SJ. Control of fetal and neonatal pulmonary circulation. In: Weir EK, Reeves JT, eds: *Pulmonary Vascular Physiology and Pathophysiology*. New York: Marcel-Dekker; 1989:33–50.
2. Rudolph AM. Fetal and neonatal pulmonary circulation. *Annu Rev Physiol* 1979;41:383–95.
3. Rudolph AM, Heymann MA, Lewis AB. Physiology and pharmacology of the pulmonary circulation in the fetus and newborn. In: Hodson W, ed: *Development of the Lung*. New York: Marcel Dekker; 1977:497–523.
4. Wallen LD, Perry SF, Alston JT, et al. Morphometric study of the role of pulmonary arterial flow in fetal lung growth in sheep. *Pediatr Res* 1990;27: 122–127.
5. Lewis AB, Heymann MA, Rudolph AM. Gestational changes in pulmonary vascular responses in fetal lambs in utero. *Circ Res* 1976;39:536–541.
6. Morin FC, Egan EA, Ferguson W, et al. Development of pulmonary vascular response to oxygen. *Am J Physiol* 1988;254:H542–H546.
7. Abman SH, Accurso FJ. Sustained fetal pulmonary vasodilation during prolonged infusion of atrial natriuretic factor and 8-bromo-guanosine monophosphate. *Am J Physiol* 1991;260:H183–H192.
8. Accurso FJ, Alpert B, Wilkening RB, et al. Time-dependent response of fetal pulmonary blood flow to an increase in fetal oxygen tension. *Respir Physiol* 1986;63:43–52.
9. Abman SH, Accurso FJ. Acute effects of partial compression of the ductus arteriosus on the fetal pulmonary circulation. *Am J Physiol* 1989;257:H626–H634.
10. Cornfield DN, McQueston JA, McMurtry IF, et al. Role of ATP-sensitive K+ channels in ovine fetal pulmonary vascular tone. *Am J Physiol* 1992; 263:H1363–H1368.
11. Hobbs AJ, Ignarro LJ. NO-cGMP signal transduction system. In: Zapol WM, Bloch K, eds: *Nitric Oxide and the Lung*. New York: Marcel Dekker; 1996:1–57.
12. Moncada S, Palmer RMJ, Higgs EA. Nitric oxide: Physiology, pathophysiology, and pharmacology. *Pharmacol Rev* 1991;43:109–142.
13. Archer SL, Huang JMC, Hampl V, et al. NO and cGMP cause vasorelaxation by activation of a charybdotoxin-sensitive K channel by cGMP-dependent protein kinase. *Proc Natl Acad Sci USA* 1994;91:7583–7587.
14. Cornfield DN, Reeve HL, Tolarova S, et al. Oxygen causes fetal pul-

monary vasodilation through activation of a calcium-dependent potassium channel. *Proc Natl Acad Sci USA* 1996;93:8089–8094.

15. Bolotina VM, Najibi S, Palacino JJ, et al. NO directly activates calcium-dependent potassium channels in vascular smooth muscle. *Nature* 1994;368: 850–853.

16. Boulanger C, Luscher TF. Release of endothelin from the porcine aorta: Inhibition by endothelium-derived nitric oxide. *J Clin Invest* 1990;85:587–590.

17. Shaul PW, Smart EJ, Robinson LJ, et al. Acylation targets endothelial NO synthase to plasmalemmel calveolae. *J Biol Chem* 1996:271:6518–6522.

18. North AJ, Star RA, Brannon TS, et al. NO synthase type I and type III gene expression are developmentally regulated in rat lung. *Am J Physiol* 1994; 266:L635–L641.

19. Kobzik L, Bredt DS, Lowenstein CJ, et al. NOS in human and rat lung: Immunocytochemical and histochemical localization. *Am J Respir Cell Mol Biol* 1993;9:371–377.

20. Bustamante SA, Pang Y, Romero S, et al. Inducible NOS and the regulation of central vessel caliber in the fetal rat. *Circulation* 1996;94:1948–1953.

21. Rairhig R, Ivy DD, Kinsella JP, et al. Inducible NOS inhibitors increase pulmonary vascular resistance in the late-gestation fetus. *J Clin Invest* 1998;101:15–21.

22. Abman SH, Chatfield BA, Rodman DM, et al. Maturation-related changes in endothelium-dependent relaxation of ovine pulmonary arteries. *Am J Physiol* 1991;260:L280–L285.

23. Kinsella JP, Ivy DD, Abman SH. Ontogeny of NO activity and response to inhaled NO in the developing ovine pulmonary circulation. *Am J Physiol* 1994;267:H1955–H1961.

24. Ziegler JW, Ivy DD, Fox JJ, et al. Dipyridamole, a cGMP phosphodiesterase inhibitor, causes pulmonary vasodilation in the ovine fetus. *Am J Physiol* 1995;269:H473–H479.

25. Hanson KA, Burns F, Rybalkin SD, et al. Developmental changes in lung cGMP phosphodiesterase-5 activity, protein and message. *Am J Resp Crit Care Med* 1995;158:279–288.

26. Hanson KA, Beavo JA, Abman SH, et al. Chronic intrauterine pulmonary hypertension increases lung cGMP hydrolytic activity and decreases cGMP kinase content in the ovine fetus. *Am J Physiol* 1998;275:L931–L941.

27. Abman SH, Chatfield BA, Hall SL, et al. Role of endothelium-derived relaxing factor during transition of pulmonary circulation at birth. *Am J Physiol* 1990;259:H1921–H1927.

28. McQueston JA, Cornfield DN, McMurtry IF, et al. Effects of oxygen and exogenous L-arginine on endothelium-derived relaxing factor activity in the fetal pulmonary circulation. *Am J Physiol* 1993;264:H865–H871.

29. Cornfield DN, Chatfield BA, McQueston JA, et al. Effects of birth-related stimuli on L-arginine-dependent pulmonary vasodilation in the ovine fetus. *Am J Physiol* 1992;262:H1474–H1481.

30. Kinsella JP, McQueston JA, Rosenberg AA, et al. Hemodynamic effects of exogenous nitric oxide in ovine transitional pulmonary circulation. *Am J Physiol* 1992;263:H875–H880.

31. Meininger GA, Davis MJ. Cellular mechanisms involved in the vascular myogenic response. *Am J Physiol* 1992;263:H647–H659.

32. Kulik TJ, Evans JN, Gamble WJ. Stretch-induced contraction in pulmonary arteries. *Am J Phsyiol* 1988;255:H1191–H1198.

33. Belik J, Stephens NL. Developmental differences in vascular smooth mus-

cle mechanics in pulmonary and systemic circulations. *J Appl Physiol* 1993;74:682–687.

33a. Storme L, Rairhig RL, Abman SH. In vivo evidence for a myogenic response in the ovine fetal pulmonary circulation. *Pediatr Res* 1999;45:425–431.

34. Beavo JA, Reifsnyder DH. Primary sequence of cyclic nucleotide phosphodiesterase isozymes and the design of selective inhibitors. *Trends Pharmacol Sci* 1990;11:150–155.

35. Braner DA, Fineman JR, Chang R, et al. M and B 22948, a cGMP phosphodiesterase inhibitor, is a pulmonary vasodilator in lambs. *Am J Physiol* 1993;264:H252–H258.

35a. Cohen AH, Hanson K, Morris K, et al. Inhibition of cGMP-specific phosphodiesterase selectively vasodilates the pulmonary circulation in chronically hypoxic rats. *J Clin Invest* 1996;97:172–179.

36. Morbidelli L, Chang C-H, Douglas JG, et al. NO mediates mitogenic effect of VEGF on coronary venular endothelium. *Am J Physiol* 1996;270:H411–H415.

37. Ziche M, Morbidelli L, Masini E, et al. NO mediates angiogenesis in vivo and endothelial cell growth and migration in vitro promoted by substance P. *J Clin Invest* 1994;94:2036–2044.

38. Halbower AC, Tuder RM, Franklin WA, et al. Maturation-related changes in endothelial NO synthase immunolocalization in the developing ovine lung. *Am J Physiol* 1994;267:L585–L591.

39. Arnal J-F, Yamin J, Dockery S, et al. Regulation of endothelial NO synthase mRNA, protein, and activity during cell growth. *Am J Physiol* 1994; 267:C1381–C1388.

40. Garg UC, Hassid A. NO-generating vasodilators and 8-bromo-cGMP inhibit mitogenesis and proliferation of cultured rat vascular smooth muscle cells. *J Clin Invest* 1989;83:17744–17747.

41. Thomae KR, Nakayama DK, Billiar TR, et al. Effect of NO on fetal pulmonary artery smooth muscle growth. *J Surg Res* 1996;270:H411–H415.

42. Fineman JR, Wong J, Morin FC, et al. Chronic NO inhibition in utero produces persistent pulmonary hypertension in newborn lambs. *J Clin Invest* 1994;93:2675–2683.

43. Cassin S. Role of prostaglandins, thromboxanes and leukotrienes in the control of the pulmonary circulation in the fetus and newborn. *Semin Perinatol* 1987;11:53–63.

44. Cassin S, Dawes GS, Mott JC, et al. Vascular resistance of the foetal and newly ventilated lung of the lamb. *J Physiol* 1964;171:61–79.

45. Davidson D, Eldemerdash A. Endothelium-derived relaxing factor: Evidence that it regulates pulmonary vascular resistance in the isolated newborn guinea pig lung. *Pediatr Res* 1991;29:538–542.

46. Leffler CW, Hessler JR, Green RS. Mechanism of stimulation of pulmonary prostacyclin synthesis at birth. *Prostaglandins* 1984;28:877–887.

47. Leffler CW, Tyler TL, Cassin S. Effect of indomethacin on pulmonary vascular response to ventilation of fetal goats. *Am J Physiol* 1978;234:H346–H351.

48. Velvis H, Moore P, Heymann MA. Prostaglandin inhibition prevents the fall in pulmonary vascular resistance as the result of rhythmic distension of the lungs in fetal lambs. *Pediatr Res* 1991;30:62–67.

49. Steudel W, Scherrer-Crosbie M, Bloch KD, et al. Sustained pulmonary hypertension and right ventricular hypertrophy after chronic hypoxia in mice with congenital deficiency of NOS III. *J Clin Invest* 1998;101:2468–2477.

50. Levin DL, Heymann MA, Kitterman JA, et al. Persistent pulmonary hypertension of the newborn. *J Pediatr* 1976;89:626–633.
51. Geggel RL, Reid LM. The structural basis of persistent pulmonary hypertension of the newborn. *Clin Perinatol* 1984;3:525–549.
52. Allen K, Haworth SG. Impaired adaptation of intrapulmonary arteries to extrauterine life in newborn pigs exposed to hypoxia: An ultrastructural study. *Fed Proc* 1986;45:879.
53. Stenmark KR, Abman SH, Accurso FJ. Etiologic mechanisms of persistent pulmonary hypertension of the newborn. In: Weir EK, Reeves JT, eds: *Pulmonary Vascular Physiology and Pathophysiology*. New York: Marcel-Dekker; 1989:335.
54. Goldberg SJ, Levy RA, Siassi B. Effects of maternal hypoxia and hyperoxia upon the neonatal pulmonary vasculature. *Pediatrics* 1971;48:528.
55. Levin DL, Hyman AI, Heymann MA. Fetal hypertension and the development of increased pulmonary vascular smooth muscle: A possible mechanism for persistent pulmonary hypertension of the newborn infant. *J Pediatr* 1978;92:265–269.
56. Abman SH, Shanley PF, Accurso FJ. Failure of postnatal adaptation of the pulmonary circulation after chronic intrauterine pulmonary hypertension in fetal lambs. *J Clin Invest* 1989;83:1849–1858.
57. Morin FC. Ligating the ductus arteriosus before birth causes persistent pulmonary hypertension in the newborn lamb. *Pediatr Res* 1989;25:245–250.
58. McQueston JA, Kinsella JP, Ivy DD, et al. Chronic pulmonary hypertension *in utero* impairs endothelium-dependent vasodilation. *Am J Physiol* 1995;268:H288–H294.
59. Villamor E, Le Cras TD, Horan M, et al. Chronic hypertension impairs endothelial NO synthase in the ovine fetus. *Am J Physiol* 1997;16:L1013–L1020.
60. Steinhorn RH, Russell JA, Morin FC. Disruption of cGMP production in pulmonary arteries isolated from fetal lambs with pulmonary hypertension. *Am J Physiol* 1995;268:H1483–H1489.
61. Hampl V, Herget J. Perinatal hypoxia increases hypoxic pulmonary vasoconsriction in adult rats recovering from chronic exposure to hypoxia. *Am Rev Resp Dis* 1990;142:619–624.
62. Sato K, Webb S, Tucker A, et al. Factors influencing the idiopathic development of pulmonary hypertension in the fawn-hooded rat. *Am Rev Resp Dis* 1992;145:793–797.
63. Fratacci M-D, Frostell CG, Chen TY, et al. Inhaled NO: A selective pulmonary vasodilator of heparin-protamine vasoconstriction in sheep. *Anesthesiology* 1991;75:990–999.
64. Roberts JD, Chen T, Kawai N, et al. Inhaled NO reverses pulmonary vasoconstriction in the hypoxic and acidotic newborn lamb. *Circ Res* 1993;72:246–254.
65. Roberts JD, Polaner DM, Lang P, et al. Inhaled nitric oxide in persistent pulmonary hypertension of the newborn. *Lancet* 1992;340:818–819.
66. Kinsella JP, Neish S, Shaffer E, et al. Low dose inhalational nitric oxide in persistent pulmonary hypertension of the newborn. *Lancet* 1992;340:819–820.
67. Kinsella JP, Neish SR, Ivy DD, et al. Clinical responses to prolonged treatment of persistent pulmonary hypertension of the newborn. *J Pediatr* 1993;123:103–108.
68. Neonatal Inhaled NO Study Group. Inhaled NO in full-term and nearly full-term infants with hypoxic respiratory failure. *N Engl J Med* 1997;336:597–604.

69. Roberts JD, Fineman JR, Morin FC, et al. Inhaled NO and PPHN. *N Engl J Med* 1997;336:605–610.
70. Roberts JD, Kinsella JP, Abman SH. Inhaled NO in neonatal pulmonary hypertension and severe RDS: Experimental and clinical studies. In: Zapol WM, Bloch K, eds: *Nitric Oxide and the Lung*. New York: Marcel Dekker; 1996:333–363.
71. Walther FJ, Bender FJ, Leighton JO. Persistent pulmonary hypertension in premature neonates with severe RDS. *Pediatrics* 1992;90:899–904.
72. Kinsella JP, Ivy DD, Abman SH. Inhaled nitric oxide improves gas exchange and lowers pulmonary vascular resistance in severe experimental hyaline membrane disease. *Pediatr Res* 1994;36:402–408.
73. Abman SH, Kinsella JP, Schaffer MS, et al. Inhaled nitric oxide therapy in a premature newborn with severe respiratory distress and pulmonary hypertension. *Pediatrics* 1993;92:606–609.
74. Kinsella JP, Halbower AC, Ziegler JW, et al. Effects of inhaled NO on pulmonary edema and lung neutrophil accumulation in severe experimental HMD. *Pediatr Res* 1997;41:457–463.

Chapter 16

Regulation of Endothelial Nitric Oxide Synthase Expression in the Developing Lung

Philip W. Shaul, MD

Introduction

The successful transition from fetal to neonatal life is dependent upon a dramatic fall in pulmonary vascular resistance, with pulmonary blood flow increasing as much as 10-fold and pulmonary arterial pressure falling from systemic levels in the fetus to one-half systemic values within hours.[1] Studies over the past decade have revealed that the signaling molecule nitric oxide (NO) produced by the enzyme NO synthase (NOS) is critically involved in this process. It is now apparent that NO also plays a role in the regulation of lung liquid production around the time of birth. This chapter will first summarize our general understanding of the regulation of NO production by NOS and the unique roles of NO in the developing lung. Mechanisms regulating the localization of the endothelial isoform of NOS (eNOS), which is the major vascular form of the enzyme, will then be addressed. In addition, the processes responsible for maturational changes in pulmonary eNOS expression will be discussed. Finally, abnormalities in eNOS expression associated with neonatal pulmonary vascular disease will be considered.

This work was supported by National Institutes of Health Grants HD-30276 and HL-58888, a Grant-in-Aid from the American Heart Association and Sanofi Winthrop, and an Established Investigatorship of the American Heart Association.

From: Weir EK, Archer SL, Reeves JT (eds). *The Fetal and Neonatal Pulmonary Circulations.* Armonk, NY: Futura Publishing Company, Inc.; ©1999.

NOS Isoforms and NO Production

In mammalian cells, NO is produced from the terminal guanidinium nitrogen of L-arginine upon its conversion to L-citrulline by NOS in a reaction that requires molecular oxygen.[2] NOS is a family of enzymes that currently includes three major isoforms known as neuronal NOS (nNOS), inducible NOS (iNOS), and endothelial NOS (eNOS).[3-9] The three isoforms, nNOS, iNOS, and eNOS, are also referred to as NOS-I, NOS-II, and NOS-III. The activity of nNOS and eNOS is calcium-dependent, whereas the activity of iNOS is calcium-independent.[2] nNOS and iNOS are primarily found in the soluble fraction, whereas eNOS is primarily in the membrane fraction.[2] All NOS isoforms are homodimers of subunits that range between 130 and 160 kD.[10] Until recently (see below), nNOS and eNOS were believed to be primarily constitutive in nature, whereas the expression of iNOS is initiated by cytokines such as tumor necrosis factor-α, interferon-γ, interferon-α, and interleukin-1β, and also by endotoxin.[2,11]

Role of NO in the Developing Lung

Role of NO in the Pulmonary Circulation

Considerable investigative efforts have been made in the past several years advancing our understanding of the physiology of NO and its capacity to relax smooth muscle in the vasculature of the late fetal and early postnatal lung. In the late-gestation fetal lamb, the intrapulmonary infusion of the NOS inhibitor nitro-L-arginine (L-NA) causes a fall in pulmonary blood flow,[12] indicating that there is basal pulmonary endothelial NO production contributing to the modulation of the pulmonary circulation. In addition, the infusion of the endothelium-dependent vasodilator acetylcholine (Ach) causes an increase in pulmonary blood flow that is negated by NOS inhibition, signifying that there is also the capacity to stimulate further NO production.[12,13] The modulation of pulmonary vascular resistance by endogenous NO is also evident earlier in gestation (0.78 term).[14] Furthermore, comparable studies in the intact newborn lamb and experiments in isolated perfused newborn guinea pig lung indicate that NO also mediates pulmonary vascular tone in the postnatal period.[15,16]

The lamb model has been used in studies of the transition of the pulmonary circulation at birth. In late-gestation fetal lambs, there is an immediate and dramatic rise in pulmonary blood flow and a fall in pulmonary artery pressure with cesarean section delivery and ventilation with 100% oxygen. These responses are markedly attenuated if delivery and ventilation take place following L-NA infusion into the pulmonary artery. These findings indicate that NO is critically involved in the birth-related decline in pulmonary vascular resistance.[12] Studies have also been done which demonstrate that NO plays a major role in the perinatal pulmonary vasodilator responses to the individual birth-related physical stimuli of ventilation, and increased oxygenation and shear stress.[17,18]

Further investigations have revealed that there are maturational changes in NO-mediated dilatation of the pulmonary circulation. In sheep, experiments with both isolated pulmonary arterial segments and perfused lung preparations indicate that there are developmental increases in NO-mediated relaxation during the late fetal and early postnatal periods.[19–21] In the pig, there is an increase in NO-mediated vasodilation during the first 2 weeks of postnatal life, followed by a decline.[22,23] These findings suggest that the capacity for NO-mediated processes increases during late fetal and early postnatal development, thereby optimizing pulmonary vasodilation at the time of transition and immediately after birth.

Role of NO in the Lung Epithelium

There is accumulating evidence that NO is also of importance as a signaling molecule modulating lung epithelial function in the perinatal period. It has been shown that Ach and bradykinin, which stimulate NO synthesis, cause marked decreases in lung liquid production in late-gestation fetal lambs.[24] In addition, the instillation of NO or cGMP, the second messenger for NO, directly into the fetal lung liquid has the same effect.[25,26] The decrease in lung liquid production, which occurs in the respiratory epithelium at the time of birth, is an essential component of the transition of the fetus from a liquid-breathing to an air-breathing status. Epithelium-derived NO is also critical to the regulation of bronchomotor tone in the developing lung, playing a role in the opposition of airway contraction, particularly in the early newborn period.[27] Furthermore, the pharmacological inhibition of NO production increases tissue resistance in the newborn lung, suggesting that endogenous NO may also regulate peripheral contractile elements.[28] Thus, NO is critical to the functions of numerous pulmonary cell types involved in cardiopulmonary transition at birth.

Localization of Pulmonary eNOS

Cell Specificity of eNOS Expression

The diversity of roles of NO in the developing lung would suggest that NOS is expressed in a variety of pulmonary cell types. Since eNOS is the principal isoform found in the vasculature, studies were performed using immunohistochemistry to delineate the distribution of eNOS in fetal (125–135 days' gestation, term = 144 days), newborn (2–4 weeks), and adult sheep lung.[29] Parallel experiments were done to reveal the distribution of iNOS and nNOS. In all age groups that were examined, eNOS protein was readily detectable in the endothelium at all levels of the vasculature. In fetal lung, eNOS expression was also readily evident in bronchial and proximal bronchiolar epithelium, but it was absent in terminal or respiratory bronchioles or alveolar epithelium. Similar to eNOS, iNOS was detected in bronchial and proximal bronchiolar epithelium, but not in alveolar epithelium. However, iNOS was also detected in the epithelium of terminal and respiratory bronchioles. nNOS was found in epithelium at all levels including the alveolar wall. In addition, iNOS and nNOS were evident in airway and vascular smooth muscle. The cellular distribution of all three isoforms was similar in fetal, newborn, and adult lung, but the intensity of eNOS staining was greatest in adult epithelium. Findings in the epithelium were confirmed by isoform-specific reverse transcription-polymerase chain reaction assays, and the observations made in all pulmonary cell types were corroborated by NADPH diaphorase histochemistry. Thus, eNOS is expressed in the vascular endothelium and proximal airway epithelium of the developing lung, and its cellular distribution differs from that of iNOS and nNOS. These observations suggest that numerous cell types besides the endothelium may be important sources of the endogenous NO that mediates both vascular and parenchymal function in the developing lung.

To begin to understand the basis of cell-specific eNOS expression in the airway epithelium, transient transfection studies were performed in human bronchiolar epithelial cells (NCI-H441) with the human eNOS promoter fused to a luciferase reporter gene (Luc).[30] Transfection with 1624 bp of the eNOS promoter sequence 5' to the initiation ATG (−1624eNOS-Luc) yielded a 19-fold increase in promoter activity relative to vector alone. Similarly, −1624eNOS-Luc yielded a 35-fold increase in promoter activity in pulmonary artery endothelial cells (PAECs). However, there was no detectable promoter activity with −1624eNOS-Luc transfected into CCD-18Lu lung fibroblasts, consistent with the cell-specific expression of pulmonary eNOS in the airway epithelium and vascular endothelium. There was 6-fold greater promoter activity in the

H441 cells, which are of Clara cell origin, compared with the non-Clara cell human airway epithelial lines BEAS-2B and NHBE. 5'deletion of the eNOS promoter from −1624 to −994, −318, and −279 did not alter basal eNOS promoter activity in the epithelial cells. However, further deletion from −279 to −248 reduced basal promoter activity by 65%, and activity was completely lost with deletion to −79. Point mutations of −1624eNOS-Luc revealed that the positive regulatory element between −279 and −248 is the consensus GATA-binding motif at −254, and that the positive regulatory element between −248 and −79 is the Sp1-binding motif at −125 (Figure 1). Parallel studies in PAECs revealed identical findings. Electrophoretic mobility shift assays (EMSA) yielded two epithelial nuclear protein-DNA complexes with the GATA site and four complexes with the Sp1 site. Immunodepletion with antisera to GATA-2 prevented formation of both GATA-nuclear protein complexes, and antisera to Sp1 supershifted the slowest migrating Sp1-nuclear protein

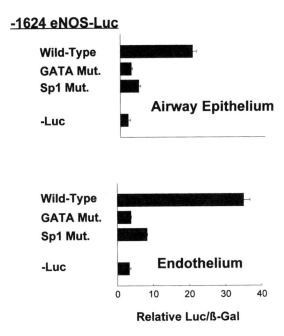

Figure 1. Activity of GATA and Sp1 site mutants of the eNOS gene promoter −1624eNOS-Luc in H441 airway epithelial cells (upper panel) and pulmonary endothelial cells (lower panel). The −1624eNOS-Luc wild-type construct, site-directed mutants of the GATA consensus site at −254, Sp1-binding motif at −125, or vector alone (−Luc) were cotransfected with SV40-driven β-galactosidase plasmid. Relative activities (Luc/β-gal) were determined in cell lysates. Values are mean ± SEM for n = 3, and the results are representative of the findings of three independent experiments.[30]

complex. Although EMSA with lung fibroblast nuclei showed complexes with the Sp1 site that were identical to those observed with epithelial nuclei, the slower-migrating GATA-nuclear protein complex seen with epithelial cells was absent. These findings suggest that the interaction of GATA-2 nuclear protein with the GATA site within the core eNOS promoter to form the slower-migrating GATA protein complex is critically involved in cell-specific eNOS expression in the airway epithelium. They also indicate that identical mechanisms most likely underlie cell-specific eNOS expression in the airway epithelium and vascular endothelium.

Subcellular Localization of eNOS

Since eNOS activity is acutely regulated by extracellular factors and the NO produced is a labile, cytotoxic messenger molecule,[31-34] the intracellular site of NO synthesis is likely to have a major influence on its biological activity. Studies were therefore designed to determine the specific subcellular location to which endothelial cell eNOS is targeted, delineating whether the enzyme is localized to plasmalemmal caveolae.[35] Caveolae are microdomains known to compartmentalize signaling molecules, including many that modulate eNOS activity.[36,37] These include G-protein-coupled receptors such as the muscarinic Ach receptor, a plasma membrane Ca^{2+} pump, an IP_3-sensitive Ca^{2+} channel, and protein kinase C.[36-38]

In the first series of experiments, caveolae membranes (CM) were isolated from highly purified plasma membrane (PM) fractions prepared from ovine fetal PAECs using a detergent-free method that takes advantage of the unique bouyant density of CM.[39] The subcellular fractions obtained were postnuclear supernatant (PNS), cytosol, PM, non-caveolae membrane PM (NCM), and CM. Using immunoblot analysis, eNOS protein was found to be highly enriched in CM, and it was not detectable in NCM. It was then determined if the localization of eNOS protein to caveolae correlates with NOS enzymatic activity. NOS activity was 7-fold greater in PM than in cytosol (Figure 2), consistent with the observations of numerous previous investigators.[40] Within the PM, NOS activity was undetectable in NCM, whereas it was 9.4-fold enriched in CM compared to whole PM. In three independent experiments, 51–86% of the total activity in PNS was recovered in PM, and 11–29% was recovered in cytosol. More importantly, 57–100% of the total activity in PM was recovered in the CM, indicating that plasmalemmal eNOS is primarily localized to caveolae. A similar distribution was demonstrated in H441 airway epithelial cells, suggesting that the subcellular localization of eNOS is identical in the two pulmonary cell types that express the enzyme. The findings in the PAECs were confirmed by

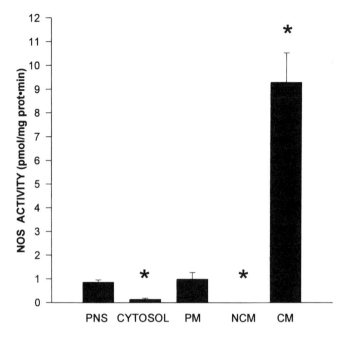

Figure 2. NOS enzymatic activity in subcellular fractions from pulmonary artery endothelial cells (PAECs). Samples of postnuclear supernatant (PNS), cytosol, plasma membrane (PM), noncaveolae membrane (NCM) and caveolae membrane (CM) were evaluated. NOS activity was determined by measurement of [^{3}H]-L-arginine conversion to [^{3}H]-L-citrulline. Enzymatic activity was undetectable in NCM. Comparable findings were obtained in three independent experiments. Mean ± SEM, *p<0.02 vs. PM.[35]

immunoelectron microscopy, which showed that eNOS heavily decorated endothelial caveolae, whereas coated pits and smooth PM were devoid of gold particles.

Further experiments were done to determine the basis for eNOS targeting to caveolae, focusing on the roles of myristoylation and palmitoylation. Myristoylation and palmitoylation are co- and post-translational processes, respectively, which couple specific lipid moieties to unique domains on the eNOS protein, enabling it to associate with cellular membranes.[41] Wild-type, myristoylation-deficient and palmitoylation-deficient mutant eNOS cDNAs were transiently transfected into COS-7 cells, which possess caveolae but do not express NOS constitutively. The subcellular distribution of wild-type eNOS in the COS-7 cells was identical to that obtained for native eNOS in endothelial cells, indicating that the eNOS protein and the CM collectively possess all of the properties necessary for this association to occur. Furthermore, the studies with the eNOS mutants revealed that both myristoylation and palmitoylation are required to target eNOS to caveolae, with each acylation process enhancing targeting by 10-fold. Thus, acylation targets eNOS to plasmalemmal caveolae, and trafficking to this microdomain is likely to optimize eNOS activation and the release of NO from both vascular endothelium and airway epithelium.[35] It is now apparent that the cellular and subcellular localization of eNOS in the lung is controlled by a variety of complex mechanisms.

Maturational Changes in Pulmonary eNOS Expression

As mentioned above, there are developmental increases in NO-mediated pulmonary vascular relaxation in the late fetal and early postnatal periods which optimize pulmonary vasodilation at the time of transition and immediately after birth.[19–21] To determine the basis for these maturational changes, endothelial NO production was investigated in ovine fetal and newborn intrapulmonary arteries.[42] It was found that basal endothelial NO production rises 2-fold from late gestation to 1 week of age, and an additional 1.6-fold from 1 to 4 weeks. Ach-stimulated NO production also increases 1.6-fold from 1 to 4 weeks. The maturational rise in NO production is evident at high PO_2 in vitro, and it is not modified by L-arginine, indicating that it is not related to changes in the availability of the substrates for NOS activity. Alternatively, it may be due to either maturational enhancement of calcium-calmodulin-mediated mechanisms, a developmental increase in eNOS abundance, or greater availability of cofactor(s) required for its activity.

To determine whether there are increases in eNOS abundance that prepare the pulmonary circulation for NO-mediated vasodilation at the time of birth, the ontogeny of eNOS expression was examined in distal lung specimens from fetal and newborn rats, thereby focusing on the endothelial expression of the isoform.[43] Maturational changes in distal lung nNOS expression were also investigated to determine if the findings for eNOS are unique to that isoform. NOS proteins were examined by immunoblot analysis, and mRNA abundance was assessed in RT-PCR assays. eNOS protein was detectable in day 16 fetal lung, its expression increased 3.8-fold to maximal levels at 20 days' gestation (term = 22 days), and fell postnatally (1–5 days) (Figure 3). nNOS protein expression also rose during late gestation (3.1-fold) and fell postnatally. In parallel with the findings for eNOS protein, eNOS mRNA increased from 16 to 20 days' gestation and fell after birth. In contrast, nNOS mRNA abundance declined during late fetal life and rose postnatally. Findings by RT-PCR were confirmed by Northern blot analyses. These observations indicate that eNOS and nNOS gene expression are devel-

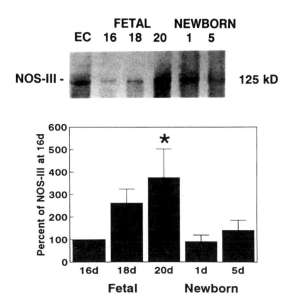

Figure 3. **Upper panel:** Immunoblot analysis for eNOS (NOS-III) in lungs from fetal rats at 16, 18, and 20 days' gestation and newborn rats at 1 and 5 days of age. Protein from endothelial cells (EC) was used as a positive control. Signal for eNOS was evident at 125–135 kD. These results are representative of six independent experiments. **Lower panel:** Summary data for quantitative densitometry for the six experiments. Mean ± SEM values are depicted for protein abundance expressed as percent of eNOS at 16 days' gestation. *p<0.05 vs. 16 days.[43]

opmentally regulated in rat lung, with maximal eNOS and nNOS protein expression near term. Furthermore, the regulation of pulmonary eNOS may primarily involve alterations in gene transcription or mRNA stability, whereas nNOS expression in the maturing lung may also be mediated by additional post-transcriptional processes. Similar developmental upregulation in eNOS expression has been demonstrated in ovine fetal lung.[44] The maximization of lung NOS expression at the time of birth may serve to optimize not only the capacity for NO-mediated pulmonary vasodilation during transition, but also the ability to decrease lung liquid production.

Mechanisms Regulating eNOS Expression During Lung Development

Studies have been performed in cultured ovine fetal PAECs to evaluate the direct effects of specific factors on eNOS gene expression. The effects of estrogen were assessed because fetal plasma estrogen levels

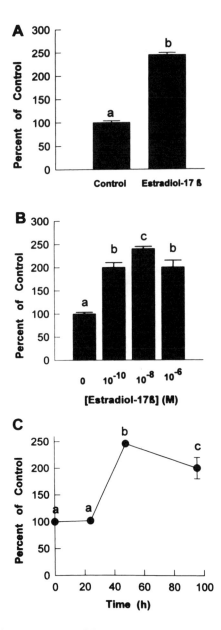

Figure 4. Effect of estrogen on NOS activity in fetal pulmonary artery endothelial cells (PAECs). A: NOS enzymatic activity was determined in lysates of control and E_2-treated cells (10^{-8} mol/L, 48 hours) by measuring [^{3}H]-L-arginine conversion to [^{3}H]-L-citrulline. B: The dose response to varying concentrations for 48 hours. C: The time course of effect of E_2 was determined in cells exposed to 10^{-8} mol/L E_2 for varying durations up to 96 hours. Results are expressed as percentage of NOS activity in control cells. The SEM for some data points was smaller than the symbol depicting the mean value (n=4). Different letters denote differences between groups by ANOVA.[46]

rise markedly during late gestation due to increased placental production of the hormone, and because there is evidence that estrogen enhances nonpulmonary NO production in adults.[45,46] It was found that NOS enzymatic activity is markedly increased in estradiol (E_2)-treated ovine fetal PAECs, and that this occurs after 48 hours in response to physiologic concentrations of the hormone (10^{-10} to 10^{-8} mol/L) (Figure 4).[46] The increase in NOS activity is related to an upregulation in eNOS protein and mRNA expression. In addition, estrogen receptor protein and mRNA expression were documented in the ovine fetal PAEC, and estrogen receptor antagonism completely inhibited E_2-mediated eNOS upregulation. Thus, physiologic levels of estrogen cause enhanced eNOS gene expression in fetal PAECs through the activation of PAEC estrogen receptors. This mechanism may be responsible for normal pulmonary eNOS upregulation during late gestation. In addition, since pregnancies complicated by placental dysfunction are characterized by attenuated placental estrogen synthesis,[47,48] it is postulated that the diminution in estrogen may lead to decreased pulmonary eNOS expression, thereby contributing to the pathogenesis of the persistent pulmonary hypertension of the newborn (PPHN) which is often associated with such pregnancies.

eNOS and Neonatal Pulmonary Vascular Disease

PPHN can also occur as a result of a variety of primary pulmonary conditions, including the lung hypoplasia which accompanies congenital diaphragmatic hernia (CDH). To determine the potential role of alterations in pulmonary eNOS expression in this process, a rat model of CDH was studied. The development of CDH can be induced in approximately 50–60% of rat fetuses following maternal ingestion of the herbicide nitrofen early in gestation. In this model, eNOS protein abundance is decreased by 42% in the lung ipsilateral to the hernia compared with lungs from control fetuses exposed to nitrofen but lacking CDH.[49] Immunoblot analysis for factor VIII-related antigen indicates that this is not due to alterations in endothelial cell density, and studies of nNOS protein reveal that this finding is unique to eNOS. eNOS mRNA abundance evaluated by RT-PCR is also decreased in CDH lung, falling to 22% of control levels (Figure 5). These findings suggest that attenuated eNOS expression may contribute to PPHN in infants with CDH.

eNOS expression has also been evaluated in a lamb model of neonatal pulmonary hypertension created by ligation of the fetal ductus arteriosus 10 days prior to delivery. Earlier studies revealed that NO-dependent relaxation is attenuated in intrapulmonary arteries from these animals.[50] It was found that eNOS protein expression is decreased

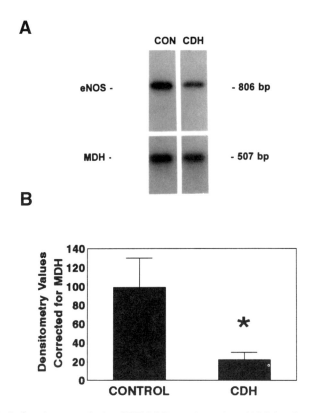

Figure 5. A: Southern analysis of RT-PCR products for eNOS (top) and malate dehydrogenase (MDH, bottom) in control (CON) and congenital diaphragmatic hernia (CDH) lungs. Band sizes were: eNOS, 806 bp; MDH, 507 bp. These data are representative of five independent experiments. B: Summary data for the five experiments is shown. eNOS densitometry values corrected for MDH are expressed as the percent in control samples (mean ± SEM). *p<0.05 vs. control.[49]

49% in the hypertensive lung and nNOS expression is unaltered. Similarly, NOS enzymatic activity is decreased 45% in the hypertensive lung. Paralleling the declines in eNOS protein and NOS enzymatic activity, eNOS mRNA abundance is decreased 64% in the hypertensive lung.[51] Similar findings have been obtained by other investigators.[44] Thus, pulmonary eNOS gene expression is attenuated in the lamb model of neonatal pulmonary hypertension.

Since chronic hypoxia is frequently an important causal factor in the development of PPHN, the effects of prolonged hypoxia on pulmonary eNOS expression have also been investigated. Previous studies revealed that chronic hypoxia attenuates both Ach-stimulated pulmonary vasodilation, and basal and Ach-stimulated NO production in the lungs of chronically hypoxic piglets.[52,53] These findings suggest that decreased pulmonary NO production contributes to the development of hypoxic pulmonary hypertension in the newborn. More recent work has demonstrated that this is due to decreased eNOS expression.[54,55] Interestingly, in adult rats chronic hypoxia causes an upregulation of both eNOS and nNOS expression in the lung.[56] This suggests that the response of pulmonary eNOS to chronic hypoxia is age-specific.

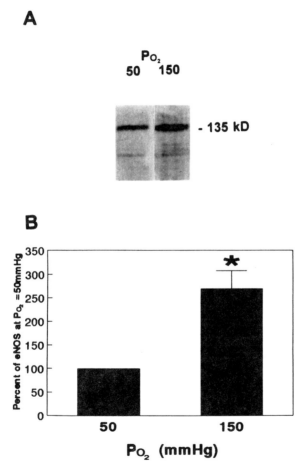

Figure 6. A: Immunoblot analysis for eNOS in fetal PAECs exposed to a P_{O_2} level of 50 or 150 mm Hg for 48 hours. Signal for eNOS was evident at 135 kD. These results are representative of six independent experiments. B: Summary data for quantitative densitometry for the six experiments. Mean ± SEM values are depicted for protein abundance expressed as the percent of eNOS at P_{O_2} = 50 mm Hg. *$p<0.05$ vs. P_{O_2} = 50 mm Hg.[57]

To determine whether hypoxia has direct effects on eNOS expression in the developing pulmonary endothelium, experiments were performed in cultured ovine fetal PAECs. It was found that eNOS protein abundance is decreased 63% in PAECs exposed to media with $PO_2 = 50$ mm Hg compared with cells exposed to $PO_2 = 150$ for 48 hours (Figure 6).[57] The fall in eNOS protein abundance is associated with 60% less NOS enzymatic activity evaluated by [^{3}H]-L-arginine to [^{3}H]-L-citrulline conversion. Steady-state levels of eNOS mRNA are also diminished by 64% at lower oxygen tension. These findings indicate that decreased oxygenation directly downregulates eNOS gene expression in fetal PAECs. Thus, there is accumulating evidence from intact animal models and cell culture studies that eNOS expression is attenuated in conditions associated with PPHN. Since NO modulates both vasodilation and vascular smooth muscle growth,[58] diminished eNOS expression may contribute to both the abnormal vasoreactivity and the excessive muscularization characteristic of many forms of the disorder.

Conclusion

It is now apparent that NO plays a critical role in modulating pulmonary vasomotor tone at the time of transition from fetal to newborn life, and that it is also involved in the regulation of lung liquid production in the perinatal period. Perhaps consistent with these multiple roles, it has been found that the endothelial isoform of NOS (eNOS) is expressed not only in the pulmonary vascular endothelium, but also in the proximal airway epithelium. In addition, iNOS is expressed in the airway epithelium and vascular and airway smooth muscle, and nNOS is found in the epithelium throughout the respiratory tract and also in vascular and airway smooth muscle. These findings suggest that numerous cell types besides the vascular endothelium may be important sources of the endogenous NO that mediates both vascular and parenchymal function in the developing lung. The cell-specific expression of eNOS in the airway epithelium and endothelium appears to involve the nuclear protein GATA-2 and a GATA-binding domain within the core eNOS promoter. Furthermore, there is specific subcellular localization of eNOS in plasmalemmal caveolae that is due to the myristoylation and palmitoylation of the protein. Thus, the cellular and subcellular localization of eNOS expression in the lung is controlled by a variety of complex mechanisms.

In addition to the processes dictating the sites of eNOS enzymatic activity in the developing lung, there are molecular events which normally occur during late gestation to enhance eNOS enzyme abundance, thereby optimizing the capacity for pulmonary NO production at birth.

Experiments in cultured ovine fetal PAECs have demonstrated that physiologic concentrations of estrogen upregulate eNOS via the activation of endothelial estrogen receptors, raising the possibility that increasing levels of placentally derived estrogen during late fetal life may mediate the maturational increase in pulmonary eNOS expression. Furthermore, studies in both intact animal models and cell culture indicate that eNOS expression is markedly attenuated in conditions associated with PPHN such as CDH and prolonged hypoxia. Continued investigation of the regulation of NOS expression in the developing lung will increase our fundamental knowledge of both successful and unsuccessful cardiopulmonary transition at birth. It is only through such an increased understanding that novel therapies will be discovered for neonatal pulmonary vascular disease.

Acknowledgment The assistance of Marilyn Dixon in the preparation of this manuscript is much appreciated.

References

1. Dawes GS, Mott JC, Widdecombe JG. Changes in the lungs of the newborn lamb. *J Physiol (Lond)* 1953;121:141–162.
2. Schmidt HHHW, Lohmann SM, Walter U. The nitric oxide and cGMP signal transduction system: Regulation and mechanism of action. *Biochim Biophys Acta* 1993;1178:153–175.
3. Bredt DS, Hwang PM, Glatt CE, et al. Cloned and expressed nitric oxide synthase structurally resembles cytochrome P-450 reductase. *Nature* 1991; 351:714–718.
4. Lyons CR, Orloff GJ, Cunningham JM. Molecular cloning and functional expression of an inducible nitric oxide synthase from a murine macrophage cell line. *J Biol Chem* 1992;267:6370–6374.
5. Xie Q, Cho HJ, Calaycay J, et al. Cloning and characterization of inducible nitric oxide synthase from mouse macrophages. *Science* 1992;256:225–228.
6. Lamas S, Marsden PA, Li GK, et al. Endothelial nitric oxide synthase: Molecular cloning and characterization of a distinct constitutive enzyme isoform. *Proc Natl Acad Sci USA* 1992;89:6348–6352.
7. Sessa WC, Harrison JK, Barber CM, et al. Molecular cloning and expression of a cDNA encoding endothelial cell nitric oxide synthase. *J Biol Chem* 1992;267:15274–15276.
8. Marsden PA, Schappert KT, Chen HS, et al. Molecular cloning and characterization of human endothelial nitric oxide synthase. *FEBS Lett* 1992; 307:287–293.
9. Nishida K, Harrison DG, Navas JP, et al. Molecular cloning and characterization of the constitutive bovine aortic endothelial cell nitric oxide synthase. *J Clin Invest* 1992;90:2092–2096.
10. Lowenstein CJ, Snyder SH. Nitric oxide, a novel biologic messenger. *Cell* 1992;70:705–707.
11. Nunokawa Y, Ishida N, Tanaka S. Promoter analysis of human inducible nitric oxide synthase gene associated with cardiovascular homeostasis. *Biochem Biophys Res Commun* 1994;200:802–807.

12. Abman SH, Chatfield BA, Hall SL, et al. Role of endothelium-derived relaxing factor during transition of pulmonary circulation at birth. *Am J Physiol* 1990;259:H1921–H1927.
13. Tiktinsky MH, Cummings JJ, Morin FC. Acetylcholine increases pulmonary blood flow in intact fetuses via endothelium-dependent vasodilation. *Am J Physiol* 1992;262:H406–H410.
14. Kinsella JP, Ivy DD, Abman SH. Ontogeny of NO activity and response to inhaled NO in the developing ovine pulmonary circulation. *Am J Physiol* 1994;267:H1955–H1961.
15. Fineman JR, Heymann MA, Soifer SJ. Nʷ-nitro-L-arginine attenuates endothelium-dependent pulmonary vasodilation in lambs. *Am J Physiol* 1991;260:H1299–H1306.
16. Davidson D, Eldemerdash A. Endothelium-derived relaxing factor: Evidence that it regulates pulmonary vascular resistance in the isolated neonatal guinea pig lung. *Pediatr Res* 1991;29:538–542.
17. Cornfield DN, Chatfield BA, McQueston JA, et al. Effects of birth-related stimuli on L-arginine-dependent pulmonary vasodilation in ovine fetus. *Am J Physiol* 1992;262:H1474–H1481.
18. Tiktinsky MH, Morin FC. Increasing oxygen tension dilates fetal pulmonary circulation via endothelium-derived relaxing factor. *Am J Physiol* 1993;265:H376–H380.
19. Abman SH, Chatfield BA, Rodman DM, et al. Maturational changes in endothelium-derived relaxing factor activity of ovine pulmonary arteries in vitro. *Am J Physiol* 1991;260:L280–L285.
20. Steinhorn RH, Morin FC, Gugino SF, et al. Developmental differences in endothelium-dependent responses in isolated ovine pulmonary arteries and veins. *Am J Physiol* 1993;264:H2162–H2167.
21. Gordon JB, Todd ML. Effects of Nʷ-nitro-L-arginine on total and segmental vascular resistances in developing lamb lungs. *J Appl Physiol* 1993;75:76–85.
22. Zellers TM, Vanhoutte PM. Endothelium-dependent relaxations of piglet pulmonary arteries augment with maturation. *Pediatr Res* 1991;30:176–180.
23. Liu SF, Hislop AA, Haworth SG, et al. Developmental changes in endothelium-dependent pulmonary vasodilatation in pigs. *Br J Pharmacol* 1992;106:324–330.
24. Cummings JJ. Pulmonary vasodilator drugs decrease lung liquid production in fetal sheep. *J Appl Physiol* 1995;79:1212–1218.
25. Cummings JJ. Nitric oxide decreases lung liquid production in fetal lambs. *J Appl Physiol* 1997;83:1538–1544.
26. Cummings JJ, Wang H. Reduction in lung liquid production caused by nitric oxide is enhanced by zaprinast. *Pediatr Res* 1998;43:279A.
27. Jakupaj M, Martin RJ, Dreshaj IA, et al. Role of endogenous NO in modulating airway contraction mediated by muscarinic receptors during development. *Am J Physiol* 1997;273:L531–L536.
28. Potter CF, Dreshaj IA, Haxhiu MA, et al. Effect of exogenous and endogenous nitric oxide on the airway and tissue components of lung resistance in the newborn piglet. *Pediatr Res* 1997;41:886–891.
29. Sherman TS, Chen Z, Yuhanna IS, et al. Nitric oxide synthase isoform expression in the developing lung epithelium. *Am J Physiol* 1999;276:L383–L390.
30. German Z, Pace MC, Michel T, et al. Molecular basis of cell-specific endothelial nitric oxide synthase expression in airway epithelium. *Pediatr Res* 1998;43:47A.

31. Bredt DS, Snyder SH. Nitric oxide: A physiologic messenger molecule. *Annu Rev Biochem* 1994;63:175–195.
32. Nathan C, Xie QW. Regulation of biosynthesis of nitric oxide. *J Biol Chem* 1994;269:13725–13728.
33. Moncada S, Higgs A. The L-arginine-nitric oxide pathway. *N Engl J Med* 1993;329:2002–2012.
34. Shaul PW. Nitric oxide in the developing lung. In: Barness LA, ed: *Advances in Pediatrics*. Chicago: Mosby-Year Book, Inc; 1995:367–414.
35. Shaul PW, Smart EJ, Robinson LJ, et al. Acylation targets endothelial nitric oxide synthase to plasmalemmal caveolae. *J Biol Chem* 1996;271:6518–6522.
36. Anderson RGW. Caveolae: Where incoming and outgoing messengers meet. *Proc Natl Acad Sci USA* 1993;90:10909–10913.
37. Smart EJ, Foster DC, Ying YS, et al. Protein kinase C activators inhibit receptor-mediated potocytosis by preventing internalization of caveolae. *J Cell Biol* 1994;124:307–313.
38. Smart EJ, Ying Y, Anderson RGW. Hormonal regulation of caveolae internalization. *J Cell Biol* 1995;131:929–938.
39. Smart EJ, Ying YS, Mineo C, et al. A detergent-free method for purifying caveolae membrane from tissue culture cells. *Proc Natl Acad Sci USA* 1995;92:10104–10108.
40. Hecker M, Mulsch A, Bassenge E, et al. Subcellular localization and characterization of nitric oxide synthase(s) in endothelial cells: Physiological implications. *Biochem J* 1994;299:247–252.
41. Casey PJ. Protein lipidation in cell signaling. *Science* 1995;268:221–225.
42. Shaul PW, Farrar MA, Magness RR. Pulmonary endothelial nitric oxide production is developmentally regulated in the fetus and newborn. *Am J Physiol* 1993;265:H1056–H1063.
43. North AJ, Star RA, Brannon TS, et al. Nitric oxide synthase Type I and Type III gene expression is developmentally regulated in rat lung. *Am J Physiol* 1994;266:L635–L641.
44. Villamor E, LeCras TD, Horan MP, et al. Chronic intrauterine pulmonary hypertension impairs endothelial nitric oxide synthase in the ovine fetus. *Am J Physiol* 1997;272:L1013–L1020.
45. Mendelsohn ME, Karas RH. Estrogen and the blood vessel wall. *Curr Opin Cardiol* 1994;9:619–626.
46. MacRitchie AN, Jun SS, Chen Z, et al. Estrogen upregulates endothelial nitric oxide synthase gene expression in fetal pulmonary artery endothelium. *Circ Res* 1997;81:355–362.
47. Gravett MG, Haluska GJ, Cook MJ, et al. Fetal and maternal endocrine responses to experimental intrauterine infection in rhesus monkeys. *Am J Obstet Gynecol* 1996;174:1725–1733.
48. Barnhart BJ, Carlson CV, Reynolds JW. Adrenal cortical function in the postmature fetus and newborn infant. *Pediatr Res* 1980;14:1367–1369.
49. North AJ, Moya FR, Mysore MR, et al. Pulmonary endothelial nitric oxide synthase gene expression is decreased in a rat model of congenital diaphragmatic hernia. *Am J Respir Cell Mol Biol* 1995;13:676–682.
50. Steinhorn RH, Russell JA, Morin FC. Disruption of cGMP production in pulmonary arteries isolated from fetal lambs with pulmonary hypertension. *Am J Physiol* 1995;268:H1483–H1489.
51. Shaul PW, Yuhanna IS, German Z, et al. Pulmonary endothelial nitric oxide synthase gene expression is decreased in fetal lambs with pulmonary hypertension. *Am J Physiol* 1997;272:L1005–L1012.

52. Fike CD, Kaplowitz MR. Chronic hypoxia alters nitric oxide-dependent pulmonary vascular responses in lungs of newborn pigs. *J Appl Physiol* 1996;81:2078–2087.
53. Fike CD, Kaplowitz MR, Thomas CJ, et al. Basal and acetylcholine stimulated nitric oxide production are decreased in lungs of chronically hypoxic newborn pigs. *Pediatr Res* 1996;39:332A.
54. Hislop AA, Springall DR, Oliveira H, et al. Endothelial nitric oxide synthase in hypoxic newborn porcine pulmonary vessels. *Arch Dis Child Fetal Neonatal Ed* 1997;77:F16–F22.
55. Fike CD, Kaplowitz MR, Thomas CJ, et al. Chronic hypoxia decreases nitric oxide production and endothelial nitric oxide synthase in newborn pig lungs. *Am J Physiol* 1998;274:L517–L526.
56. Shaul PW, North AJ, Brannon TS, et al. Prolonged in vivo hypoxia enhances nitric oxide synthase Type I and Type III gene expression in adult rat lung. *Am J Respir Cell Mol Biol* 1995;13:167–174.
57. North AJ, Lau KS, Brannon TS, et al. Oxygen upregulates nitric oxide synthase gene expression in ovine fetal pulmonary artery endothelial cells. *Am J Physiol* 1996;270:L643–L649.
58. Garg UC, Hassid A. Nitric oxide-generating vasodilators and 8-bromo-cyclic guanosine monophosphate inhibit mitogenesis and proliferation of cultured rat vascular smooth muscle cells. *J Clin Invest* 1989;83:1774–1777.

Chapter 17

The Role of Endothelin in Perinatal Pulmonary Vasoregulation

D. Dunbar Ivy, MD, and Steven H. Abman MD

Introduction

Pulmonary vascular resistance (PVR) is elevated in the normal fetal lung, as pulmonary blood flow accounts for less than 8–10% of the combined ventricular output of blood from the heart.[1] Mechanisms responsible for the maintenance of high PVR in the fetus may include physical factors, such as lack of an air-liquid interface or ventilation, relative low oxygen tension, decreased vasodilator activity, or perhaps increased vasoconstrictor activity.[2-4] Endothelium-derived products, including vasodilator stimuli such as endothelium-derived relaxing factor-nitric oxide (EDRF-NO) and prostacyclin (PGI$_2$), and vasoconstrictor stimuli, such as leukotrienes and endothelin-1 (ET-1), contribute to vascular tone in the fetal lung.[2-8] These endothelial products may not only contribute to basal tone in the fetal lung, but also may modulate responses to physiologic stimuli, such as increases in pressure and shear stress.[5,9,10] Intrauterine mechanisms of altered pulmonary vascular structure and function may be an important determinant of successful postnatal adaptation.

At birth, pulmonary blood flow dramatically increases 8- to 10-fold with a progressive fall in pulmonary pressure. With the initiation of ventilation, PVR initially falls, and continues to decline until adult levels are reached at 2–6 weeks of age.[11-13] Mechanisms that contribute to the decline in PVR at birth remain incompletely understood. Both structural and functional changes occur at birth. During the early newborn period, small pulmonary arteries show an initial decrease in wall thickness.[14,15] Following the initial decrease in wall thickness, peripheral muscularization

From: Weir EK, Archer SL, Reeves JT (eds). *The Fetal and Neonatal Pulmonary Circulations.*
Armonk, NY: Futura Publishing Company, Inc.; ©1999.

of small pulmonary arteries occurs until the adult pattern of muscularization of small pulmonary arteries is achieved. Within minutes of birth, the endothelium becomes flattened[16] secondary to vascular dilation and distension. Functional changes of the endothelium may accompany these structural changes. In addition to increases in oxygen tension, establishment of a gas-liquid interface, and ventilation, altered production of endothelium-derived mediators likely plays an important role in the normal transition.[3,4,6,17–19] Bradykinin, PGI_2, and, recently, EDRF-NO have been shown to contribute to the postnatal adaptation of the pulmonary circulation at birth.[4,17] In contrast, the role of ET-1 during the transition remains less clear.[20]

Biology of Endothelin

First detected by Hickey et al[21] and O'Brien and McMurtry,[22] and characterized by Yanagisawa et al,[23] ET-1 is a 21 amino acid peptide with potent vasoactive properties. ET-1 is initially synthesized as a 203 amino acid prepropeptide (preproET-1), which is then cleaved by an endopeptidase to proET-1 ("big ET-1").[24] The in vitro vasoconstrictor activity of big ET-1 is much lower (<100-fold) than that of ET-1. Big ET-1, a 38 amino acid peptide, is then converted to ET-1 by an endothelin-converting enzyme (ECE), which is a membrane-bound metalloprotease present in endothelial and smooth muscle cells.[25–27] Two isoenzymes of ECE have been described: ECE-1 and ECE-2.[26–28] ECE-1 is associated with the plasma membrane and has optimum activity at neutral pH, whereas ECE-2 is intracellular and active at an acidic pH.[26] ECE-1 has two isoforms: ECE-1a and ECE-1b.[25,29] No functional differences between the ECE-1a and ECE-1b isoforms have been identified. ET-1 may inhibit ECE-1 expression.[30]

ET-1 is the major isopeptide produced by endothelial cells, and has been the most extensively studied in various experimental and clinical settings. ET-1 is involved in the normal development of the heart and great arteries.[31] Subsequent studies have also characterized two other endothelin isopeptides, ET-2 and ET-3.[24] ET-2 expression has been identified in human kidney and jejunum.[32] Although ET-3 was thought to be mainly a neuroactive peptide, it has also been detected in human endothelial cells[33] and lung.[34] Each member of the endothelin family is represented by a separate gene[35] on different chromosomes[36] that encodes a specific precursor for the mature isopeptide. Endothelin peptides share sequence homology and bioactivity with sarafotoxins (including S6c), which are closely related to snake venom toxins.

Endothelin isopeptides have potent hemodynamic effects, which are due to slow dissociation from its receptors. In vivo and in vitro studies have demonstrated that infusions of ET-1 cause progressive and sustained vasoconstriction in most vascular beds, often following a transient dilator response. This brief vasodilatation may be due to transient NO or PGI_2 release[37–43] or to direct activation of smooth muscle K^+ channels.[40–42,44–46] ET-1 is a more potent constrictor than other known vasoconstrictors, such as angiotensin II and norepinephrine, and subthreshold amounts appear to augment vasoconstrictor activity of other agonists.[47] ET-1 stimulates vasoconstriction through complex signal transduction pathways in vascular smooth muscle cells after binding to specific receptors. ET-1 activates phospholipase C (PLC) though a pertussis toxin-insensitive G-protein,[36,48] causing a rapid in-crease of inositol triphosphate[49] and mobilization of intracellular calcium.[36] PLC stimulation also activates protein kinase C through diaclyglycerol,[49] causing entry of extracellular calcium, transcription of growth-promoting genes, and mitogenesis.[50] Several investigators, however, have failed to attenuate its constrictor effects with calcium channel blockers. In contrast with ET-1, ET-2 and ET-3 have less potent constrictor activities. This probably reflects differences in affinity for different endothelin receptors, and differences in activity of these receptors in various vascular beds.

Recent studies have demonstrated at least two distinct endothelin receptors (ET_A and ET_B), that may mediate different endothelin activities in endothelium and vascular smooth muscle cells.[51–54] ET_A receptors have high affinity for ET-1 and ET-2, but not ET-3.[49] The ET_A receptors are located on smooth muscle cells, and mediate vasoconstriction in most vascular beds.[55] It has been suggested that ET_A receptors may also be present on some endothelial cells, leading to PGI_2 release with stimulation.[43] ET_B receptors are mostly present on endothelial cells, have equal affinity for all three isopeptides, and may release NO with stimulation.[7,37,40,41,45,46,56–60] Some studies have shown ET_B receptors on vascular smooth muscle mediating vasoconstriction[54,61–64]; therefore some reports have classified the ET_B receptor as ET_{B1} for ET_B-mediated vasodilation, and ET_{B2} for ET_B-mediated vasoconstriction.[61,65] However, only one gene for the ET_B receptor has been identified.[36,66] Furthermore, recent studies suggest that the ET_B receptor may act as a clearance receptor for circulating ET-1.[67]

Physiologic studies have suggested that ET-1 release is induced by various stimuli, including stretch, increased pressure, thrombin, norepinephrine, transforming growth factor-β, A23187 (a calcium ionophore), and phorbol ester.[22] Despite past controversy, recent studies have demonstrated that prolonged hypoxia is a potent stimulus to preproET-1 messinger RNA (mRNA) expression in cultured human endothelial cells[68] and perfused rat mesenteric arteries.[69] Several stimuli including increased flow, NO activity and atrial natriuretic factor (ANF) decrease endothelin production.[70,71] Some reports have found that ET-1 is not rapidly released, and therefore may have an important role in long-term modulation of vascular tone. In these reports, ET-1 is thought to be generated by de novo synthesis and not stored intracellularly, with regulation of ET-1 production at the level of mRNA transcription.[24] However, recent studies have shown that endothelial cells can store ET-1 and release pre-formed stores of ET-1 acutely.[72,73] In response to stretch, bovine aortic endothelial cells rapidly release ET-1 that is unaffected by actinomycin D or cyclohexamide and is therefore not dependent on new synthesis of the peptide.[73] HPLC analysis showed that ET-1 was stored in endothelial cells in amounts 20 times greater than big ET-1.[73] These findings support the interpretation that mature ET-1 may be stored in endothelial cells in a form available for acute release. Phosphoramidon, an inhibitor of neutral endopeptidases, effectively blocks ECE-1 activity in vitro[74] and inhibits the pressor effects of big ET-1 in anesthetized rats, indicating that a neutral endopeptidase-like converting enzyme system may be involved in ET-1 production in vivo.[75] Phosphoramidon generally has no effect on basal tone in fetal and adult animals, but markedly attenuates the response to exogenous big ET-1 in dose-related fashion.[76] Hemodynamic effects of big ET-1 are thought to be due to the local and not systemic conversion to ET-1.[77] Thus, the physiologic activity of ET-1 is related not only to stimulation of the different receptors but also to its production.

Endothelin in the Perinatal Pulmonary Circulation

The physiologic role of endothelin in the normal ovine fetal pulmonary circulation has been controversial.[7,40,46,78–81] ET-1 is present in the perinatal lung,[82] and is vasoactive in the fetus.[7,79,80,83] Many studies have examined exogenous infusion of ET-1 to determine its physiologic role in the perinatal lung; however, exogenous infusion of ET-1 may not accurately describe the hemodynamic effects of endogenous production of ET-1 in the fetal lung. Circulating plasma concentrations of ET-1 are lower than those reported to be biologically active,[84] and secretion of ET-1 by endothelial cells is polar and directed in an abluminal direction toward the interstitial region.[85] Brief infusion of ET-1 in the normal ovine fetal lung causes acute fetal pulmonary vasodilation[40,79]; however, hypertension develops during prolonged infusion (Figure 1).[79] Although ET-1 infusions cause vasodilation in the presence of high pulmonary vascular tone, similar infusions cause vasoconstriction when the pulmonary vascular tone is decreased during acute ventilation.[78] Several studies suggest that the predominant role of endogenous ET-1 in the normal ovine fetus is stimulation of the ET_A receptor mediating vasoconstriction.[7,81,86] Infusion of big ET-1, the precursor of ET-1, causes only

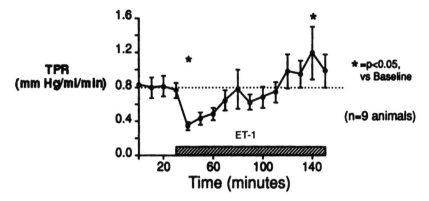

Figure 1. Prolonged infusion of endothelin-1 (ET-1) in the late-gestation fetal lamb causes a transient fall in total pulmonary resistance (TPR) followed by sustained vasoconstriction.

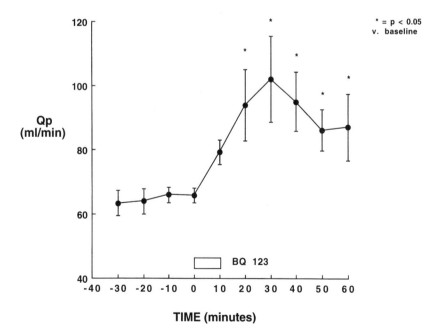

Figure 2A. Brief intrapulmonary infusion of BQ 123, a selective ET_A receptor antagonist, in the late-gestation fetal lamb causes a sustained and progressive increase in Qp (left pulmonary artery flow) suggesting that the ET_A receptor contributes to basal tone in the fetal lung.

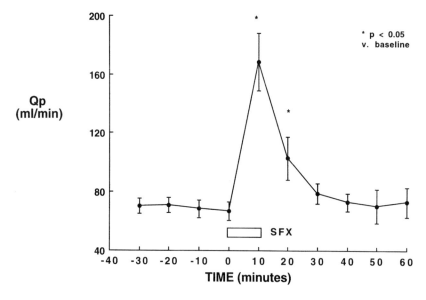

Figure 2B. Brief intrapulmonary infusion of sarafotoxin S6c (SFX), a selective ET$_B$ receptor agonist, rapidly increases Qp in the late-gestation fetal lamb.

hypertension without vasodilation,[7,80] suggesting that stimulation of endogenous ET-1 may have very different effects than brief exogenous infusions of ET-1. Selective ET$_A$ receptor blockade with BQ 123 causes sustained vasodilation in the normal ovine fetus (Figure 2A).[7]

Selective ET$_B$ blockade of the ET$_{B1}$ (vasodilation) or ET$_{B2}$ (vasoconstriction) receptors does not change basal pulmonary tone in the ovine fetus, suggesting that ET$_A$ receptor-mediated vasoconstriction is more prominent than ET$_B$ receptor-mediated vasodilation. However, brief and prolonged stimulation of the ET$_B$ receptors with sarafotoxin S6c causes only vasodilation, suggesting the presence of only ET$_{B1}$ receptors in the normal ovine fetal lung (Figure 2B).[7] This is confirmed by in situ hybridization studies revealing the mRNA for the ET$_B$ receptor only on the vascular endothelium (Figure 3). In contrast, a study in newborn piglets suggests the presence of both ET$_{B1}$ (vasodilation) and ET$_{B2}$ (vasoconstriction) receptors in the neonatal lung.[61] Therefore, it is likely that the balance of endothelin receptor activity favors vasoconstriction in the normal late-gestation ovine fetal lung (Figure 4).

ET-1 not only modulates basal pulmonary tone in the fetus, but also modulates responses to physiologic stimuli, such as increases in pressure and shear stress.[9] Partial ductus arteriosus compression in the late-gestation ovine fetus has been used to evaluate the response of the fetal pulmonary vasculature to these stimuli. During a constant increase in pulmonary artery pressure using a vascular occluder, pulmonary blood

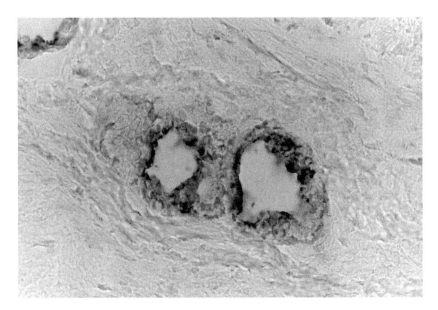

Figure 3. The mRNA of the ET_B receptor is localized to the vascular endothelium of small pulmonary arteries in the late-gestation fetal lamb by in situ hybridization.

flow initially increases, but then steadily declines, and by 2 hours is not different from baseline values. PVR initially falls during the first 30 minutes of partial compression, but then steadily increases and remains elevated above baseline values for at least 30 minutes after the release of the occluder. The ET-1 antagonists, BQ 123 (a selective ET_A receptor antagonist) and phosphoramidon (a nonselective ET-1 converting enzyme inhibitor), augment the peak vasodilator response and prolong the increase in flow during ductus arteriosus compression. Thus, ET-1 activity regulates acute and prolonged responses of the fetal pulmonary circulation to physiologic stimuli.

Little is known of the role of ET-1 during the transition from intrauterine to newborn life. Studies in humans have revealed increased circulating ET-1 levels in the fetus and newborn in comparison with maternal controls.[87,88] In some studies, fetal ET-1 levels are greater than those found in the newborn period. However, Radunovic et al showed that fetal plasma ET-1 levels were significantly lower than neonatal umbilical vein ET-1 levels.[88] As some authors consider that the primary role of ET-1 in the ovine fetal lung is vasodilation,[42,83,89] combined ET_A and ET_B receptor blockade was studied in the ovine lamb during in utero oxygen ventilation. Bosentan, a nonselective ET_A and ET_B receptor antagonist, did not change the increase in pulmonary blood flow or

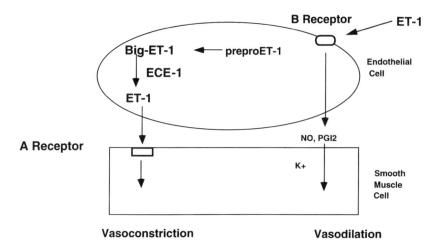

Figure 4. The role of endothelin-1 (ET-1) in the normal late-gestation ovine fetal lamb lung. ET-1 is produced via cleavage of its precursor proendothelin-1 (big-ET-1) by endothelin-converting enzyme (ECE-1). The mature peptide can then act locally at vascular smooth muscle cell ET_A receptors to mediate vasoconstriction, or at endothelial cell ET_B receptors to stimulate production of vasodilators. ET_B-mediated vasodilation may occur via endothelial production of nitric oxide (NO) or prostacyclin (PGI2) or stimulate potassium channels (K+). The ET_B receptor may be located on smooth muscle cells in other vascular sites and species.

decrease in PVR with in utero oxygen ventilation. Therefore, endogenous ET-1 activity may not play a critical role in the increased pulmonary blood flow during the normal transitional circulation at birth.[20]

Endothelin in Experimental Perinatal Pulmonary Hypertension

Mechanisms that regulate high PVR in the normal fetus and contribute to postnatal adaptation of the pulmonary circulation remain incompletely understood, but are vital to understanding of disease states characterized by an abnormal transition to postnatal life, such as the clinical syndrome of persistent pulmonary hypertension of the newborn (PPHN). PPHN is a clinical syndrome characterized by elevated PVR resulting in right-to-left shunting across the foramen ovale and ductus arteriosus with severe hypoxemia.[90] Although mechanisms contributing to PPHN are poorly understood, clinical and experimental studies suggest that chronic pulmonary hypertension in utero leads to failure of the normal transition at birth.[90–93] Chronic intrauterine pulmonary hypertension due to ligation of the ductus arteriosus in fetal lambs causes marked elevation of intrauterine pulmonary artery pressure, right ventricular hypertrophy, hypertensive lung structural changes, as well as abnormal pulmonary vasoreactivity and the failure to achieve the normal decline in pulmonary resistance at birth.[91–94] Attenuation of pulmonary vasodilation to small increases in fetal PO_2,[91] and impairment of endothelium-dependent vasodilation to acetylcholine, also characterize this experimental model of pulmonary hypertension.[95] Ligation of the ductus arteriosus in late-gestation fetal lambs has provided an experimental model for studying mechanisms that contribute to structural and functional changes associated with perinatal pulmonary hypertension.[91,92,94,95]

Several studies suggest that ET-1 may contribute to vasoconstriction and altered vasoreactivity in experimental PPHN.[78–81,86] An imbalance in the NO-cGMP system and ET-1 system likely contributes to pulmonary hypertensive states. Diminished NO production and altered smooth muscle cell responsiveness are known to contribute to pulmonary hypertension.[5,95–98] The decrease in NO production may lead to increased ET-1 production.[99] Increased ET-1 activity also stimulates smooth muscle proliferation, which may further increase PVR.[100] ET-1 has been shown to contribute to the development of pulmonary hypertension due to chronic hypoxia or monocrotaline-induced hypertension.[101–104] Blockade of ET_A receptor activity attenuates the development of pulmonary hypertension and right ventricular hypertrophy in adult models of pulmonary hypertension caused by chronic hypoxia or monocrotaline.[101–105] Furthermore, adult animal models of pulmonary hypertension demonstrate increased expression of the ET_A receptor[106] and decreased expression of the ET_B receptor.[107] Increased production of ET-1 has also been shown in adult pulmonary hypertension models.[107–109]

Chronic intrauterine pulmonary hypertension caused by ductus arteriosus ligation changes the activity of the endothelin receptors.[110] To examine the effects of experimental perinatal pulmonary hypertension on activity of the ET_A and ET_B receptors, the hemodynamic effects of ET-3 (a selective ETB receptor agonist, ET-1 (a nonselective ET_A and ET_B receptor agonist), and BQ 123 (a selective ET_A receptor antagonist) was studied in the chronically prepared late gestation fetal lamb after ligation of the ductus arteriosus. Serial changes in the pulmonary vascular effects of these agents were measured early (1–3 days) and late (7–10 days) after ductus arteriosus ligation (Figure 5A). Left lung total pulmonary resistance (TPR) in the normal late-gestation fetus was 0.62 ± 0.01 mm Hg/mL/min. After partial ductus arteriosus ligation, TPR increased to 1.2 ± 0.3 (early), and progressively rose to 1.9 ± 0.2 mm Hg/mL/min (late). Intrapulmonary infusion of ET-3 increased pulmonary blood flow in the normal fetus, but had no effect during late pulmonary hypertension. Infusions of ET-1 caused transient pulmonary vasodilation

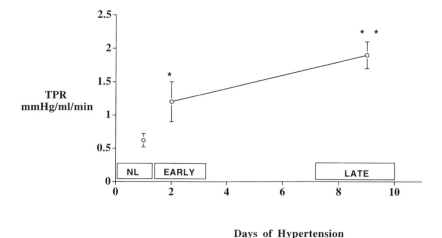

Days of Hypertension

Figure 5A. Ductus arteriosus ligation causes progressive pulmonary hypertension. Total pulmonary resistance (TPR) increased 2-fold above normal (NL) values at 1–3 days (EARLY) of ductus arteriosus ligation (*p<0.05). TPR doubled again at 7–10 days of ligation (LATE) (**p<0.05, EARLY vs. LATE).

followed by vasoconstriction during early pulmonary hypertension. During late pulmonary hypertension, however, infusion of ET-1 caused predominantly vasoconstriction. Pulmonary vasodilation to BQ 123 was greater during late than early pulmonary hypertension (Figure 5B). It appears that that diminished ET_B receptor-mediated vasodilation in combination with enhanced ET_A receptor-mediated vasoconstriction contributes to high PVR in perinatal pulmonary hypertension.

Several mechanisms may explain the attenuation of ET_B receptor vasodilation during chronic pulmonary hypertension. NO production,[7,44] ATP-sensitive potassium channels,[44] or PGI_2 production[43] may mediate ET_B receptor-induced vasodilation. Chronic pulmonary hypertension may decrease ET-1-induced production of these vasodilating stimuli by decreasing NOS or PGI_2 synthesis. Furthermore, chronic pulmonary hypertension may alter ET receptor expression leading to altered vasoreactivity. Decreased ET_B receptor mRNA expression has been shown in the fetal model of pulmonary hypertension due to ductus arteriosus ligation,[111] and in monocrotaline-induced pulmonary hypertension.[107] Enhanced ET_A receptor activity may also contribute to diminished ET_B receptor activity as has been shown in hypoxia-induced pulmonary hypertension[101,105,106] and the monocrotaline model.[102] Finally, diminished ET_B receptor numbers may lead to decreased clearance of ET-1 in the lung leading to increased circulating ET-1.[67]

Molecular analysis of the endothelin system has also revealed al-

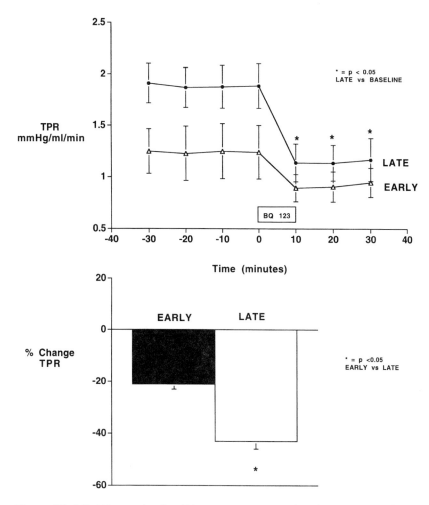

Figure 5B. BQ 123, a selective ET_A receptor antagonist, decreases total pulmonary resistance (TPR) at 7–10 days (LATE) of pulmonary hypertension caused by ductus arteriosus ligation. The fall in TPR to BQ 123 was greater during LATE than EARLY pulmonary hypertension suggesting an increase in ET_A receptor activity during pulmonary hypertension in this model.

tered expression in chronic intrauterine pulmonary hypertension.[111] Lung mRNA expression of preproET-1, ECE-1, and the ET_A and ET_B receptors has been studied in normal and hypertensive fetal lambs after ductus arteriosus ligation. Northern blot analysis revealed a $71 \pm 24\%$ increase in steady-state preproET-1 mRNA and a $62 \pm 5\%$ decrease in ET_B mRNA expression in ductus arteriosus ligation. ECE-1 and ET_A receptor mRNA expression did not change. Ductus arteriosus ligation

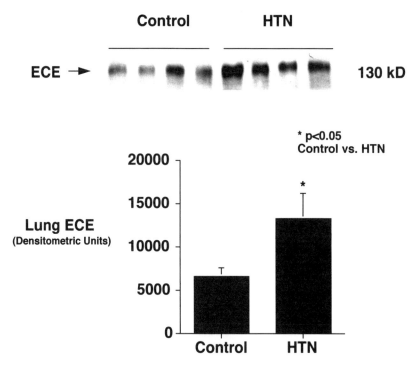

Figure 6. Lung endothelin-converting enzyme (ECE) protein content is increased after pulmonary hypertension (HTN) caused by ductus arteriosus ligation.

also increased immunoreactive ET-1 content in whole lung tissue 3-fold in comparison with control lungs.[110] Although ECE-1 mRNA expression did not change after ductus arteriosus ligation, Western blot analysis revealed an increase in lung ECE-1 protein content (Figure 6). It appears that increased preproET-1 mRNA and ET-1 protein production, decreased ET_B receptor mRNA expression, and increased ECE-1 protein contribute to increased vasoconstrictor tone in this experimental model of neonatal pulmonary hypertension (Figure 7).

As chronic intrauterine pulmonary hypertension was characterized by increased ET_A receptor activity, prolonged ET_A receptor blockade with BQ 123 was studied during ductus arteriosus ligation.[112] Chronic blockade of the ET_A receptor with BQ 123 lowered fetal pulmonary artery pressure, enhanced vasodilation at delivery, decreased right ventricular hypertrophy, and decreased distal muscularization of small pulmonary arteries during the development of intrauterine pulmonary hypertension by ductus arteriosus ligation (Figure 8). In response to birth-related stimuli, including rhythmic lung distention and ventilation with 100% oxygen, PVR fell to lower levels in lambs chronically treated with BQ 123.

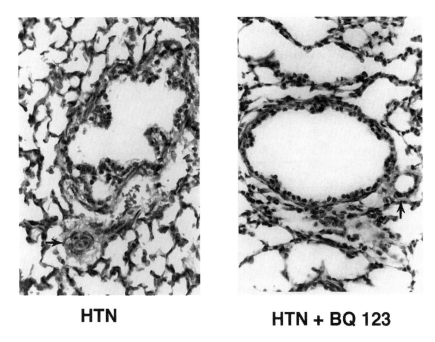

HTN HTN + BQ 123

Figure 7. Prolonged ET_A receptor blockade with BQ 123 decreases distal muscularization of small pulmonary arteries. BQ 123 (right) attenuated the medial hypertrophy of small pulmonary arteries < 100 μm (arrow) adjacent to terminal bronchioles in comparison with hypertensive controls (left).

Furthermore, selective ET_A receptor blockade acutely lowered PVR in control animals ventilated with 100% oxygen and inhaled NO demonstrating that ET_A-mediated vasoconstriction contributes to residual high tone even after rhythmic distension and vasodilation with 100% oxygen and inhaled NO. These findings support the hypothesis that increased ET_A receptor activity contributes to the maintenance of high PVR in utero, the failure of the normal transition at birth, the right ventricular hypertrophy, and the structural changes in the pulmonary vascular bed during chronic fetal pulmonary hypertension.

The role of ET-1 in the development of ventricular hypertrophy is under active investigation. Cultured rat neonatal ventricular cardiomyocytes express a low level of ET-1 mRNA in the unstimulated state, but ET-1 mRNA expression increases in response to the α-adrenergic agonist phenylephrine.[113] Catecholamines increase expression of ET-1 mRNA by cultured ventricular myocytes in vitro and in vivo,[113,114] and exogenous ET-1 induces hypertrophy of cultured myocytes. Increased pressure load to the myocardium also increases ET-1 mRNA expression.[115] The ET_A receptor mediates the hypertrophic effects of ET-1 on

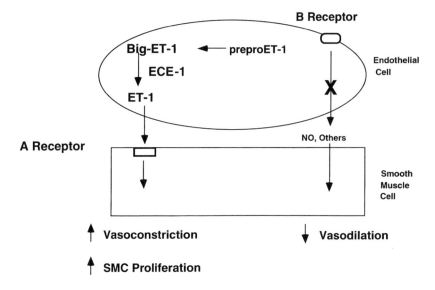

Figure 8. Chronic intrauterine pulmonary hypertension caused by ductus arteriosus ligation causes increased preproET-1 mRNA expression, increased endothelin-converting enzyme (ECE) protein content, increased lung ET-1 protein content, and increased ET_A receptor activity. Expression of the mRNA for the ET_B receptor and ET_B receptor activity is decreased as well. These changes contribute to increased vasoconstriction, decreased vasodilation, and increased smooth muscle cell (SMC) hypertrophy.

cultured adult and neonatal ventricular myocytes.[116] Although adult myocytes do not express ET_B receptors, angiotensin II may increase expression of ET_B receptors in neonatal rat cardiomyocytes.[117] Expression of ET-1, ECE-1, the ET_A and ET_B receptors, has not been examined in the myocardium after chronic intrauterine pulmonary hypertension from ductus arteriosus ligation.

Endothelin in the Premature Lamb with Respiratory Distress Syndrome

ET-1 contributes to pulmonary hypertension in other models of pulmonary hypertension, such as pulmonary hypertension associated with respiratory distress syndrome (RDS). After premature birth, respiratory failure is the result of both structural and functional immaturity. Surfactant deficiency is a primary defect in RDS, and treatment with exogenous surfactant can cause dramatic improvement in oxygenation. However, exogenous surfactant results in suboptimal responses in up to 50% of human newborns with RDS, suggesting that other mechanisms may contribute to failure of postnatal adaptation after premature birth. Human neonates with severe or fatal RDS often have pulmonary hypertension and poor gas exchange. Mechanisms that lead to an increase in PVR and the role of pulmonary hypertension in outcome are uncertain.

Premature delivery and ventilation of the ovine fetus has provided a useful animal model for the study of RDS.[118] Severe RDS in premature lambs is characterized by elevated PVR, impaired gas exchange, pulmonary edema, and inflammation.[118–120] Past studies have emphasized the effects of acute lung injury on epithelial and airway function; however, few studies have examined mechanisms of increased PVR. Vasoactive mediators, such as endogenous NO or ET-1, may contribute to changes in PVR in the fetal lung. Endogenous NO production contributes to maintenance of pulmonary vascular tone as early as 0.78 term gestation and contributes to the rise in pulmonary blood flow after delivery.[5,17,121] Inhaled NO improves oxygenation, increases pulmonary blood flow without increasing pulmonary edema, lowers PVR, and decreases lung neutrophil accumulation in severe experimental hyaline membrane disease.[119,120]

Based on past studies which demonstrated progressive increases in PVR in lambs that were ventilated after premature delivery,[119,122] it was hypothesized that high PVR and poor gas exchange may be due to ET-1-induced pulmonary vasoconstriction and that this may be mediated by increased ET_A receptor activity. To test this hypothesis, serial measurements of circulating ET-1 levels were measured in severely premature lambs, and the response to treatment with the selective ET_A receptor antagonist, BQ 123, was studied. Plasma ET-1 levels increased after delivery of premature fetal lambs. BQ 123 increased left pulmonary artery blood flow, decreased PVR (Figure 9), and improved oxygenation after premature delivery and prolonged ventilation.[123] These studies suggest that ET-1 contributes to the hemodynamic and gas exchange abnormalities in this model of pulmonary hypertension and severe RDS.

Although ET-1 was originally thought to contribute only to vasoconstriction and smooth muscle proliferation, accumulating evidence indicates that ET-1 also contributes to inflammation and acute lung injury.[124] ET-1 may act as a cytokine,[125] promote neutrophil adhesion, and increase lung vascular permeability.[126] Similarly, the pathophysiology of RDS is also characterized by increased lung vascular permeability and lung neutrophil accumulation,[119] as well as altered production of inflammatory cytokines. Circulating ET-1 levels are found in humans with acute lung injury and the adult RDS.[127] ET-1, through stimulation of the ET_A receptor, may also contribute to acute lung injury in this model of severe respiratory failure caused by premature delivery and RDS in the ovine fetus.[123]

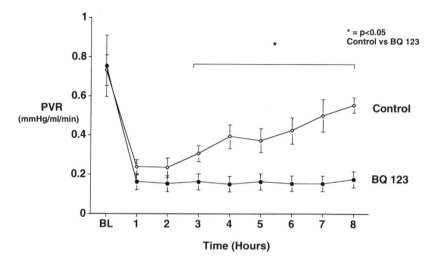

Figure 9. Prolonged ETA receptor blockade with BQ 123, a selective ET_A receptor antagonist, causes a sustained fall in left lung pulmonary vascular resistance (PVR) after acute delivery and ventilation of premature lambs with respiratory distress syndrome.

Endothelin in Human Pulmonary Hypertension

ET-1 levels are increased in many human disorders of pulmonary hypertension. Elevated immunoreactive ET-1 levels have been found in primary pulmonary hypertension, Eisenmenger syndrome,[128] PPHN,[129] children with pulmonary hypertension associated with congenital heart disease and bronchopulmonary dysplasia,[130] and children with congenital heart disease and increased pulmonary blood flow.[131,132] Increased expression of ET-1 in vascular endothelial cells has been reported in adult patients with primary pulmonary hypertension, suggesting that the local production of ET-1 may contribute to the altered vascular reactivity and structural changes seen in pulmonary hypertension.[133] Recently, acute infusion of the combined ET_A and ET_B receptor antagonist, bosentan, has been shown to lower PVR and increase cardiac output in congestive heart failure and pulmonary hypertension.[134]

Conclusion

In summary, ET-1, a potent vasoactive peptide, is present in the fetal lung, contributes to regulation of vascular tone in utero, and modulates responses to physiologic stimuli, such as increases in pressure and shear stress. ET-1 contributes to pulmonary hypertension in models of pulmonary hypertension caused by ductus arteriosus ligation and in severe experimental RDS. The development of antagonists to the endothelin receptors may provide novel therapies for disorders associated with pulmonary hypertension.

References

1. Heymann MA, Creasy RK, Rudolph AM. *Quantitation of Blood Flow Patterns in the Foetal Lamb in Utero.* Cambridge, UK: Cambridge University Press; 1973.
2. Enhorning G, Adams FH, Norman A. Effect of lung expansion on the fetal lamb circulation. *Acta Paediatr Scand* 1966;55:441–451.
3. Soifer SJ, Loitz RD, Roman C, et al. Leukotriene end organ antagonists increase pulmonary blood flow in fetal lambs. *Am J Physiol* 1985;249:H570–H576.
4. Cassin S. Role of prostaglandins, thromboxanes, and leukotrienes in the control of the pulmonary circulation in the fetus and newborn. *Semin Perinatol* 1987;11(1):53–63.
5. Cornfield DN, Chatfield BA, McQueston JA, et al. Effects of birth-related stimuli on L-arginine-dependent pulmonary vasodilation in ovine fetus. *Am J Physiol* 1992;262:H1474–H1481.
6. Davidson D. Pulmonary hemodynamics at birth: Effect of acute cyclooxygenase inhibition in lambs. *J Appl Physiol* 1988;64:1676–1682.
7. Ivy DD, Kinsella JP, Abman SH. Physiologic characterization of endothelin A and B receptor activity in the ovine fetal pulmonary circulation. *J Clin Invest* 1994;93:2141–2148.
8. Wang Y, Coceani F. Isolated pulmonary resistance vessels from fetal lambs: Contractile behavior and responses to indomethacin and endothelin-1. *Circ Res* 1992;71:320–330.
9. Ivy DD, Kinsella JP, Abman SH. Endothelin blockade augments pulmonary vasodilation in the ovine fetus. *J Appl Physiol* 1996;81:2481–2487.
10. Abman SH, Accurso FJ. Acute effects of partial compression of ductus arteriosus on fetal pulmonary circulation. *Am J Physiol* 1989;257:H626–H634.
11. Krovetz LJ, Goldbloom J. Normal standards for cardiovascular data II: Pressure and vascular resistances. *Johns Hopkins Med J* 1972;130:187–195.
12. Rudolph AM, Auld PA, Golinko RJ. Pulmonary vascular adjustments in the neonatal period. *Pediatrics* 1961;28:28–34.
13. Rudolph AM. The changes in the circulation after birth: Their importance in congenital heart disease. *Circulation* 1970;41:343–359.
14. Meyrick B, Reid L. Pulmonary arterial and alveolar development in normal postnatal rat lung. *Am Rev Respir Dis* 1982;125:468–473.
15. Reid LM. The pulmonary circulation: Remodeling in growth and disease. The 1978 J. Burns Amberson lecture. *Am Rev Respir Dis* 1979;119:531–546.
16. Haworth SG. Pulmonary vascular remodeling in neonatal pulmonary hypertension: State of the art. *Chest* 1988;93:133S–138S.
17. Abman SH, Chatfield BA, Hall SL, et al. Role of endothelium-derived relaxing factor during transition of pulmonary circulation at birth. *Am J Physiol* 1990;259:H1921–H1927.
18. Heymann MA, Rudolph AM, Nies AS, et al. Bradykinin production associated with oxygenation of the fetal lamb. *Circ Res* 1969;25:521–534.

19. Leffler CW, Tyler TL, Cassin S. Effect of indomethacin on pulmonary vascular response to ventilation of fetal goats. *Am J Physiol* 1978;234:H346–H351.
20. Winters JW, Wong J, Van Dyke D, et al. Endothelin receptor blockade does not alter the increase in pulmonary blood flow due to oxygen ventilation in fetal lambs. *Pediatr Res* 1996;40:152–157.
21. Hickey KA, Rubanyi G, Paul RJ, et al. Characterization of a coronary vasoconstrictor produced by cultured endothelial cells. *Am J Physiol* 1985;248: C550–C556.
22. O'Brien RF, McMurtry IF. Endothelial cell supernatants contract bovine pulmonary artery rings. *Am Rev Respir Dis* 1984;129:A337.
23. Yanagisawa M, Kurihara H, Kimura S, et al. A novel potent vasoconstrictor peptide produced by vascular endothelial cells. *Nature* 1988;332:411–415.
24. Simonson MS, Dunn MJ. Cellular signaling by peptides of the endothelin gene family. *FASEB J* 1990;4:2989–3000.
25. Valdenaire O, Rohrbacher E, Mattei MG. Organization of the gene encoding the human endothelin-converting enzyme (ECE-1). *J Biol Chem* 1995; 270:29794–29798.
26. Emoto N, Yanagisawa M. Endothelin-converting enzyme-2 is a membrane-bound, phosphoramidon-sensitive metalloprotease with acidic pH optimum. *J Biol Chem* 1995;270:15262–15268.
27. Xu D, Emoto N, Giaid A, et al. ECE-1: A membrane-bound metalloprotease that catalyzes the proteolytic activation of big endothelin-1. *Cell* 1994;78:473–485.
28. Ikura T, Sawamura T, Shiraki T, et al. cDNA cloning and expression of bovine endothelin converting enzyme. *Biochem Biophys Res Commun* 1994; 203:1417–1422.
29. Shimada K, Takahashi M, Ikeda M, et al. Identification and characterization of two isoforms of an endothelin-converting enzyme-1. *FEBS Lett* 1995;371:140–144.
30. Naomi S, Iwaoka T, Disashi T, et al. Endothelin-1 inhibits endothelin-converting enzyme-1 expression in cultured rat pulmonary endothelial cells. *Circulation* 1998;97:234–236.
31. Kuirhara Y, Kurihara H, Oda H, et al. Aortic arch malformations and ventricular septal defect in mice deficient in endothelin-1. *J Clin Invest* 1995;96: 293–300.
32. Masaki T. Endothelins: Homeostatic and compensatory actions in the circulatory and endocrine systems. *Endocr Rev* 1993;14:256–268.
33. Suzuki N, Matsumoto H, Miyauchi T, et al. Endothelin-3 concentrations in human plasma: The increased concentrations in patients undergoing haemodialysis. *Biochem Biophys Res Commun* 1990;169:809–815.
34. Bloch KD, Eddy RL, Shows TB, et al. cDNA cloning and chromosomal assignment of the gene encoding endothelin 3. *J Biol Chem* 1989;264:18156–18161.
35. Inoue A, Yanagisawa M, Kimura S, et al. The human endothelin family: Three structurally and pharmacologically distinct isopeptides predicted by three separate genes. *Proc Natl Acad Sci USA* 1989;86:2863–2867.
36. Rubanyi GM, Polokoff MA. Endothelins: Molecular biology, biochemistry, pharmacology, physiology, and pathophysiology. *Pharmacol Rev* 1994;46:325–415.
37. Fujitani Y, Ueda H, Okada T, et al. A selective agonist of endothelin type B receptor, IRL 1620, stimulates cyclic GMP increase via nitric oxide formation in rat aorta. *J Pharmacol Exp Ther* 1993;267:683–689.
38. Lang D, Lewis MJ. Endothelium-derived relaxing factor inhibits the

endothelin-1-induced increase in protein kinase C activity in rat aorta. *Br J Pharmacol* 1991;104:139–144.

39. Pinheiro JM, Malik AB. Mechanisms of endothelin-1-induced pulmonary vasodilatation in neonatal pigs. *J Physiol (Lond)* 1993;469:739–752.
40. Wong J, Vanderford PA, Fineman JR, et al. Endothelin-1 produces pulmonary vasodilation in the intact newborn lamb. *Am J Physiol* 1993;265: H1318–H1325.
41. Wong J, Vanderford PA, Fineman JR, et al. Developmental effects of endothelin-1 on the pulmonary circulation in sheep. *Pediatr Res* 1994;36: 394–401.
42. Wong J, Vanderford PA, Winters J, et al. Endothelin B receptor agonists produce pulmonary vasodilation in intact newborn lambs with pulmonary hypertension. *J Cardiovasc Pharmacol* 1995;25:207–215.
43. D'Orleans-Juste P, Telemaque S, Claing A, et al. Human big-endothelin-1 and endothelin-1 release prostacyclin via the activation of ET1 receptors in the rat perfused lung. *Br J Pharmacol* 1992;105:773–775.
44. Hasunuma K, Rodman DM, O'Brien RF, et al. Endothelin 1 causes pulmonary vasodilation in rats. *Am J Physiol* 1990;259:H48–H54.
45. Wong J, Fineman JR, Heymann MA. The role of endothelin and endothelin receptor subtypes in regulation of fetal pulmonary vascular tone. *Pediatr Res* 1994;35:664–670.
46. Wong J, Fineman JR, Heymann MA. The role of endothelin and endothelin receptor subtypes in regulation of fetal pulmonary vascular tone. *Pediatr Res* 1994;35:664–670.
47. Miller RC, Pelton JT, Huggins JP. Endothelins: From receptors to medicine. *Trends Pharmacol Sci* 1993;14:54–60.
48. Takuwa Y, Kasuya N, Takuwa N. Endothelin receptor is coupled to phospholipase C via a pertussis toxin-insensitive guanine nucleotide-binding regulatory protein in vascular smooth muscle cells. *J Clin Invest* 1990;85: 653–658.
49. Resink TJ, Scott-Burden T, Buhler FR. Endothelin stimulates phospholipase C in cultured vascular smooth muscle cells. *Biochem Biophys Res Commun* 1988;157:1360–1368.
50. Komuro I, Kurihara H, Sugiyama T, et al. Endothelin stimulates c-fos and c-myc expression and proliferation of vascular smooth muscle cells [published erratum appears in FEBS Lett 1989 Feb 27;244(2):509]. *FEBS Lett* 1988;238:249–252.
51. Arai H, Hori S, Aramori I, et al. Cloning and expression of a cDNA encoding an endothelin receptor. *Nature* 1990;348:730–732.
52. Arai H, Nakao K, Hosoda K, et al. Molecular cloning of human endothelin receptors and their expression in vascular endothelial cells and smooth muscle cells. *Jpn Circ J* 1992;56(suppl 5):1303–1307.
53. Arai H, Nakao K, Takaya K, et al. The human endothelin-B receptor gene: Structural organization and chromosomal assignment. *J Biol Chem* 1993; 268:3463–3470.
54. Warner TD, Allcock GH, Corder R, et al. Use of the endothelin antagonists BQ-123 and PD 142893 to reveal three endothelin receptors mediating smooth muscle contraction and the release of EDRF. *Br J Pharmacol* 1993; 110:777–782.
55. Ihara M, Fukuroda T, Saeki T, et al. An endothelin receptor (ETA) antagonist isolated from Streptomyces misakiensis. *Biochem Biophys Res Commun* 1991;178:132–137.
56. Ghoneim MA, Yamamoto T, Hirose S, et al. Endothelium localization of

ETB receptor revealed by immunohistochemistry. *J Cardiovasc Pharmacol* 1993;22(suppl 8):S111–S112.

57. Hirata Y, Emori T, Eguchi S, et al. Endothelin receptor subtype B mediates synthesis of nitric oxide by cultured bovine endothelial cells. *J Clin Invest* 1993;91:1367–1373.

58. Kohan DE, Padilla E, Hughes AK. Endothelin B receptor mediates ET-1 effects on cAMP and PGE2 accumulation in rat IMCD. *Am J Physiol* 1993;265:F670–F676.

59. McMurdo L, Thiemermann C, Vane JR. The endothelin ETB receptor agonist, IRL 1620, causes vasodilatation and inhibits ex vivo platelet aggregation in the anaesthetised rabbit. *Eur J Pharmacol* 1994;259:51–55.

60. Zellers TM, McCormick J, Wu Y. Interaction among ET-1, endothelium-derived nitric oxide, and prostacyclin in pulmonary arteries and veins. *Am J Physiol* 1994;267:H139–H147.

61. Perreault T, Baribeau J. Characterization of endothelin receptors in newborn piglet lung. *Am J Physiol* 1995;268:L607–L614.

62. Clozel M, Gray GA, Breu V, et al. The endothelin ETB receptor mediates both vasodilation and vasoconstriction in vivo. *Biochem Biophys Res Commun* 1992;186:867–873.

63. Sumner MJ, Cannon TR, Mundin JW, et al. Endothelin ETA and ETB receptors mediate vascular smooth muscle contraction. *Br J Pharmacol* 1992; 107:858–860.

64. Seo B, Oemar BS, Siebenmann R, et al. Both ETA and ETB receptors mediate contraction to endothelin-1 in human blood vessels. *Circulation* 1994;89:1203–1208.

65. Bax WA, Saxena PR. The current endothelin receptor classification: Time for reconsideration? *Trends Pharmacol Sci* 1994;15:379–386.

66. Masaki T, Vane JR, Vanhoutte PM. International Union of Pharmacology nomenclature of endothelin receptors. *Pharmacol Rev* 1994;46:137–142.

67. Fukuroda T, Fujikawa T, Ozaki S, et al. Clearance of circulating endothelin-1 by ETB receptors in rats. *Biochem Biophys Res Commun* 1994;199:1461–1465.

68. Kourembanas S, Marsden PA, McQuillan LP, et al. Hypoxia induces endothelin gene expression and secretion in cultured human endothelium. *J Clin Invest* 1991;88:1054–1057.

69. Rakugi H, Tabuchi Y, Nakamaru M, et al. Evidence for endothelin-1 release from resistance vessels of rats in response to hypoxia. *Biochem Biophys Res Commun* 1990;169:973–977.

70. Boulanger C, Luscher TF. Release of endothelin from the porcine aorta: Inhibition by endothelium-derived nitric oxide. *J Clin Invest* 1990;85:587–590.

71. Sharefkin JB, Diamond SL, Eskin SG, et al. Fluid flow decreases preproendothelin mRNA levels and suppresses endothelin-1 peptide release in cultured human endothelial cells. *J Vasc Surg* 1991;14:1–9.

72. McClellan G, Weisberg A, Rose D, et al. Endothelial cell storage and release of endothelin as a cardioregulatory mechanism. *Circ Res* 1994;75:85–96.

73. Macarthur H, Warner TD, Wood EG, et al. Endothelin-1 release from endothelial cells in culture is elevated both acutely and chronically by short periods of mechanical stretch. *Biochem Biophys Res Commun* 1994;200:395–400.

74. Pollock DM, Opgenorth TJ. Evidence for metalloprotease involvement in the in vivo effects of big endothelin 1. *Am J Physiol* 1991;261:R257–R263.

75. Takada J, Okada K, Ikenaga T, et al. Phosphoramidon-sensitive endothelin-converting enzyme in the cytosol of cultured bovine endothelial cells. *Biochem Biophys Res Commun* 1991;176:860–865.

76. Gardiner SM, Compton AM, Kemp PA, et al. The effects of phosphoramidon on the regional haemodynamic responses to human proendothelin [1–38] in conscious rats. *Br J Pharmacol* 1991;103:2009–2015.
77. Hisaki K, Matsumura Y, Ikegawa R, et al. Evidence for phosphoramidon-sensitive conversion of big endothelin-1 to endothelin-1 in isolated rat mesenteric artery. *Biochem Biophys Res Commun* 1991;177:1127–1132.
78. Cassin S, Kristova V, Davis T, et al. Tone-dependent responses to endothelin in the isolated perfused fetal sheep pulmonary circulation in situ. *J Appl Physiol* 1991;70:1228–1234.
79. Chatfield BA, McMurtry IF, Hall SL, et al. Hemodynamic effects of endothelin-1 on ovine fetal pulmonary circulation. *Amer J Physiol* 1991;261: R182–R187.
80. Jones OW, Abman SH. Systemic and pulmonary hemodynamic effects of big endothelin-1 and phosphoramidon in the ovine fetus. *Am J Physiol* 1994;266:R929–R955.
81. Wang Y, Coe Y, Toyoda O, et al. Involvement of endothelin-1 in hypoxic pulmonary vasoconstriction in the lamb. *J Physiol* 1995;482:421–434.
82. MacCumber MW, Ross CA, Glaser BM, et al. Endothelin: Visualization of mRNAs by in situ hybridization provides evidence for local action. *Proc Natl Acad Sci USA* 1989;86:7285–7289.
83. Tod ML, Cassin S. Endothelin-1-induced pulmonary arterial dilation is reduced by N-omega-nitro-L-arginine in fetal lambs. *J Appl Physiol* 1992;72: 1730–1734.
84. Creminon C, Frobert Y, Habib A, et al. Enzyme immunometric assay for endothelin using tandem monoclonal antibodies. *J Immunol Methods* 1993; 162:179–192.
85. Wagner OF, Christ G, Wojta J, et al. Polar secretion of endothelin-1 by cultured endothelial cells. *J Biol Chem* 1992;267:16066–16068.
86. Wang Y, Coceani F. Isolated pulmonary resistance vessels from fetal lambs: Contractile behavior and responses to indomethacin and endothelin-1. *Circ Res* 1992;71:320–330.
87. Nakamura T, Kasai K, Konuma S, et al. Immunoreactive endothelin concentrations in maternal and fetal blood. *Life Sci* 1990;46:1045–1050.
88. Radunovic N, Lockwood CJ, Alvarez M, et al. Fetal and maternal plasma endothelin levels during the second half of pregnancy. *Am J Obstet Gynecol* 1995;172:28–32.
89. Wong J, Vanderford PA, Fineman JR, et al. Endothelin-1 produces pulmonary vasodilation in the intact newborn lamb. *Am J Physiol* 1993;265: H1318–H1325.
90. Levin DL, Heymann MA, Kitterman JA, et al. Persistent pulmonary hypertension of the newborn infant. *J Pediatr* 1976;89:626–630.
91. Abman SH, Shanley PF, Accurso FJ. Failure of postnatal adaptation of the pulmonary circulation after chronic intrauterine pulmonary hypertension in fetal lambs. *J Clin Invest* 1989;83:1849–1858.
92. Morin FCd. Ligating the ductus arteriosus before birth causes persistent pulmonary hypertension in the newborn lamb. *Pediatr Res* 1989;25:245–250.
93. Murphy JD, Rabinovitch M, Goldstein JD, et al. The structural basis of persistent pulmonary hypertension of the newborn infant. *J Pediatr* 1981;98: 962–967.
94. Belik J, Halayko AJ, Rao K, et al. Fetal ductus arteriosus ligation: Pulmonary vascular smooth muscle biochemical and mechanical changes. *Circ Res* 1993;72:588–596.

95. McQueston JA, Kinsella JP, Ivy DD, et al. Chronic pulmonary hypertension in utero impairs endothelium-dependent vasodilation. *Am J Physiol* 1995;268:H288–H294.
96. Belik J. Myogenic response in large pulmonary arteries and its ontogenesis. *Pediatr Res* 1994;36:34–40.
97. Belik J. The myogenic response of arterial vessels is increased in fetal pulmonary hypertension. *Pediatr Res* 1995;37:196–201.
98. Fineman JR, Wong J, Morin FC, et al. Chronic nitric oxide inhibition in utero produces persistent pulmonary hypertension in newborn lambs. *J Clin Invest* 1994;93:2675–2683.
99. Kourembanas S, McQuillan LP, Leung GK, et al. Nitric oxide regulates the expression of vasoconstrictors and growth factors by vascular endothelium under both normoxia and hypoxia. *J Clin Invest* 1993;92:99–104.
100. Zamora MA, Dempsey EC, Walchak SJ, et al. BQ123, an ETA receptor antagonist, inhibits endothelin-1-mediated proliferation of human pulmonary artery smooth muscle cells. *Am J Respir Cell Mol Biol* 1993;9:429–433.
101. Bonvallet ST, Zamora MR, Hasunuma K, et al. BQ123, an ETA-receptor antagonist, attenuates hypoxic pulmonary hypertension in rats. *Am J Physiol* 1994;266:H1327–H1331.
102. Miyauchi T, Yorikane R, Sakai S, et al. Contribution of endogenous endothelin-1 to the progression of cardiopulmonary alterations in rats with monocrotaline-induced pulmonary hypertension. *Circ Res* 1993;73:887–897.
103. Chen SJ, Chen YF, Meng QC, et al. Endothelin-receptor antagonist bosentan prevents and reverses hypoxic pulmonary hypertension in rats. *J Appl Physiol* 1995;79:2122–2131.
104. DiCarlo VS, Chen SJ, Meng QC, et al. ETA-receptor antagonist prevents and reverses chronic hypoxia-induced pulmonary hypertension in rat. *Am J Physiol* 1995;269:L690–L697.
105. Eddahibi S, Raffestin B, Braquet P, et al. Pulmonary vascular reactivity to endothelin-1 in normal and chronically pulmonary hypertensive rats. *J Cardiovasc Pharmacol* 1991;17(suppl 7):S358–S361.
106. Li H, Elton TS, Chen YF, et al. Increased endothelin receptor gene expression in hypoxic rat lung. *Am J Physiol* 1994;266:L553–L560.
107. Yorikane R, Miyauchi T, Sakai S, et al. Altered expression of ETB-receptor mRNA in the lung of rats with pulmonary hypertension. *J Cardiovasc Pharmacol* 1993;22(suppl 8):S336–S338.
108. Stelzner TJ, O'Brien RF, Yanagisawa M, et al. Increased lung endothelin-1 production in rats with idiopathic pulmonary hypertension. *Am J Physiol* 1992;262:L614–L620.
109. Li H, Chen SJ, Chen YF, et al. Enhanced endothelin-1 and endothelin receptor gene expression in chronic hypoxia. *J Appl Physiol* 1994;77:1451–1459.
110. Ivy DD, Ziegler JW, Dubus MF, et al. Chronic intrauterine pulmonary hypertension alters endothelin receptor activity in the ovine fetal lung. *Pediatr Res* 1996;39:435–442.
111. Ivy DD, Le Cras TD, Horan MP, et al. Increased lung preproET-1 and decreased ETB-receptor gene expression in fetal pulmonary hypertension. *Am J Physiol* 1998;274:L535–L541.
112. Ivy DD, Parker TA, Ziegler JW, et al. Prolonged endothelin A receptor blockade attenuates chronic pulmonary hypertension in the ovine fetus. *J Clin Invest* 1997;99:1179–1186.
113. Kaddoura S, Firth JD, Fuller SJ, et al. Ventricular myocytes in culture ex-

press endothelin-1 but not ET-2 or ET-3 mRNA in response to the hypertrophic agonists phenylephrine and ET-1. *J Am Coll Cardiol* 1995:415A.

114. Kaddoura S, Firth JD, Boheler KR, et al. Endothelin-1 is involved in norepinephrine-induced ventricular hypertrophy in vivo. *Circulation* 1996;93: 2068–2079.

115. Ito H, Hiroe M, Hirata Y, et al. Endothelin ETA receptor antagonist blocks cardiac hypertrophy provoked by hemodynamic overload. *Circulation* 1994;89:2198–2203.

116. Ito H, Hirata Y, Adachi S, et al. Endothelin-1 is an autocrine/paracrine factor in the mechanism of angiotensin II-induced hypertrophy in cultured rat cardiomyocytes. *J Clin Invest* 1993;92:398–403.

117. Kanno K, Hirata Y, Tsujino M, et al. Up-regulation of ETB receptor subtype mRNA by angiotensin-II in rat cardiomyocytes. *Biochem Biophys Res Commun* 1993;194:1282–1287.

118. Jobe A, Ikegami M, Jacobs H, et al. Surfactant and pulmonary blood flow distributions following treatment of premature lambs with natural surfactant. *J Clin Invest* 1984;73:848–856.

119. Kinsella JP, Parker TA, Galan H, et al. Effects of inhaled nitric oxide on pulmonary edema and lung neutrophil accumulation in severe experimental hyaline membrane disease. *Pediatr Res* 1997;41:457–463.

120. Kinsella JP, Ivy DD, Abman SH. Inhaled nitric oxide improves gas exchange and lowers pulmonary vascular resistance in severe experimental hyaline membrane disease. *Pediatr Res* 1994;36:402–408.

121. Kinsella JP, Ivy DD, Abman SH. Ontogeny of NO activity and response to inhaled NO in the developing ovine pulmonary circulation. *Am J Physiol* 1994;267:H1955–H1961.

122. Kinsella JP, Ivy DD, Abman SH. Inhaled nitric oxide improves gas exchange and lowers pulmonary vascular resistance in severe experimental hyaline membrane disease. *Pediatr Res* 1994;36:402–408.

123. Ivy DD, Parker TA, Kinsella JP, et al. Endothelin A receptor blockade decreases pulmonary vascular resistance in premature lambs with hyaline membrane disease. *Pediatr Res* 1998;44:175–180.

124. Michael JR, Markewitz BA. Endothelins and the lung. *Am J Respir Crit Care Med* 1996;154:555–581.

125. McMillen MA, Sumpio BE. Endothelins: Polyfunctional cytokines. *J Am Coll Surg* 1995;180:621–637.

126. Rodman DM, Stelzner TJ, Zamora MR, et al. Endothelin-1 increases the pulmonary microvascular pressure and causes pulmonary edema in salt solution but not blood-perfused rat lungs. *J Cardiovasc Pharmacol* 1992;20: 658–663.

127. Langleben D, DeMarchie M, Laporta D, et al. Endothelin-1 in acute lung injury and the adult respiratory distress syndrome. *Am Rev Respir Dis* 1993;148:1646–1650.

128. Cacoub P, Dorent R, Maistre G, et al. Endothelin-1 in primary pulmonary hypertension and the Eisenmenger syndrome. *Am J Cardiol* 1993;71:448–450.

129. Rosenberg AA, Kennaugh J, Koppenhafer SL, et al. Elevated immunoreactive endothelin-1 levels in newborn infants with persistent pulmonary hypertension. *J Pediatr* 1993;123:109–114.

130. Allen SW, Chatfield BA, Koppenhafer SA, et al. Circulating immunoreactive endothelin-1 in children with pulmonary hypertension. Association with acute hypoxic pulmonary vasoreactivity. *Am Rev Respir Dis* 1993;148: 519–522.

131. Komai H, Adatia IT, Elliott MJ, et al. Increased plasma levels of endothe-
     lin-1 after cardiopulmonary bypass in patients with pulmonary hyper-
     tension and congenital heart disease. *J Thorac Cardiovasc Surg* 1993;106:
     473–478.
132. Vincent JA, Ross RD, Kassab J, et al. Relation of elevated plasma en-
     dothelin in congenital heart disease to increased pulmonary blood flow.
     Am J Cardiol 1993;71:1204–1207.
133. Giaid A, Yanagisawa M, Langleben D, et al. Expression of endothelin-1 in
     the lungs of patients with pulmonary hypertension. *N Engl J Med* 1993;
     328:1732–1739.
134. Kiowski W, Sutsch G, Hunziker P, et al. Evidence for endothelin-1-mediated
     vasoconstriction in severe chronic heart failure. *Lancet* 1995;346:732–736.

Chapter 18

O_2-Sensitive K^+ Channel Activity in the Ovine Pulmonary Circulation Shifts with Maturation

David N. Cornfield, MD, Helen L. Reeve, PhD, and E. Kenneth Weir, MD

Background

The physiologic environment of the pulmonary vasculature during fetal life is unique. It is characterized by low blood flow, high pulmonary vascular resistance (PVR), and low O_2 tension.[1] At birth, the pulmonary circulation undergoes a dramatic transition. Pulmonary blood flow increases 8- to 10-fold and pulmonary artery (PA) pressure declines steadily over the first several hours of life.[2,3] Investigations surrounding the physiologic mechanisms responsible for the transition of the pulmonary circulation at birth have been ongoing for over 40 years. In 1953, Dawes and coworkers published a seminal manuscript demonstrating that ventilation and establishment of an air-liquid interface caused an immediate increase in pulmonary blood flow and a decrease in PA blood pressure.[3] Evidence for an integral role for O_2 in the postnatal adaptation of the pulmonary circulation came first with the finding that, while ventilation with N_2 caused pulmonary vasodilation, ventilation with O_2 caused even greater pulmonary vasodilation.[2] Clear evidence that an increase in fetal O_2 tension, in the absence of any other physiologic stimulus, could cause fetal pulmonary vasodilation came from

D.N. Cornfield is supported by an American Heart Association Clinician Scientist Award and the University of Minnesota Children's Foundation. H.L. Reeve is supported by National Heart, Lung and Blood Institute Grant R29-HL-59182. E.K. Weir is supported by the Department of Veteran's Affairs Merit Review funding.

From: Weir EK, Archer SL, Reeves JT (eds). *The Fetal and Neonatal Pulmonary Circulations.* Armonk, NY: Futura Publishing Company, Inc.; ©1999.

experiments wherein pulmonary blood flow increased by more than 3-fold when pregnant ewes were placed in a hyperbaric chamber.[4]

Several factors contribute to the increase in pulmonary blood flow at birth: ventilation of the lung;[5] increased shear stress; and an increase in O_2 tension.[4] One of the mechanisms whereby these stimuli cause perinatal pulmonary vasodilation is through the elaboration of vasoactive mediators such as prostacyclin[6] and nitric oxide (NO), from the pulmonary endothelium. NO has been shown to mediate the increase in pulmonary blood flow that results from ventilation,[7] elevation of O_2,[8,9] and increased shear stress.[10] Inhibition of NO synthesis can attenuate the postnatal adaptation of the pulmonary circulation.[7,11] The observation that endothelial nitric oxide synthase (eNOS) expression is diminished in models of congenital diaphragmatic hernia[12] and neonatal pulmonary hypertension[13,14] emphasizes the central importance of NO in both normal and abnormal perinatal pulmonary vasoreactivity.

Though K^+ channels have been shown to play a critical role in the regulation of pulmonary vascular tone in the adult, the role of K^+ channels in the perinatal circulation remains largely unknown. In the adult pulmonary circulation, a decrease in O_2 tension inactivates a K^+ channel, depolarizes PA smooth muscle cells (SMCs) to a threshold that opens voltage-operated Ca^{2+} channels (VOCC), and increases intracellular Ca^{2+} concentration ($[Ca^{2+}]_i$) to cause vasoconstriction.[15–18] Through K^+ channel inhibition, hypoxia causes pulmonary vasoconstriction, which optimizes the perfusion of well-ventilated lung units, preventing intrapulmonary shunting. Altered K^+ channel activity has been implicated in the pathogenesis of cardiovascular diseases such as primary pulmonary hypertension[19,20] and systemic arterial hypertension.[21,22] Recent work has identified a critically important role for the Ca^{2+}-sensitive K^+ (K_{Ca}) channel in the prevention of cerebrovascular disease during chronic hypertension in rats.[23]

K^+ channels are expressed in virtually all excitable and nonexcitable cells.[24] Using electrophysiological techniques, three different types of K^+ channels have been identified in PA SMCs: K_{Ca}; voltage-gated K^+ (K_v); and ATP-sensitive (K_{ATP}).[25] In the adult pulmonary circulation, several reports indicate that the K_v channel regulates resting membrane potential (E_m) and is inactivated by an acute decrease in O_2 tension. Thus, in the adult pulmonary circulation, the K_v channel is likely to be at least one of the key O_2 sensors,[17] although the K_{Ca} channel has also been implicated as a potential O_2 sensor.[16] Alternatively, the K_{Ca} channel may function to limit PA constriction, as a small elevation in Ca^{2+} in the region of the K_{Ca} channel allows for a large increase in K^+ efflux through the K_{Ca} channel, resulting in E_m hyperpolarization, closing VOCC, and leading to SMC relaxation.[26]

O₂ Sensing

The ability to sense changes in O_2 tension is of fundamental biological importance. While the exact identity of the O_2 sensor has not been definitively established, there is increasing evidence that K^+ channels play a central role in mediating responses to alterations in O_2 tension. Carotid bodies are the main arterial O_2 sensor in mammals. Glomus cells of the carotid body have been thought to act as the primary O_2 sensor. Direct proof for the chemoreceptive properties of the glomus cells have come from patch-clamp experiments demonstrating that these cells contain K^+ channels whose activity can be inhibited by lowering O_2 tension.[27] Further experiments have strongly suggested that hypoxia inactivates O_2-sensitive K^+ channels, resulting in membrane depolarization and an increase in $[Ca^{2+}]_i$ to trigger the release of neurotransmitters.[28,29]

While there is general consensus that hypoxia causes inhibition of K^+ channels in carotid glomus cells, it remains unclear which subtype of K^+ channel is inhibited. Perhaps, the divergence of results can be explained, in part, by a developmental change in the O_2−sensitive K^+ channels of the carotid body. In adult rabbit type I cells, hypoxia inhibits a 4-aminopyridine-sensitive (4AP), Ca^{2+}-independent K_v channel.[27,30] This observation is in direct contrast with the results obtained in neonatal rat type I cells, where the K_{Ca} channel is selectively inhibited by hypoxia.[31,32] Thus, there is a precedent, in the carotid body, for the concept of a developmental change in the K^+ channel that is the O_2 sensor. If such a developmental shift is present in the pulmonary circulation as well as in the carotid body, it might represent the mechanism whereby the pulmonary circulation of the normal newborn infant is adapted to respond to an acute increase in O_2 tension, while the pulmonary circulation of the adult is adapted to respond to an acute decrease in O_2 tension.

Data suggest that vascular SMCs (VSMCs), as well as glomus cells of the carotid body, are capable of directly sensing changes in O_2 tension. The response of VSMCs to alterations in O_2 tension is contingent upon the vascular bed of origin.[33] In the systemic vasculature, a decrease in O_2 tension results in vasodilation, which acts to improve perfusion. In the lung, hypoxia causes pulmonary vasoconstriction (HPV). During postnatal life, HPV directs blood away from poorly ventilated portions of the lung. Without HPV, ventilation and perfusion would not be well matched and poorly oxygenated blood would enter the systemic circulation, resulting in systemic hypoxemia. Thus, HPV is an essential adaptive response that is intrinsic to the PA SMCs.[34]

Identification of the PA SMC K^+ channel that is sensitive to alterations in O_2 tension has been derived from patch-clamp experiments.

In single channel experiments using amphotericin-perforated vesicles, hypoxia caused reversible K^+ channel inhibition; similar results were obtained during hypoxia in cell-attached patch-clamp studies, despite the presence of pharmacological blockers of K_{Ca} and chloride channel activity. These data implicate the K_v channel as the O_2-sensitive K^+ channel in SMCs from the resistance PA of the rat.[35] Furthermore, whole-cell current-clamp studies show that hypoxia and 4AP (a blocker of K_v channels), depolarizes E_m from -37 to -22 mV. In the adult pulmonary circulation, a decrease in O_2 tension inactivates the K_v channel, depolarizes PA SMCs, opens VOCC, and increases $[Ca^{2+}]_i$ to cause vasoconstriction.[36]

PA SMCs isolated from the late-gestation ovine fetus can directly sense an acute decrease in O_2 tension. Specifically, a change in O_2 tension from 125 to 30 torr causes PA SMCs $[Ca^{2+}]_i$ to increase by more than 100%. Since verapamil, a VOCC antagonist, attenuates, and BAY K 8644, a facilitator of VOCC, potentiates the hypoxia-induced increase in $[Ca^{2+}]_i$, it seems likely that acute hypoxia causes fetal PA SMC membrane depolarization and an increase in the rate of Ca^{2+} entry into PA SMCs via VOCC.[37] This effect is specific to PA SMCs derived from the distal pulmonary vasculature, as hypoxia causes a decrease in $[Ca^{2+}]_i$ in carotid artery SMCs and no change in SMCs derived from the proximal PA.[38] The observation that charybdotoxin (CTX), a K_{Ca} channel antagonist,[39] mimics the effect of hypoxia on fetal PA SMCs $[Ca^{2+}]_i$ (Figure 1)[37] provides support for the hypothesis that a subset of K^+ channels are involved in the maintenance of Ca^{2+} homeostasis under normoxic conditions (Figure 1). CTX blocks not only K_{Ca} channels, but also K_v 1.2, 1.3,[40] and 1.6.[41] However, the use of a more specific K_{Ca} channel blocker, iberi-

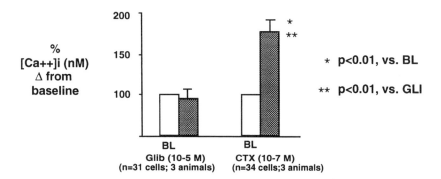

Figure 1. Effect of K^+ channel antagonists (shaded boxes), glibenclamide (GLI), and charybdotoxin (CTX) on basal (BL) $[Ca^{2+}]_i$ (open boxes) in PA SMCs. Charybdotoxin increased $[Ca^{2+}]_i$ from baseline, while glibenclamide had no effect on basal $[Ca^{2+}]_i$.

otoxin (IBTX), discussed later, makes it seem likely that K_{Ca} channels may serve as O_2 sensors in fetal PA SMCs.

K+ Channels and Perinatal Pulmonary Vasodilation

Pharmacological Studies

The observation that pharmacological blockade of NO production attenuates the decrease in PVR resulting from both ventilation alone and ventilation with 100% O_2 (Figure 2) provides direct evidence that NO production plays a key role in O_2-induced fetal pulmonary vasodilation.[10] Two separate studies have found that O_2-induced pulmonary vasodilation is either attenuated or prevented by pharmacological blockade of NO in the chronically instrumented fetal lamb.[8,9] These findings, which are consistent with the observation that O_2 tension is capable of modulating NO production in fetal PA endothelial cells,[42] imply that the increase in O_2 tension that occurs at birth may contribute to sustained and progressive pulmonary vasodilation by providing a stimulus for augmented NO production by the pulmonary endothelium.

Along with the emergence of data demonstrating a critically important role for NO in the transition of the perinatal pulmonary circulation,

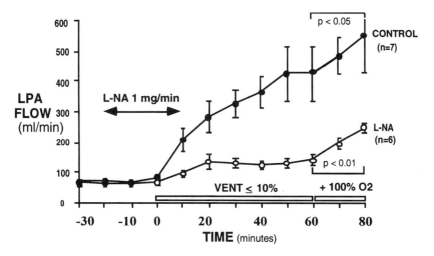

Figure 2. Hemodynamic effects of nitro-L-arginine (L-NA), a competitive inhibitor of nitric oxide production, on left pulmonary artery blood (LPA) flow, and during sequential ventilation with low and high F_{IO_2}. In comparison with control animals (closed circles; n=6 animals), L-NA treatment (open circles; n=7 animals) markedly attenuated the rise in LPA flow during ventilation with low F_{IO_2} (<0.10) and with high F_{IO_2} (1.00).

other studies indicated a link between the vasodilation caused by NO and K$^+$ channel activation in VSMCs. Robertson et al[43] demonstrated that, in cerebral artery SMCs, cyclic guanosine 3',5'-monophosphate (cGMP)-dependent protein kinase acts to phosphorylate the large conductance K_{Ca} channel. In PA SMCs, NO-induced increases in intracellular levels of cGMP cause activation of a cGMP-sensitive kinase and this, in turn, activates a K_{Ca} channel, resulting in vasodilation.[44] NO has also been shown to directly activate K_{Ca} channels.[45] If NO caused pulmonary vasodilation through K$^+$ channel activation, then blockade of K$^+$ channel activation would prevent the postnatal adaptation of the pulmonary circulation.

To test the hypothesis that K$^+$ channels modulate the changes in pulmonary hemodynamics associated with birth, the effect of K$^+$ channel inhibition on two physiologic stimuli essential for the transitional pulmonary circulation was studied in the acutely prepared late-gestation fetal lamb. These physiologic stimuli were: (1) mechanical ventilation with low inspired O$_2$ concentrations (designed to maintain normal fetal blood gas tensions), and (2) mechanical ventilation with high inspired O$_2$ concentrations. Acutely instrumented fetal lambs were treated with tetraethylammonium (TEA; a preferential K_{Ca} channel blocker[25]), glibenclamide (GLI; a blocker of K_{ATP} channels[46]), or saline. Lambs were ventilated with 0.10 inspired O$_2$ concentration (FIO$_2$) for 60 minutes, followed by 1.0 FIO$_2$ for 20 minutes. Neither TEA nor GLI had an effect on basal pulmonary tone. TEA attenuated and GLI had no effect on the increase in left pulmonary artery (LPA) flow and decrease in PVR in response to

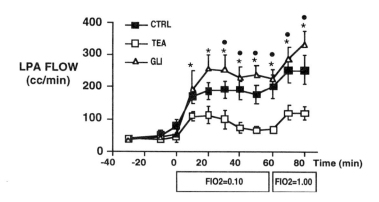

Figure 3. Effect of tetraethylammonium (TEA) and glibencamide (GLI) on left pulmonary artery blood (LPA) flow in response to sequential ventilation with low and high O$_2$. LPA flow in the TEA group was attenuated compared to control (CTRL) in response to both low and high O$_2$. LPA flow did not differ in CTRL and GLI groups. FIO$_2$ = fractional inspired O$_2$ concentration. * p<0.01, all groups compared to baseline value. • p<0.01 CTRL vs. TEA.

mechanical ventilation with 0.10 and 1.0 FIO_2 (Figure 3). While flow did increase in response to ventilation with low O_2 in the presence of K^+ channel inhibition, the increase was significantly attenuated compared to control. These results demonstrate that K^+ channel activation is required for postnatal adaptation of the pulmonary circulation. LPA flow is similarly attenuated in the presence of endothelium-derived NO (EDNO) inhibition, suggesting that EDNO may act, in part, through K^+ channel activation.[47] These data demonstrate that K^+ channel activation plays a central and critically important role in the pulmonary vasodilation that occurs at birth.

In the perinatal pulmonary circulation, the response of the pulmonary circulation to an acute increase in O_2 tension is biologically essential. If K_{Ca} channel activation is required for O_2-induced fetal pulmonary vasodilation, pharmacological blockade of the K_{Ca} channel should prevent the pulmonary vasodilation. To test this hypothesis, acutely instrumented late-gestation ovine fetuses were studied. O_2-induced fetal pulmonary vasodilation was blocked by TEA and IBTX, a specific K_{Ca} channel antagonist, but unaffected by GLI (Figure 4). This suggests that O_2 causes fetal pulmonary vasodilation through K_{Ca} channel activation. Inhibitors of either guanylate cyclase or cyclic nucleotide-dependent kinases, at doses that block the effect of cGMP, also attenuated O_2-dependent fetal pulmonary vasodilation, implying that elevated fetal O_2 acts to increase guanylate cyclase activity and cGMP concentra-

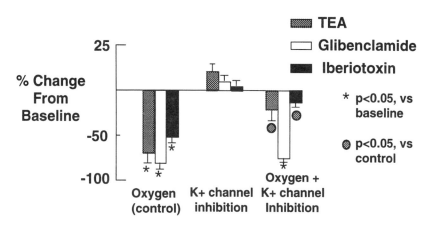

Figure 4. The effect of K^+ channel inhibition on O_2-induced fetal pulmonary vasodilation. In each of the control periods, O_2 caused a decrease in PVR ($p<0.05$). K^+ channel inhibition had no effect on basal PVR. Tetraethylammonium (TEA) blocked ($p<0.05$) and glibenclamide had no effect on O_2-induced fetal pulmonary vasodilation. Iberiotoxin, a specific K_{Ca} channel blocker, attenuated O_2-induced fetal pulmonary vasodilation ($p<0.05$).

tion. These in turn activate cyclic nucleotide-dependent kinases in fetal PA SMCs causing K_{Ca} channel activation and vasodilation.[48]

Electrophysiological Studies

The electrophysiological properties of fetal PA SMCs were further characterized using whole-cell, patch-clamp techniques and pharmacological probes. Initial studies were performed in external K^+ concentrations of 4.2 mmol/L, 8.4 mmol/L, and 16.8 mmol/L. Reversal potentials were calculated as -83.1 ± 1.5 mV (n=4), -67.1 ± 1.7 mV (n=3), and -50.5 ± 1.1 mV (n=3), respectively. These values approximate those calculated by the Nernst equation (at 30°C), -91.6 mV, -73.5 mV, and -55.4 mV, confirming that these were primarily K^+ conductances.

Under hypoxic conditions, outward currents recorded from PA SMCs were small (400 $\pm$ 47 pA at +40 mV; n=19) and showed brief bursts of superimposed outward current characteristic of spontaneously transient outward currents (STOCs). STOCs, defined as a transient, rapid increase in outward current carried by a K_{Ca} channel, were also observed when the cells were held at -30 mV (Figure 5). Whole-cell K^+ current and STOC activity was inhibited by TEA and CTX. It is thought that STOCs are initiated by the localized release of Ca^{2+} from a ryanodine (RyR)-sensitive Ca^{2+} pool in the sarcoplasmic reticulum. This release (termed a Ca^{2+} "spark") then activates plasmalemmal K_{Ca}

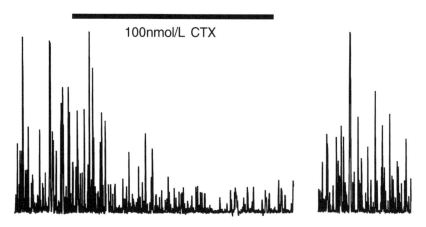

Figure 5. Representative recording of spontaneous transient outward currents (STOCS) in a fetal PA SMCs in hypoxia (30 torr). Currents were recorded at a steady-state potential of -30 mV. Application of 100 nmol/L charybdotoxin (CTX), indicated by the bar, decreased the current. Break in baseline indicates a 15-minute washout period.

channels closely associated with the release site. Thus, Ca^{2+} sparks stimulate an outward K^+ current causing membrane hyperpolarization and inhibition of Ca^{2+} entry into the cell. Ca^{2+} sparks, have been measured in VSMCs where they have been shown to activate 10–100 nearby plasmalemmal K_{Ca} channels to cause the spontaneously transient outward current or STOC.[26] Blocking Ca^{2+} sparks or decreasing their frequency will lead to membrane depolarization and vasoconstriction through a decrease in K_{Ca} channel activity. Conversely, increasing amplitude or frequency of Ca^{2+} sparks might lead to vasodilation through activation of K_{Ca} channel activity.[49] STOCs have been demonstrated in fetal PA SMCs (Figure 5), but not in PA SMCs from neonatal lambs or adult sheep. Consistent with a role for STOC activity in the regulation of fetal pulmonary vascular tone is previous work that demonstrated the presence of an internal RyR-sensitive Ca^{2+} store in fetal PA SMCs.

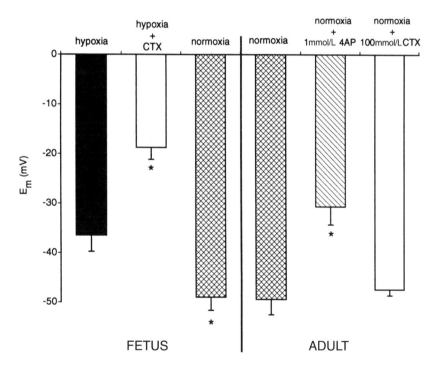

Figure 6. Mean (± SEM) membrane potentials (E_m) recorded from fetal and adult PA SMCs as indicated. Fetal membrane potentials were recorded in hypoxia (filled bar), after exposure to 100 nmol/L charybdotoxin (CTX) (open bar), and following exposure to normoxia (cross-hatched bar). Adult membrane potentials were recorded in normoxia (cross-hatched bar), and following exposure to either 1 mM 4-aminopyridine (4AP; diagonal-striped bar) or 100 nmol/L CTX (open bar). *p<0.05 from hypoxic control in fetus and normoxic controls in adult.

With the application of RyR, $[Ca^{2+}]_i$ increased immediately, indicating a role for the RyR-sensitive stores in the maintenance of Ca^{2+} homeostasis.[37] The presence of STOCs may reflect the high tone environment of the fetal pulmonary vasculature since they are also found in other high resistance beds such as the adult cerebral circulation. The physiologic significance for STOCs in the developing fetal pulmonary circulation is unknown but may provide a moderating influence that prevents fetal PVR from rising too high.

To determine the effect of an increase in O_2 tension on K^+ currents, whole-cell K^+ currents (I_K) were recorded from fetal PA SMCs in hypoxia ($\approx$30 torr) and then exposed to acute normoxia ($\approx$160 torr). Normoxia increased I_K (376 $\pm$ 80% at +40 mV; n=6; p<0.05) and this increase was reversed by 100 nmol/L CTX. The cGMP-dependent kinase inhibitor KT 5823 had no effect on basal, hypoxic I_K but prevented the normoxia-induced increase in I_K (n=3). NO caused a 253 $\pm$ 28% increase in I_K at +40 mV, an increase similar to that caused by normoxia (n=4). Hypoxic fetal PA SMCs had an E_m of -37.2 $\pm$ 1.9 mV (n=14). Normoxia hyperpolarized the membrane by 11.9 $\pm$ 2.6 mV, while CTX depolarized the membrane potential by 17.6 $\pm$ 3.1 mV (Figure 6). Thus, the pharmacological profile was consistent with the K_{Ca} channel being the major determinant of PA SMC resting membrane potential. These experiments suggest that increases in K_{Ca} channel activity may mediate the pulmonary vasodilation caused by elevation of O_2 tension in the perinatal pulmonary circulation. The increase in K^+ channel activity is likely to be mediated through a cGMP-dependent kinase. In these studies, O_2 appears to act through an intracellular second messenger system rather than directly on the channel.

Electrophysiological Comparison of Fetal and Adult PA SMCs

Additional experiments were done to investigate changes in functional expression of K^+ channels between the fetal and adult pulmonary circulations. Using the whole-cell patch-clamp technique, K^+ channel current was measured in freshly dispersed PA SMCs, from late gestation fetal and adult sheep. As previously shown, whole-cell K^+ currents recorded from fetal PA SMCs in hypoxia were small and characteristic of STOCs (Figure 5). Average E_m was -36 ± 3 mV and could be depolarized by CTX or TEA, but not by 4AP or GLI. In hypoxia, chelation of intracellular Ca^{2+} by 5 mmol/L BAPTA further reduced the amplitude of the whole-cell K^+ current and prevented STOC activity. Under these conditions, the remaining current was partially inhibited by 1 mmol/L 4AP. K$^+$ currents of fetal PA SMCs maintained in normoxia, were not significantly reduced by acute hypoxia. In contrast, in normoxic adult PA SMCs, whole-cell K$^+$ currents were large and resting membrane potential (RMP) was significantly more hyperpolarized (-49 ± 3 mV; Figure 6). These 4AP-sensitive K$^+$ currents, were partially inhibited by exposure to acute hypoxia. Thus, the K$^+$ channel regulating RMP in the ovine pulmonary circulation changes, following birth, from a K_{Ca} channel to a K_V channel. These observations provide evidence for the concept that maturational-dependent differences in the response of PA SMCs to changes in O$_2$ tension may be due to differences in K$^+$ channel activity.[50]

Molecular Assessment of Developmental Changes in PA SMC K$^+$ Channel Expression

K_{Ca} Channel Expression

If the overall hypothesis that K_{Ca} channel activity is greatest in the fetus and newborn and decreases with maturation is correct, then PA SMCs from the fetal pulmonary circulation should express the K_{Ca} channel and this expression might decrease with maturation. To determine K_{Ca} channel expression in the pulmonary circulation, vascular tissue was isolated from the lung of fetal and neonatal sheep. Tissue was obtained from the proximal and distal (fourth generation or greater intralobar pulmonary vessel) PAs. Western blotting was performed with 20 μg of crude protein per lane. Protein samples were subjected to sodium dodecyl sulfate-polyacrylamide gel electroporesis (SDS-PAGE) according to the method of Laemmli[51] in a minigel system (Biorad). Proteins were transferred onto PVDF membranes for 60 minutes at 100 V constant voltage using a mini-trans-blot cell. After protein transfer, the PVDF membranes were rinsed in TBS and incubated for 60 minutes in TBS with 5% dry milk. The K_{Ca} channel antibody (kindly provided by Irwin Levitan, PhD, Brandeis University) was diluted in TBS-milk and incubated overnight with the blots at 4°C. After 2 washes with TBS, the secondary antibody, goat anti-rabbit IgG, was added for 2 hours. Following washing, blots were exposed to X-ray film for time periods ranging from 2 minutes to overnight.

We have found that protein extract from the fetal and neonatal pulmonary vasculature expresses both a 62-kD fragment and a 135-kD band. The 135-kD band is consistent with full length alpha subunit of the K_{Ca} channel and the 62-kD band is consistent with an alpha subunit fragment.[52] The antibody used is directed against amino acids 455–477 of the

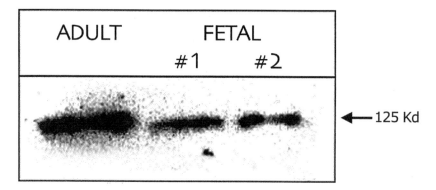

Figure 7. Western blot of the K_v 2.1 channel in distal pulmonary artery from adult and fetal sheep. Intensity of the band indicates increasing channel protein levels of the K_v2.1 channel with postnatal maturation. The 125-kD band is consistent with previously published reports. Each lane was loaded with 20 μg of protein.

alpha subunit. Our data support the notion that the K_{Ca} channel is abundantly expressed in the fetal and neonatal pulmonary circulations.

To test whether K_v channel expression increases with maturation, the expression of one K_v channel which has been shown to be O_2-sensitive (K_v 2.1[53]) was evaluated using protein extract from fetal, newborn, and adult distal pulmonary circulations. Consistent with the physiologic increase in HPV that occurs with maturation, K_v 2.1 channel expression increases with maturation (Figure 7). To perform these experiments, the antibody directed against the K_v 2.1 channel was obtained from Upstate Laboratories (Lake Placid, NY). These data provide evidence that developmentally regulated alterations in PA SMC K^+ channel expression are present, and may represent an adaptation that allows the pulmonary circulation to respond to specific physiologic signals that are relevant to a particular developmental stage.

In summary, these studies show that there are maturational changes in K^+ channel activity in the pulmonary circulation, and that the change in channel-controlling RMP between the low O_2 tension environment of the normal fetus and the normoxic environment of the adult circulation may parallel the different O_2-sensing mechanisms of each bed. The mechanism whereby a maturation-related change in K_{Ca} and K_v channel activity occurs remains unknown. Definitive identification of the O_2 sensor in the developing pulmonary vasculature may provide a specific molecular target for treatment of pulmonary vascular disease in newborn infants.

Acknowledgments   Jean Herron is acknowledged for excellent technical assistance.

References

1. Rudolph A. Distribution and regulation of blood flow in the fetal and neonatal lamb. *Circ Res* 1985;57:811–821.
2. Cassin S, Dawes GS, Mott JC, et al. The vascular resistance of the fetal and newly ventilated lung of the lamb. *J Physiol* 1964;171:61–79.
3. Dawes GS, Mott JC, Widdicombe JG, et al. Changes in the lungs of the newborn lamb. *J Physiol (Lond)* 1953;121:141–162.
4. Cassin S, Dawes GS, Ross BB. Pulmonary blood flow and vascular resistance in immature fetal lambs. *J Physiol* 1964;171:80–89.
5. Assali NS, Kirchbaum TH, Dilts PV. Effects of hyperbaric oxygen on utero placental and fetal circulation. *Circ Res* 1968;22:573–588.
6. Leffler CW, Hessler JR, Green RS. The onset of breathing at birth stimulates pulmonary vascular prostacyclin synthesis. *Ped Res* 1984;18:938–942.
7. Abman SH, Chatfield BA, Hall SL, et al. Role of endothelium-derived relaxing factor during transition of pulmonary circulation at birth. *Am J Physiol* 1990;259:H1921-H1927.
8. McQueston JA, Cornfield DN, McMurtry IF, et al. Effects of oxygen and exogenous L-arginine on EDRF activity in fetal pulmonary circulation. *Am J Physol* 1993;264:H865-H871.
9. Tiktinsky MH, Morin FC III. Increasing oxygen tension dilates fetal pulmonary circulation via endothelium-derived relaxing factor. *Am J Physiol* 1993;265:H376-H380.
10. Cornfield D, Chatfield B, McQueston J, et al. Effects of birth-related stimuli on L-arginine-dependent pulmonary vasodilation in ovine fetus. *Am J Physiol* 1992;262:H1474-H1481.
11. Moore P, Velvis H, Fineman JR, et al. EDRF inhibition attenuates the increase in pulmonary blood flow due to oxygen ventilation in fetal lambs. *J Appl Physiol* 1992;73:2151–2157.
12. North AJ, Moya FR, Mysore MR, et al. Pulmonary endothelial nitric oxide synthase gene expression is decreased in a rat model of congenital diaphragmatic hernia. *Am J Respir Cell Mol Biol* 1995;13:676–682.
13. Shaul PW, Yuhanna IS, German Z, et al. Pulmonary endothelial NO synthase gene expression is decreased in fetal lambs with pulmonary hypertension. *Am J Physiol* 1997;272:L1005-L1012.
14. Tajchman UW, Tuder RM, Horan M, et al. Persistent eNOS in lung hypoplasia caused by left pulmonary artery ligation in the ovine fetus. *Am J Physiol* 1997;272:L969-L978.
15. McMurtry IF, Davidson AB, Reeves JT, et al. Inhibition of hypoxic pulmonary vasoconstriction by calcium antagonists in isolated rat lungs. *Circ Res* 1976;38:99–104.
16. Post JM, Hume JR, Archer SL, et al. Direct role for potassium channel inhibition in hypoxic pulmonary vasoconstriction. *Am J Physiol* 1992;262: C882-C890.
17. Yuan X-J, Goldman WF, Tod ML, et al. Hypoxia reduces potassium currents in cultured rat pulmonary but not mesenteric arterial myocytes. *Am J Physiol* 1993;264:L116-L123.
18. Salvaterra CG, Goldman W. Acute hypoxia increases cytosolic calcium in cultured pulmonary arterial myocytes. *Am J Physiol* 1993;264:L323-L328.
19. Yuan XJ, Wang J, Juhaszova M, et al. Attenuated K⁺ channel gene transcription in primary pulmonary hypertension. *Lancet* 1998;351:726–727.
20. Wang J, Juhaszova M, Rubin LJ, et al. Hypoxia inhibits gene expression of

voltage-gated K$^+$ channel alpha subunits in pulmonary artery smooth muscle cells. *J Clin Invest* 1997;100:2347–2353.

21. Rusch NJ, Runnels AM. Remission of high blood pressure reverses arterial potassium channel alterations. *Hypertension* 1994;23:941–945.

22. Martens JR, Gelband CH. Alterations in rat interlobar artery membrane potential and K$^+$ channels in genetic and nongenetic hypertension. *Circ Res* 1996;79:295–301.

23. Liu Y, Hudetz AG, Knaus H-G, et al. Increased expression of Ca^{2+}-sensitive K$^+$ channels in the cerebral microcirculation of genetically hypertensive rats. *Circ Res* 1998;82:729–737.

24. Rudy B. Diversity and ubiquity of K$^+$ channels. *Neuroscience* 1988;25:729–749.

25. Nelson MT, Quayle JM. Physiological roles and properties of potassium channels in arterial smooth muscle. *Am J Physiol* 1995;268:C799-C822.

26. Nelson MT, Cheng H, Rubart M, et al. Relaxation of arterial smooth muscle by arterial sparks. *Science* 1995;270:633–637.

27. López-Barneo J, López-López JR, Ureña J, et al. Chemotransduction in the carotid body: K$^+$ current modulated by PO$_2$ in type I chemoreceptor cells. *Science* 1988;241:580–582.

28. Montoro RJ, Urena J, Fernandez-Chacon R, et al. Oxygen sensing by ion channels and chemoreception in single glomus cells. *J Gen Physiol* 1996; 107:133–143.

29. Urena J, Fernandez-Chacon R, Benot AR, et al. Hypoxia induces voltage dependent Ca^{2+} entry and quantal dopamine secretion in carotid body glomus cells. *Proc Natl Acad Sci USA* 1994;91:10208-10211.

30. Ganforina MD, Lopez-Barneo J. Single K$^+$ channels in membrane paths of arterial chemoreceptor cells are modulated by O$_2$ tension. *Proc Natl Acad Sci USA* 1991;88:2927–2930.

31. Peers C. Hypoxic suppression of K$^+$ currents in type I carotid body cells: Selective effect on the Ca^{2+}-activated K$^+$ current. *Neurosci Lett* 1990;119: 253–256.

32. Hatton CJ, Carpenter E, Pepper DR, et al. Developmental changes in isolated rat type I carotid body cell K$^+$ currents and their modulation by hypoxia. *J Physiol* 1997;501:49–58.

33. Yuan X-J, Tod ML, Rubin LJ, et al. Contrasting effects of hypoxia on tension in rat pulmonary and mesenteric arteries. *Am J Physiol* 1990;259: H281-H289.

34. Weir EK, Archer SL. The mechanism of hypoxic pulmonary vasoconstriction: The tale of two channels. *FASEB J* 1995;9:183–189.

35. Archer SL, Huang JMC, Reeve HL, et al. The differential distribution of electrophysiologically distinct myocytes in conduit and resistance arteries determines their response to nitric oxide and hypoxia. *Circ Res* 1996;78: 431–442.

36. Yuan XJ. Voltage-gated K$^+$ currents regulate resting membrane potential and [Ca^{2+}]i in pulmonary arterial myocytes. *Circ Res* 1995;77:370–378.

37. Cornfield DN, Stevens T, McMurtry IF, et al. Acute hypoxia causes membrane depolarization and calcium influx in fetal pulmonary artery smooth muscle cells. *Am J Physiol* 1994;266:L469-L475.

38. Cornfield DN, Stevens T, McMurtry IF, et al. Acute hypoxia increases cytosolic calcium in fetal pulmonary artery smooth muscle cells. *Am J Physiol* 1993;265:L53-L56.

39. Miller C, Moczydlowski E, Latorre R, et al. Charybdotoxin, a protein in-

hibitor of single Ca^{2+}-activated K$^+$ channels from mammalian skeletal muscle. *Nature* 1985;313:316–318.

40. Grissmer S, Nguyen AN, Aiyar J, et al. Pharmacological characterization of five cloned voltage-gated K$^+$ channels, types Kv1.1, 1.2, 1.5, and 3.1, stably expressed in mammalian cell lines. *Mol Pharmacol* 1994;45:1227–1234.

41. Garcia ML, Garcia-Calvo M, Hidalgo P, et al. Purification and characterization of three inhibitors of voltage-dependent K$^+$ channels from *Leiurus quinquestriatus* var. *herbraeus* venom. *Biochemistry* 1994;33:6834–6839.

42. Shaul PW, Wells LB. Oxygen modulates nitric oxide production selectively in fetal pulmonary endothelial cells. *Am J Respir Cell Mol Biol* 1994;11:432–438.

43. Robertson BE, Schubert R, Hescheler J, et al. cGMP-dependent protein kinase activates Ca^{2+}-activated K$^+$ channels in cerebral artery smooth muscle cells. *Am J Physiol* 1993;265:C299-C303.

44. Archer SL, Huang JM-C, Hampl V, et al. Nitric oxide and cGMP cause vasorelaxation by activation of a charybdotoxin-sensitive K channel by cGMP-dependent protein kinase. *Proc Natl Acad Sci USA* 1994;91:7583–7587.

45. Bolotina VM, Najibi S, Palacino JJ, et al. Nitric oxide directly activates calcium-dependent potassium channels in vascular smooth muscle. *Nature* 1994;368:850–853.

46. Standen NB, Quayle JM, Davies NW, et al. Hyperpolarizing vasodilators activate ATP-sensitive K$^+$ channels in arterial smooth muscle. *Science* 1989;245:177–180.

47. Tristani-Firouzi M, Martin EB, Tolarova S, et al. Ventilation-induced pulmonary vasodilation at birth is modulated by potassium channel activity. *Am J Physiol* 1996;271:H2353-H2359.

48. Cornfield DN, Reeve HL, Tolarova S, et al. L. Oxygen causes fetal pulmonary vasodilation through activation of a calcium-dependent potassium channel. *Proc Natl Acad Sci USA* 1996;93:8089–8094.

49. Porter VA, Bonev AD, Knot HJ, et al. Frequency modulation of Ca^{2+} sparks is involved in regulation of arterial diameter by cyclic nucleotides. *Am J Physiol* 1998;274:C1346-C1355.

50. Reeve HL, Archer SL, Weir EK, et al. Maturational changes in K$^+$ channel activity and oxygen sensing in the ovine pulmonary vasculature. *Am J Physiol* 1998;275:L1019-L1025.

51. Laemmli UK. Cleavage of structural proteins during the assembly of the head of bacteriophage T4. *Nature* 1970;227:680–685.

52. Garcia-Calvo M, Knaus H-G, McManus OB, et al. Purification and reconstitution of the high conductance, calcium-activated potassium channel from tracheal smooth muscle. *J Biol Chem* 1994;269:676–682.

53. Patel A, Lazdunski M, Honore E. Kv2.1/Kv9.3 a novel ATP-dependent delayed rectifier channel in oxygen-sensitive pulmonary artery myocytes. *EMBO J* 1997;16:6615–6625.

Chapter 19

Regulation of Ion Channels in the Ductus Arteriosus

Helen L. Reeve, PhD, and E. Kenneth Weir, MD

The ductus arteriosus (DA) is an essential fetal structure that diverts deoxygenated blood from the main pulmonary artery directly into the descending aorta. This allows the high resistance fetal pulmonary circulation to be bypassed. At birth, the pulmonary circulation dilates and the DA gradually constricts, thus removing the right to left shunt.[1] The process of closure occurs in two stages: the oxygen (O_2)-induced functional closure that occurs within 48 hours of birth in the human, and permanent anatomic closure (necrosis and fibrosis of intimal and medial layers), which occurs by 2–3 weeks of age.[2] The processes involved in the functional closure of the DA are poorly understood, although it seems clear that two separate mechanisms are involved—removal of the dilator influence of prostaglandins, and active constriction of the smooth muscle.[3] Numerous theories regarding functional closure have been proposed, but to date none of these fully explain the phenomenon.[4] One important aspect is that an increase in O_2 levels is required (at birth, PaO_2 levels increase from approximately 20 to 100 mm Hg), because while lung inflation with nitrogen is sufficient to dilate the constricted pulmonary circulation,[5] it will not activate ductal closure.[6,7] This dependency on the O_2 level may explain the higher incidence of patent ductus (where the DA fails to constrict at birth) at high altitude, where the air has lower O_2 levels.[8] The O_2 response was demonstrated to be intrinsic to the DA by Kovalcik,[9] who showed that raising O_2 levels constricted DA strips but had no effect on strips taken from the adjacent pulmonary artery or aorta. Fay[10] showed

This work was supported by National Institutes of Health Grant R29 HL59182–01 (H.L. Reeve) and Veterans Administration Merit Review Funding (E.K. Weir).

From: Weir EK, Archer SL, Reeves JT (eds). *The Fetal and Neonatal Pulmonary Circulations.* Armonk, NY: Futura Publishing Company, Inc.; ©1999.

that the O_2-dependent constriction did not require the presence of either the adventitia or the endothelium, and consequently was a function of the DA smooth muscle. A rise in intracellular Ca^{2+} has also been shown to be necessary for DA constriction. Kovalcik,[9] showed that in isolated DA rings, chelating extracellular Ca^{2+} with EGTA prevented O_2-induced constriction, while normal constriction could be restored by returning Ca^{2+} to the medium.

The most common clinical treatment at present for patent ductus is the administration of the cyclooxygenase inhibitor, indomethacin.[11] Prostaglandins, in particular PGE_2, have been shown to play a role in maintaining the patency of the ductus during development.[12-20] In the rabbit, this dilation is mediated through the EP_4 receptor.[21] Furthermore, EP_4-deficient mice show less ductal constriction, demonstrating an active role for prostaglandins in constriction.[22] The cellular mechanism for the action of PGE_2 is likely to involve its inhibition of contractile protein Ca^{2+} sensitivity.[23] Despite the importance of prostaglandins, the closure of the DA is mediated by more than just the withdrawal of a dilator influence.[4] The increase in O_2 tension at birth is likely to be the major factor controlling the mechanism of active ductal constriction.

There is a large body of data from other O_2-sensitive tissues such as the pulmonary artery[24-26] and carotid body[27,28] indicating that K^+ channels play an essential role in their responsiveness to changes in O_2. The activity of K^+ channels, at least partially, determines the resting membrane potential (RMP) of most cells, and so modulation of their activity can produce profound cellular effects. Inhibition of a K^+ channel that sets the RMP in a vascular smooth muscle cell will cause depolarization of the cell membrane, which in turn will open voltage-dependent Ca^{2+} channels, increase intracellular Ca^{2+}, and induce constriction. In contrast, activation of K^+ channels will hyperpolarize the cell membrane and either oppose vasoconstriction or induce vasodilatation. The adult pulmonary artery constricts to decreased O_2 (hypoxia) via inhibition of a 4-amino-pyridine (4AP)-sensitive, voltage-gated K^+ (K_v) channel whose activity underlies the RMP of the pulmonary artery smooth muscle cells.[26,29] In the carotid body, hypoxic inhibition of K^+ channels can lead to a change in respiratory rate.[30] Data obtained from adult carotid body type I cells show that low levels of O_2 inhibit a K_v channel to initiate the associated release of dopamine.[27,30] Systemic vessels, which dilate to a decrease in O_2, may also do so through modulation of K^+ channels. Hypoxia has been shown to activate Ca^{2+}-dependent K^+ channels (K_{Ca}) and ATP-dependent K^+ channels (K_{ATP}) to cause vasodilatation in cerebral[31] and coronary[32] blood vessels, respectively. It is therefore clear that ion channels and O_2 are intimately linked. Studies by Roulet and Coburn[33] showed that O_2-induced contraction of the DA was associated with smooth muscle cell depolarization, suggesting that there may be a role for ion channels in modulation of DA vasoconstriction.

K⁺ Channels in DA Smooth Muscle

Studies using pharmacological antagonists of K⁺ channels have given indirect evidence for the presence of different K⁺ channels in DA smooth muscle cells. Nakanishi et al[34] demonstrated that rabbit DA rings could be constricted in hypoxia by glibenclamide (GLI), a blocker of K_{ATP} channels. Furthermore, O_2-induced contraction could be overcome by cromakalim, a K_{ATP} opener. More recently, Tristani-Firouzi et al[35] showed that fetal rabbit rings were more likely to constrict to the K_v channel blocker 4AP (1 mmol/L) than GLI, indicating a K_v channel may be controlling RMP. Whole-cell and single channel patch-clamp studies identified several types of K⁺ channel in DA smooth muscle cells. Whole-cell currents recorded from a holding potential of −70 mV in hypoxic DA smooth muscle cells could be inhibited by both 1 mmol/L 4AP and 1 mmol/L tetraethylammonium (a blocker of K_{Ca} channels) indicating the presence of both K_v channels and K_{Ca} channels

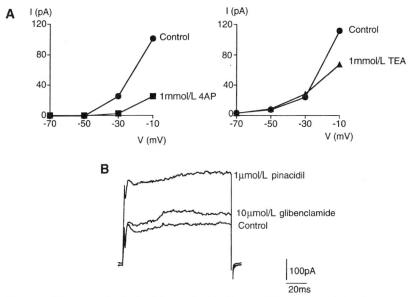

Figure 1. Pharmacological evidence for K_v, K_{Ca}, and K_{ATP} channels in ductus arteriosus (DA) smooth muscle. **A:** Representative current-voltage (I-V) curves recorded from a DA smooth muscle cell from a holding potential of −70 mV. Outward currents were partially inhibited by 1 mmol/L 4-aminopyridine (4AP) at all potentials positive to −50 mV (left panel). Following washout of 4AP, the cell was exposed to 1 mmol/L tetraethylammonium (TEA) and inhibition was observed at potentials more positive than −10 mV (right panel). **B:** Actual current traces recorded from a DA smooth muscle cell by stepping from −70 mV to +30 mV. Currents were recorded during control, after exposure to 1 μmol/L pinacidil and (in the continued presence of pinacidil) after 10 μmol/L glibenclamide.

(Figure 1A). Activity of K_v channels could be completely abolished by holding the cell at a more depolarized membrane potential (-10 mV), indicating that they were open at more negative potentials and therefore likely to be the channels at the RMP of the cell. This was confirmed by membrane potential measurements which showed that cells could be depolarized by 4AP, but not by tetraethylammonium or glibenclamide. While it is unlikely that K_{ATP} channels are open under normal conditions (glibenclamide has no effect on outward K^+ current recorded from the hypoxic ductus[35]), they are present in DA smooth muscle cells. Whole-cell K^+ currents treated with 1 μmol/L pinacidil (an activator of K_{ATP} channels) show an increase in outward and inward current such that total current becomes voltage-independent, consistent with activation of K_{ATP} channels. This activation can be completely overcome by 10 μmol/L glibenclamide (Figure 1B). Coupled with cromakalim's dilation of O_2-constricted rings[34] there is strong evidence for the presence of K_{ATP} channels in DA smooth muscle cells, although at present their function is not known. Single channel studies have shown the presence of at least three different con-

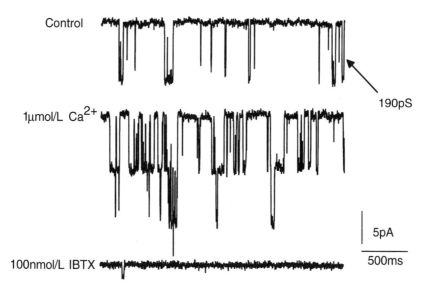

Figure 2. Single channel evidence for K_{Ca} channels in DA smooth muscle cells. Single channels were recorded using the inside-out configuration of the patch-clamp technique at a potential of -30 mV. Activity was shown under control conditions (nominal Ca^{2+}), following addition of 1 μmol/L Ca^{2+} to the bath, and after addition of 100 nmol/L iberiotoxin (IBTX). Note the presence of a small conductance channel following IBTX.

ductance channels: 30 pS, 54–58 pS, and 150–190 pS. The large con-ductance channel is activated by Ca^{2+} and inhibited by iberiotoxin in inside-out patches, indicating it to be a K_{Ca} channel (Figure 2). The mid-conductance channel is inhibited by 1 mmol/L 4AP and so likely to be of the K_v family, despite its unusually large single channel conductance. These data show that DA smooth muscle cells, like other vascular smooth muscle cells,[36] have K_v, K_{Ca}, and K_{ATP} channel activity, with the K_v channel controlling RMP and therefore, tone.

Ca^{2+} Channels in DA Smooth Muscle Cells

The dependence of ductal constriction on extracellular Ca^{2+} was demonstrated by Kovalcik,[9] who temporarily abolished constriction with EGTA. More recent data has shown that DA constriction can be prevented or reversed by L-type Ca^{2+} channel antagonists such as nisoldipine and verapamil, but not by T-type Ca^{2+} channel blockers.[34,35] As yet, there are no reports of Ca^{2+} channels recorded from DA smooth muscle using direct, electrophysiological techniques.

O_2 and Ion Channels

The interactions of O_2 and ion channels have become the focus of a large body of work in a variety of tissues including the carotid body,[27,28,37] the neuroepithelial body,[38] pulmonary artery smooth,[24–26] and systemic smooth muscle.[31,32] All of these tissues have a commonality in that they seem to respond to changes in O_2 tension through modulation of ion channel activity and, in particular, K^+ channel activity. O_2 also modifies K^+ channels in DA smooth muscle cells. DA rings constricted with 4AP have no additional response to O_2. Whole-cell outward K^+ current is significantly reduced in DA smooth muscle cells maintained in normoxia following digestion, as compared to hypoxia (506 ± 137 pA, n=9, in hypoxia compared with 170 ± 20 pA in normoxia, n=13, both at +30 mV). Similarly, hypoxic K^+ current could be partially inhibited by acute exposure to O_2.[35] Furthermore, in single channel studies, a 4AP-sensitive K_v channel was inhibited by normoxia, while the larger conductance K_{Ca} channel was not. Recordings of membrane potential also suggest that acute O_2 can depolarize the membrane of hypoxic DA smooth muscle cells.[35] Together, these data indicate that the increase in O_2 levels that occurs at birth may initiate ductal constriction, at least in part through inhibition of a K_v channel, membrane depolarization, and subsequent influx of Ca^{2+} through L-type Ca^{2+} channels.

Modulation of K^+ Channels by Catalase in DA Smooth Muscle Cells

The mechanism by which ion channel activity is modulated by changes in O_2 remains controversial. It has been proposed that the change in O_2 can alter the redox status of the cell and that this change can then influence the activity of ion channels.[39] There is substantial evidence that K^+ channels can be redox-modulated. Ruppersburg et al[40] showed that the redox status of glutathione could determine the gating of some mammalian K^+ channels by modifying a critical cysteine residue in the N-terminal region. In addition, there are several reports that oxidizing and reducing agents can change the activity of K^+ channels in cells as diverse as bacteria and smooth muscle.[41-43] As reducing equivalents such as NADH are oxidized to form ATP molecules in mitochondrial oxidative phosphorylation, reactive O_2 species including superoxide and hydrogen peroxide (H_2O_2) are formed in proportion to the level of cellular O_2. H_2O_2 has also been shown to modulate K^+ channel activity, although its effects have been to either increase or decrease endogenous channel activity depending on the cell being studied.[44-47] While it is known that exogenous H_2O_2 can change the activity of K^+ channels, the effect of endogenous H_2O_2 is more difficult to study. Cellular degradation of H_2O_2 to H_2O and O_2 occurs through the activity of catalase. Preliminary electrophysiological studies in DA smooth muscle cells suggest that modulation of endogenous levels of H_2O_2 may have an effect on K^+ channel activity. In normoxic cells, inclusion of catalase in the patch-clamp pipette causes a gradual increase in whole-cell outward K^+ current over 20 minutes (Figure 3A). This increase is not mimicked by dialysis of the cells for 20 minutes without catalase in the pipette or with boiled catalase, Na citrate (catalase buffer), or a millimolar equivalent concentration of albumin. This suggests that endogenous H_2O_2 levels inhibit K^+ channel activity, and that this inhibition is lost when H_2O_2 is removed by catalase. Pharmacological and voltage studies suggest that the increase in current may be due to activation of both K_v and K_{Ca} channels. Ten $\mu mol/L$ glibenclamide is unable to prevent the increase in current that occurs in the presence of intracellular catalase, while 1 mmol/L 4AP brings the current almost back to control levels (Figure 3B). Currents recorded at a holding potential of -10 mV (to inactivate K_v channels) are significantly smaller, but are also enhanced following catalase dialysis, with the increased current being inhibited by 100 nmol/L iberiotoxin (Figure 3C). While these data do not remove the possibility that loss of reactive O_2 species further down the reaction pathway from H_2O_2 (such as the hydroxyl radical) may account for the changes in K^+ current, they do provide the

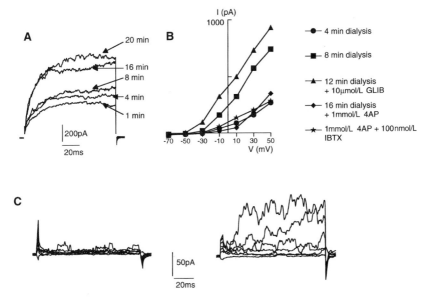

Figure 3. Catalase activation of K$^+$ currents in DA smooth muscle cells. **A:** Actual current traces recorded from a DA smooth muscle cell by stepping from −70 mV to +50 mV. The intracellular pipette solution contained 200 U/mL catalase. Currents were recorded at 1, 4, 8, 16, and 20 minutes (min) after achieving the whole-cell configuration as indicated. **B:** Representative I-V plot of currents recorded from a holding potential of -70 mV with 200 U/mL catalase in the pipette. Currents were recorded following 4 min dialysis (●), 8 min dialysis (■), 12 min dialysis in the presence of 10 μmol/L glibenclamide (GLIB;▲), at 16 min plus 1 mmol/L 4AP (in the continued presence of GLIB; ♦) and following 100 nmol/L IBTX (★). **C:** Actual current traces were recorded from a DA smooth muscle cell using a holding potential of -10 mV to inactivate K$_v$ channels. Traces on the left were recorded with 200U/mL catalase in the pipette at 1 min after achieving whole-cell configuration, and on the right at 20 min of dialysis (note smaller pA scale).

first evidence that modulating endogenous H$_2$O$_2$ levels can alter channel activity. A schema of the mechanism by which endogenous H$_2$O$_2$ may control K$^+$ channel activity and, hence, tone in the ductus, is shown in Figure 4. During development in utero, where O$_2$ levels, and hence, H$_2$O$_2$ levels, are low, K$^+$ channels are open, the membrane is hyperpolarized, and the ductus is dilated. As O$_2$ levels increase at birth, the rise in H$_2$O$_2$ inhibits K$^+$ channel activity resulting in membrane depolarization and constriction. There is some circumstantial data in isolated ductal rings supporting this mechanism. Rings constricted by normoxia can be dilated by NMPG, a reducing agent that decreases H$_2$O$_2$ levels to a similar extent as hypoxia.[48] It has previously been suggested that reactive O$_2$ species may be important in control of ductal

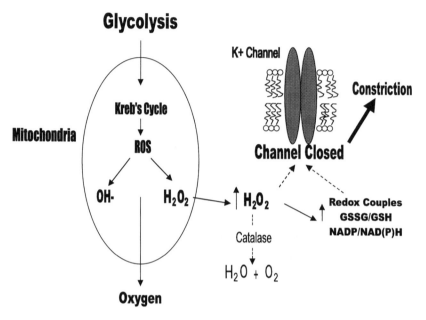

Figure 4. Schematic representation of mechanism by which changes in O_2 may be sensed by K^+ channels in DA smooth muscle cells. OH− = superoxide; H_2O_2 = hydrogen peroxide; ROS = reactive O_2 species.

tone. Clyman et al[49] demonstrated that high concentrations (1 mmol/L) of t-butyl H_2O_2 could dilate intact, O_2-constricted ductal rings. On reflection, this observed dilator effect is not likely to be part of the physiologic response of the ductus to O_2. In vivo, an increase in H_2O_2 would occur concomitant with the rise in O_2 at birth. According to Clyman's model, this increase in H_2O_2 should cause dilation of the ductus while, in fact, increasing O_2 levels causes constriction. It is more likely that the observed dilation is an anomaly of exposing the rings to high extracellular levels of an oxidizing agent.

In conclusion, it appears that regulation of ion channels may play a significant role in regulation of tone in the DA. The mechanism of ductal constriction that occurs on exposure to high levels of O_2 at birth may include inhibition of the activity of a K_v channel by the increased levels of cytosolic H_2O_2. We should not forget that O_2 may also directly or indirectly modulate the activity of other ion channels, such as Ca^{2+} and Cl^-, which in turn may influence ductal tone. In the pulmonary artery, Ca^{2+} channels have been shown to be O_2-sensitive,[50,51] while

Ca^{2+}-dependent Cl^- channels can be activated[52,53] and K_v channels inhibited by, endothelin-1.[54,55] This may be of importance in the DA since endothelin-1 is released from the ductus in an O_2-dependent manner and thought to play a part in ductal constriction.[56–58] As with other vascular tissues, it is likely that multiple pathways control ductal tone and future experiments should include the investigation of other ion channels.

References

1. Heymann MA, Rudolph AM. Control of the ductus arteriosus. *Physiol Rev* 1975;55:62–78.
2. Eldridge FL, Hultgre HN. The physiologic closure of the ductus arteriosus in the newborn infant. *J Clin Invest* 1955;34:987–996.
3. Coceani F, Olley PM. Eicosanoids in the fetal and transitional pulmonary circulation. *Chest* 1988;93:112S-117S.
4. Smith GC. The pharmacology of the ductus arteriosus. *Pharm Rev* 1998;50:35–58.
5. Dawes GS, Mott JC, Widdicombe JG, et al. Changes in the lungs of the newborn lamb. *J Physiol (Lond)* 1953;121:141–162.
6. Kennedy JA, Clark, SL. Observations on the ductus arteriosus of the guinea pig in relation to its method of closure. *Anat Rec* 1941;79:349–371.
7. Kennedy JA, Clark SL. Observations on the physiological reactions of the ductus arteriosus. *Am J Physiol* 1942;136:140–147.
8. Alzamora V. On the possible influence of great altitudes on the determination of certain cardiovascular anomalies. *Pediatrics* 1953;12:259–263.
9. Kovalcik V. The response of the isolated ductus arteriosus to oxygen and anoxia. *J Physiol (Lond)* 1963;169:185–197.
10. Fay FS. Guinea pig ductus arteriosus I: Cellular and metabolic basis for oxygen sensitivity. *Am J Physiol* 1971;221:470–479.
11. Gersony WM. Effects of indomethacin in premature infants with patent ductus arteriosus: Results of a national collaborative study. *J Pediatr* 1983;102:895–906.
12. Coceani F, Olley PM. The response of the ductus arteriosus to prostaglandins. *Can J Physiol Pharmacol* 1973;51:220–223. 13.
13. Coceani F, Olley PM, Bodach E. Lamb ductus arteriosus: Effect of prostaglandin synthesis inhibitors on the muscle tone and the response to prostaglandin E2. *Prostaglandins* 1975;9:299–308.
14. Coceani F, Olley PM, Lock JE. Prostaglandins, ductus arteriosus, pulmonary circulation: Current concepts and clinical potential. *Eur J Clin Pharmacol* 1980;18:75–81.
15. Olley PM, Bodach E, Heaton J, et al. Further evidence implicating E-type prostaglandins in the patency of the lamb ductus arteriosus. *Eur J Pharmacol* 1975;34:247–250.
16. Sharpe GL, Larsson KS. Studies on closure of the ductus arteriosus. X. In vivo effects of prostaglandins. *Prostaglandins* 1975;9:703–709.
17. Starling MB, Elliott RB. The effects of prostaglandins, prostaglandin inhibitors and oxygen on the closure of the ductus arteriosus, pulmonary arteries and umbilical vessels in vitro. *Prostaglandins* 1974;8:187–203.
18. Clyman RI, Heymann MA, Rudolph AM. Ductus arteriosus responses to

prostaglandin E1 at high and low oxygen concentrations. *Prostaglandins* 1977;13:219–223.

19. Clyman RI, Mauray F, Koerper MA, et al. Formation of prostacyclin (PGI2) by the ductus arteriosus of fetal lambs at different stages of gestation. *Prostaglandins* 1978;16:633–642.

20. Clyman RI, Mauray F, Heymann MA, et al. Ductus arteriosus: Developmental response to oxygen and indomethacin. *Prostaglandins* 1978;15:993–998.

21. Smith GC, Coleman RA, McGrath JC. Characterization of dilator prostanoid receptors in the fetal rabbit ductus arteriosus. *J Pharmacol Exp Ther* 1994;271:390–396.

22. Nguyen MT, Camenisch T, Snouwaert JN, et al. The prostaglandin receptor EP4 triggers remodeling of the cardiovascular system at birth. *Nature* 1997;390:78–81.

23. Crichton CA, Smith GCS, Smith GL. Alpha-toxin permeabilized rabbit fetal ductus arteriosus is more sensitive to Ca^{2+} than aorta or main pulmonary artery. *Cardiovasc Res* 1997;33:223–229.

24. Post JM, Hume JR, Archer SL, et al. Direct role for potassium channel inhibition in hypoxic pulmonary vasoconstriction. *Am J Physiol* 1992;262: C882-C890.

25. Yuan X-J, Goldman WF, Tod ML, et al. Hypoxia reduces potassium currents in cultured rat pulmonary but not mesenteric arterial myocytes. *Am J Physiol* 1993;264:L116-L123.

26. Archer SL, Huang JMC, Reeve HL, et al. Differential distribution of electrophysiologically distinct myocytes in conduit and resistance arteries determines their response to nitric oxide and hypoxia. *Circ Res* 1996;78:431–442.

27. Lopez-Barneo J, Lopez-Lopez JR, Urena J, et al. Chemotransduction in the carotid body: K^+ current modulated by pO_2 in type I chemoreceptor cells. *Science* 1989;241:580–582.

28. Peers C. Hypoxic suppression of K^+ currents in type I carotid body cells: Selective effect on the Ca^{2+}-activated K^+ current. *Neurosci Lett* 1990;119: 253–256.

29. Yuan X-J. Voltage-gated K^+ currents regulate resting membrane potential and $[Ca^{2+}]_i$ in pulmonary arterial myocytes. *Circ Res* 1995;77:370–378.

30. Urena J, Fernanadez-Chacon R, Benot AR, et al. Hypoxia induces voltage-dependent Ca^{2+} entry and quantal dopamine secretion in carotid body glomus cells. *Proc Natl Acad Sci USA* 1994;91:10208-10211.

31. Gebremedhin D, Bonnet P, Greene AS, et al. Hypoxia increases the activity of Ca^{2+}-sensitive K^+ channels in cat cerebral arterial muscle cell membranes. *Pflügers Arch* 1994;428:621–630.

32. Dart C, Standen NB. Activation of ATP-dependent K^+ channels by hypoxia in smooth muscle cells isolated from the pig coronary artery. *J Physiol (Lond)* 1995;483:29–39.

33. Roulet MJ, Coburn RF. Oxygen-induced contraction in guinea-pig neonatal ductus arteriosus. *Circ Res* 1981;49:997–1002.

34. Nakanishi T, Gu H, Hagiward N, et al. Mechanism of oxygen-induced contraction of ductus arteriosus isolated from fetal rabbit. *Circ Res* 1993;72: 1218–1228.

35. Tristani-Firouzi M, Reeve HL, Tolarova SL, et al. Oxygen-induced constriction of rabbit ductus arteriosus occurs via inhibition of a 4-aminopyridine voltage-sensitive potassium channel. *J Clin Invest* 1996;98:1959–1965.

36. Nelson MT, Quayle JM. Physiological roles and properties of potassium channels in arterial smooth muscle. *Am J Physiol* 1995;37:C799-C822.
37. Buckler KJ. A novel oxygen-sensitive potassium current in rat carotid body type I cells. *J Physiol (Lond)* 1997;498:649–662.
38. Youngson C, Nurse C, Yeger H, et al. Oxygen sensing in airway chemoreceptors. *Nature* 1993;365:153–155.
39. Weir EK, Archer SL. The mechanism of acute hypoxic pulmonary vasoconstriction: The tale of two channels. *FASEB J* 1995;9:183–189.
40. Ruppersburg J, Stocker M, Pongs O, et al. Regulation of fast inactivation of cloned mammalian IK(A) channels by cysteine oxidation. *Nature* 1991; 352:711–714.
41. Meury J, Robin A. Glutathione-gated K$^+$ channels of *Escherichia coli* carry out K$^+$ efflux controlled by the redox status of the cell. *Arch Microbiol* 1990;154:475–482.
42. Archer S, Huang J, Henry T, et al. A redox based O$_2$ sensor in rat pulmonary vasculature. *Circ Res* 1993;73:1100–1112.
43. Reeve HL, Weir EK, Nelson DA, et al. Opposing effects of oxidants and antioxidants on K$^+$ channel activity and tone in vascular tissue. *Exp Physiol* 1995;80:825–834.
44. Filipovic DM, Reeves WB. Hydrogen peroxide activates glibenclamide-sensitive K$^+$ channels in LLC-PK1 cells. *Am J Physiol* 1997;272:C737-C743.
45. Sobey CG, Heistad DD, Faraci FM. Mechanisms of bradykinin-induced cerebral vasodilatation in rats: Evidence that reactive oxygen species activate K$^+$ channels. *Stroke* 1997;28:2290–2294.
46. Szabo I, Nilius B, Zhang X, et al. Inhibitory effects of oxidants on n-type K$^+$ channels in Xenopus oocytes. *Pflügers Arch* 1997;433:626–632.
47. Vega-Saenz de Miera E, Rudy B. Modulation of K$^+$ channels by hydrogen peroxide. *Biochem Biophys Res Commun* 1992;186:1681–1687.
48. Kroll SL, Czyzyk-Krzeska MF. Role of H$_2$O$_2$ and heme-containing O$_2$ sensors in hypoxic regulation of tyrosine hydroxylase gene expression. *Am J Physiol* 1998;274:C167-C174.
49. Clyman RI, Saugstad OD, Mauray F. Reactive oxygen species relax the lamb ductus arteriosus by stimulating prostaglandin production. *Circ Res* 1989;64:1–8.
50. Franco-Obregon A, Urena J, Lopez-Barneo J. Oxygen-sensitive calcium channels in vascular smooth muscle and their possible role in hypoxic arterial relaxation. *Proc Natl Acad Sci USA* 1995;92:4715–4719.
51. Franco-Obregon A, Lopez-Barneo J. Differential oxygen sensitivity of calcium channels in rabbit smooth muscle cells of conduit and resistance pulmonary arteries. *J Physiol (Lond)* 1996;491:511–518.
52. Salter KJ, Koslowski RZ. Endothelin receptor coupling to potassium and chloride channels in isolated rat pulmonary arterial myocytes. *J Pharmacol Exp Ther* 1996;279:1053–1062.
53. Hyvelin JM, Guibert C, Marthan R, et al. Cellular mechanisms and role of endothelin-1-induced calcium oscillations in pulmonary arterial myocytes. *Am J Physiol* 1998;275:L269-L282.
54. Shimoda LA, Sylvester JT, Sham JS. Inhibition of voltage-gated K$^+$ current in rat intrapulmonary arterial myocytes by endothelin-1. *Am J Physiol* 1998;274:L842-L853.
55. Salter KJ, Wilson CM, Kato K, et al. Endothelin-1, delayed rectifier K channels and pulmonary arterial smooth muscle. *J Cardiovasc Pharmacol* 1998;31:S81-S83.

56. Coceani F, Armstrong C, Kelsey L. Endothelin is a potent constrictor of the lamb ductus arteriosus. *Can J Physiol Pharmacol* 1989;67:902–904.
57. Coceani F, Kelsey L. Endothelin-1 release from lamb ductus arteriosus: Relevance to postnatal closure of the vessel. *Can J Physiol Pharmacol* 1991; 69:218–221.
58. Coceani F, Kelsey L, Seidlitz E. Evidence for an effector role of endothelin in closure of the ductus arteriosus at birth. *Can J Physiol Pharmacol* 1992; 70:1061–1064.

Chapter 20

Cytochrome P450 in the Contractile Tone of the Ductus Arteriosus:
Regulatory and Effector Mechanisms

Flavio Coceani, MD

The ductus arteriosus (DA) is a large muscular shunt connecting the pulmonary artery in the fetus with the aorta, and allowing blood to bypass the unexpanded lungs. At birth, as the lungs acquire their ventilatory function and blood PO_2 rises to extrauterine values, the DA constricts and within hours undergoes functional closure. While there is good evidence implicating prostaglandin E_2 (PGE_2)[1-3] alone or in combination with nitric oxide (NO),[4,5] and possibly carbon monoxide (CO),[6,7] in DA patency, the mechanism of DA closure continues to be debated.[3,7] Several schemes have been suggested through the years, all in agreement on the idea of oxygen as the trigger for ductal constriction at birth, but in disagreement on the identity of the effector.[3,7-10] In that respect, the present volume is not an exception, and seemingly conflicting explanations are provided for this transitional event.

We have proposed that DA closure takes place through a multistep process in which oxygen is the trigger, a cytochrome P450 (CYP450)-based monooxygenase reaction is the signal transducer, and endothelin-1 (ET-1), acting via the ET_A receptor subtype, is the effector.[9,11,12] Subsidence of the relaxing influence of PGE_2 at birth, secondary to the fall in blood levels of the prostaglandins and the lesser sensitivity of the oxygen-primed ductal muscle to the compound,[1-3] is an additional, and reportedly important,[13] factor contributing to closure.

This work was supported by the Heart and Stroke Foundation of Ontario (Grant no. T-3329).

From: Weir EK, Archer SL, Reeves JT (eds). *The Fetal and Neonatal Pulmonary Circulations.* Armonk, NY: Futura Publishing Company, Inc.; ©1999.

The purpose of this chapter is twofold: to examine the data supporting the involvement of a CYP450/ET-1 system in the generation of contractile tone in the DA, specifically its oxygen-dependent component; and to discuss the possible modulation of this vasoconstrictor mechanism. In the process, an attempt will be made to resolve apparent inconsistencies in our scheme.

A Cytochrome P450 Mechanism as Oxygen Sensor

Different lines of evidence coincide in pointing to a CYP450 hemoprotein as the target for oxygen in the DA, as summarized in Table 1. Particularly significant is the fact that CO relaxation is reversed by monochromatic light with a maximum at 450 nm.[15] Other hemoproteins that could account for this relaxation either by being inhibited (cytochrome oxidase)[20] or activated (guanylate cyclase)[12] by CO would instead provide a spectral peak between 420 and 430 nm. An additional, noteworthy finding is that photoreversal can take place only if oxygen is combined with CO in the medium. In its absence, light, whether polychromatic[14] or monochromatic (unpublished data), is marginally effective, or not effective at all, against the CO relaxation. While this linkage with oxygen could be fortuitous, it may also mean that CO has two components in its action, only one of which is directed toward a target, such as CYP450, common to oxygen. We take the latter position, noting that oxygen does not bind to guanylate cyclase[21] and that, consequently, this enzyme cannot be the site for any oxygen/CO competition. This issue will be considered again later in this chapter.

As experiments with CO involve a CYP450 in the generation of contractile tone, those with 1-aminobenzotriazole (ABT) imply that this hemoprotein operates as a catalytic factor in a monooxygenase reaction.[11] The alternative possibility of CYP450 functioning as a signaling agent through a conformational change is not in accord with the ABT data[11] or, moreover, with the notion that CO and oxygen exert opposite effects on ductal tone when their binding with CYP450 elicits identical, or nearly identical, changes.[22] An apparent difficulty with our reasoning is that the ABT effect is rapidly reversible when inhibition of CYP450-based monooxygenase reactions is expected to be long-lasting. In fact, this incongruence has been taken as an argument against the specificity of ABT action in another, potentially CYP450-mediated, process.[23] However, it must be noted that our scheme calls for the existence of a special CYP450 hemoprotein operating in a dynamic fashion over a physiologic range of P_{O_2} values. Hence, the hemoprotein in question is intrinsically different from the conventional CYP450 isozymes associated with the metabolism of xenobiotics and certain hormones. Among its attributes,

Table 1

Arguments Supporting the Involvement of a Distinct CYP450 Hemoprotein in the Generation of Contractile Tone in the Ductus Arteriosus

Finding	Reference
• CO is a relaxant agent and the target site in the muscle has greater affinity for the CO than oxygen.	14, 15
• CO is only effective on ductus muscle cells with an intact plasma membrane.	16
• CO relaxation is reversed by monochromatic light with a peak at 450 nm.	15
• CYP450 inhibitors of diverse chemical structure relax the ductus.	14, 15
• ABT, a mechanism-based inactivator of CYP450, is a relaxant agent on the ductus.	11
• A CYP450 belonging to the 3A (glucocorticoid-inducible) subfamily is present in the plasma membrane of ductus muscle cells.	17
• Treatment of lambs in utero with activators of glucocorticoid-inducible CYP450 results in ductus constriction. Accordingly, glucocorticoids are beneficial in the prevention and treatment of a persistent ductus in premature infants.	17–19

one may well envisage the rapid turnover. An analogous distinction has been made by another group when defining the properties of an allied hemoprotein located in the systemic vasculature.[24] With the same argument, it is also possible to explain our failure to measure, with conventional probes,[17] monooxygenase activity in ductal tissue. The putative signaling hemoprotein, which is appropriately located in the plasma membrane,[17] may be too scarce to sustain measurable catalytic activity or the reaction itself may utilize a distinct, and still unknown, substrate.

Endothelin–1 as the Oxygen Effector

Several data have been obtained in recent years implicating ET-1 as the oxygen messenger in the DA (Table 2). Collectively, they form a

Table 2

Arguments Supporting an Effector Role of ET-1 in the Constrictor Response of the Ductus Arteriosus to Oxygen

Finding	Reference
• ET-1 is a singularly potent ductus constrictor acting via the ETA receptor subtype.	25
• ET-1 is formed in the ductus; its synthesis has been localized not only in endothelial, but also in muscle cells.	26,27
• Oxygen increases ET-1 release from the ductus.	27 unpublished data
• Oxygen constriction is curtailed by inhibitors of ET-1 synthesis (phosphoramidon) and action (BQ123).	27

convincing case; nevertheless, there are difficulties in the study of this compound that require discussion and may be responsible for certain inconsistencies in the results. ET-1 release, though originating from appropriate regions of the DA wall, is exceedingly small and not amenable to quantification over a short interval.[26,27] This has complicated any correlation of ET-1 output with changes in tone secondary to physiologic stimuli or pharmacological interventions. Leaving aside this practical problem, one may raise questions about the functional significance of ET-1 and wonder, for example, whether there is a contradiction between the modest ET-1 release and the role being assigned to the compound in the generation of contractile tone. In comparison, PGE_2, the prime agent responsible for DA patency, is released at a rate that is 2–3 orders of magnitude higher.[28,29] No direct answer can be provided with the available data. However, it must be pointed out that tissues, and vascular smooth muscle in particular, have active mechanisms for binding/internalization and catabolism of ET-1.[30–32] Hence, any ET-1 measured in the medium likely represents only a fraction of the compound being formed in the DA and acting therein. In addition, ET-1 is liable to autoinduction (via both ET_A and ET_B receptor subtypes[33,34]) and, if existent in the DA, this phenomenon could also account for the low yield. In fact, with its tendency to become irreversible through repeated challenges,[35] the DA constriction to oxygen would well qualify as a process sustained by a positive feedback mechanism.

Table 3

Arguments Supporting a Functional Linkage Between CYP450 and ET-1 Systems in the Ductus Arteriosus

Finding	Reference
• ET-1 reverses the ductus relaxation brought about by CO.	25
• Reversal of CO relaxation by monochromatic light at 450 nm is curtailed by inhibitors of ET-1 synthesis (phosphoramidon) and action (BQ123).	unpublished data
• CO inhibits ET-1 release from the ductus.	27 unpublished data
• ABT tends to reduce ET-1 release from the ductus.	11

Another potential complication in studying ET-1 release relates to the varied effect of oxygen-derived free radicals on the synthetic system and the peptide itself. Reactive oxygen species may stimulate or inhibit ET-1 formation, depending on the study,[36,37] and may also structurally alter the compound with resulting loss of immunoreactivity.[38] If these events take place in the DA, an uncontrollable variable is introduced in experimental procedures expectedly facilitating (eg, exposure to oxygen) or curtailing (eg, treatment with ABT) the generation of free radicals. For example, the failure of ABT to cause a significant reduction in ET-1 release from the DA (see Table 3) could be explained by this methodological factor. Lack of specificity in some of the drugs being used to manipulate the ET-1 system is also a possible cause for inconsistencies. We have shown that phosphoramidon attenuates the constrictor response of the DA to oxygen at submaximal, but not maximal, PO_2 values.[27] While this finding could simply reflect an inadequacy of the agent, deriving from either limited accessibility of the ET-1-converting enzyme or overriding activation by oxygen, the possibility of some accessory effect interfering with the main effect should also be considered. According to Gandhi,[32] phosphoramidon not only inhibits the synthesis but also the breakdown of ET-1, and these two actions combined could lead to spurious results.

In brief, despite some shortcomings, the concept that ET-1 functions as an effector for oxygen in the DA appears to be well founded. It is also in accord with the dynamic role in cellular events that is assigned to the peptide by other studies.[39,40]

Functional Linkage Between Cytochrome P450 and Endothelin–1

Although distant in their usual function, the CYP450 and ET-1 systems are seemingly joined in a causal relationship in the DA. Several findings, cited in Table 3, support this view. Nevertheless, key questions need to be addressed on the actual operation of this proposed linkage. Specifically, it would be important to know, for conceptual and practical reasons, the identity of both substrate and endproduct in the CYP450-based monooxygenase reaction functioning as a signal transducer for oxygen. Our early attempt to identify the active principle with an arachidonate epoxide or some related metabolite from the epoxygenase pathway has failed.[15] Interestingly, one of the compounds that we tested and found not to be suitable (ie, 20-hydroxy arachidonic acid; unpublished data) has subsequently been assigned a messenger role in an allied, CYP450-based oxygen-sensing system located in the systemic vasculature.[24]

Regulation of the CYP450/ET–1 Complex

Several agents, originating from within and outside the DA, could exert a modulatory effect on the CYP450/ET-1 complex and its proposed oxygen-sensing function. Cortisol is one such agent, and supporting evidence has been presented earlier in this chapter. We have focused our attention on CO and NO, both of which are formed in the DA and exert therein a relaxant effect.[4–6] Despite these common features, however, the two agents differ in their mode of action. Both of them inhibit ET-1 release from the DA (Table 3; unpublished data); however, only NO (tested as the NO donor, sodium nitroprusside) promotes accumulation of cyclic GMP (cGMP) proportional to the magnitude of the relaxation (Figure 1). In contrast, CO causes complete relaxation with only a marginal increase in cGMP content (Figure 2). Any endogenously formed CO is likely to act as the exogenous CO. We have found that endotoxin, a potential inducer of both NO- and CO-forming enzymes (ie, NO synthase and heme oxygenase), relaxes the ductus without altering cGMP levels.[6] Still, it decreases ET-1 release (unpublished data), and the relaxation is reversed by the heme oxygenase inhibitor, zinc protoporphyrin IX.[6]

It thus seems evident that CO relaxes the DA primarily by inhibiting the CYP450/ET-1 system, while NO is effective on both this system and guanylate cyclase. This arrangement, however, is likely to change under different physiologic conditions or with intervening pathologi-

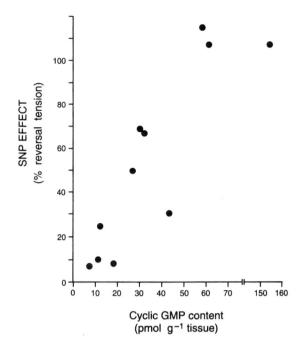

Cyclic GMP content
(pmol g^{-1} tissue)

Figure 1. In vitro preparation of lamb ductus arteriosus. Relationship between reversal of contractile tone and cyclic GMP accumulation during treatment with sodium nitroprusside (SNP; concentration range, 0.003–1 μmol/L). Krebs medium was gassed with 30% oxygen and contained indomethacin (2.8 μmol/L). Each point refers to a different experiment and the correlation coefficient is 0.72 (p=0.01). (Reproduced with permission from Reference 12.)

cal states. For example, it is interesting to speculate on the functional state of the CYP450/ET-1 system during hypoxia. We have shown that ABT,[11] unlike CO,[14] is without effect on the hypoxic DA. Equally ineffective under the same condition is the ET-1 antagonist, BQ123[27]; moreover, photoreversal of the CO relaxation is very small or absent.[14] In brief, based on these findings, hypoxia would appear as a condition in which the CYP450/ET-1 system is not functional. This is not surprising, perhaps, if one considers that oxygen is rate-limiting for monooxygenase reactions and may even be more acutely so with a reaction, as envisaged in our scheme, expectedly operating over a higher range of PO_2 values. Intrinsic in this reasoning is the assumption that any rise in DA tone under hypoxia results primarily from the withdrawal of relaxing influences (specifically, PGE_2 and NO) which, like the contractile mechanism under examination, necessitate oxygen for their expression. A corollary assumption is that CO relaxation under hypoxia is brought about by activation of guanylate cyclase. The only incongruence in this

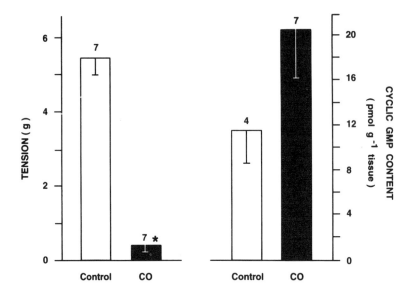

Figure 2. In vitro preparation of lamb ductus arteriosus. Contractile tension (left panel) and cyclic GMP content (right panel) under control conditions (open bar) and during treatment with CO (65 μmol/L) (solid bar). Krebs medium was gassed with 30% oxygen and contained indomethacin (2.8 μmol/L). The number of experiments appears above each column, and a significant difference between control and treatment groups is indicated by the asterisk (p<0.01). (Modified with permission from Reference 12.)

line of speculation is that drugs directly inhibiting CYP450 behave differently from ABT and relax the hypoxic DA.[15] Further work is required to resolve this issue, bearing in mind that the hypoxic DA in vitro may be a model for the behavior of the vessel in cyanotic infants. Significantly, these infants are able to close their DA, albeit more slowly compared to normally oxygenated infants.

Conclusion

Our studies document the key role of a CYP450/ET-1 system in the oxygen-triggered constriction of the DA and, by extension, in postnatal closure of the vessel. The precise mechanism by which the two elements of this system are joined in an operational sequence is not known, but evidence points to a monooxygenase reaction yielding an, as yet unknown, ET-1-activating product. The hemoprotein in question may be the member of a new class of signaling agents,[24] sensing variations in oxygen concentration and causing appropriate adjustments in vascular tone. The relation of our findings to those implicating K^+ channel activities in oxygen sensing[7,8,10] is not clear. However, there are intriguing data linking the operation of K^+ channels with both ET-1[41] and CYP450[24] functions. Advances in this area may provide new approaches for the pharmacological manipulation of the DA in infants.

References

1. Clyman RI. Ductus arteriosus: Current theories of prenatal and postnatal regulation. *Semin Perinatol* 1987;11:64–71.
2. Coceani F, Olley PM. The control of cardiovascular shunts in the fetal and perinatal period. *Can J Physiol Pharmacol* 1988;66:1129–1134.
3. Smith GCS. The pharmacology of the ductus arteriosus. *Pharmacol Rev* 1998;50:35–58.
4. Coceani F, Kelsey L, Seidlitz E. Occurrence of endothelium-derived relaxing factor/nitric oxide in the lamb ductus arteriosus. *Can J Physiol Pharmacol* 1994;72:82–88.
5. Bustamante SA, Pang Y, Romero S, et al. Inducible nitric oxide synthase and the regulation of central vessel caliber in the fetal rat. *Circulation* 1996;94:1948–1953.
6. Coceani F, Kelsey L, Seidlitz E, et al. Carbon monoxide formation in the ductus arteriosus in the lamb: Implications for the regulation of muscle tone. *Br J Pharmacol* 1997;120:599–608.
7. Wang R. Resurgence of carbon monoxide: An endogenous gaseous vasorelaxing factor. *Can J Physiol Pharmacol* 1998;76:1–15.
8. Nakanishi T, Gu H, Hagiwara N, et al. Mechanisms of oxygen-induced contraction of ductus arteriosus isolated from the fetal rabbit. *Circ Res* 1993;72:1218–1228.
9. Coceani F. Control of the ductus arteriosus: A new function for cytochrome P450, endothelin and nitric oxide. *Biochem Pharmacol* 1994;48:1315–1318.
10. Tristani-Firouzi M, Reeve HL, Tolarova S, et al. Oxygen-induced constriction of rabbit ductus arteriosus occurs via inhibition of a 4-aminopyridine-, voltage-sensitive potassium channel. *J Clin Invest* 1996;98:1959–1965.
11. Coceani F, Kelsey L, Seidlitz E, et al. Inhibition of the contraction of the ductus arteriosus to oxygen by 1-aminobenzotriazole, a mechanism-based inactivator of cytochrome P450. *Br J Pharmacol* 1996;117:1586–1592.
12. Coceani F, Kelsey L, Seidlitz E. Carbon monoxide induced relaxation of the ductus arteriosus in the lamb: Evidence against the prime role of guanylyl cyclase. *Br J Pharmacol* 1996;118:1689–1696.
13. Nguyen M, Camenish T, Snouwaert JN, et al. The prostaglandin receptor EP_4 triggers remodelling of the cardiovascular system at birth. *Nature* 1997;390:78–81.
14. Coceani F, Hamilton NC, Labuc J, et al. Cytochrome P_{450}-linked monooxygenase: Involvement in the lamb ductus arteriosus. *Am J Physiol* 1984;246: H640-H643.
15. Coceani F, Breen CA, Lees JG, et al. Further evidence implicating a cytochrome P-450-mediated reaction in the contractile tension of the lamb ductus arteriosus. *Circ Res* 1988;62:471–477.
16. Coceani F, Wright J, Breen C. Ductus arteriosus: Involvement of a

sarcolemmal cytochrome P-450 in O_2 constriction? *Can J Physiol Pharmacol* 1989;67:1448–1450.

17. Coceani F, Kelsey L, Ackerley C, et al. Cytochrome P450 during ontogenic development: Occurrence in the ductus arteriosus and other tissues. *Can J Physiol Pharmacol* 1994;72:217–226.

18. Clyman RI, Ballard PL, Sniderman S, et al. Prenatal administration of betamethasone for prevention of patent ductus arteriosus. *J Pediatr* 1981;98: 123–125.

19. Heyman E, Ohlsson A, Shennan AT, et al. Closure of patent ductus arteriosus after treatment with dexamethasone. *Acta Paediatr Scand* 1990;79: 698–700.

20. Fay FS. Guinea pig ductus arteriosus. I. Cellular and metabolic basis for oxygen sensitivity. *Am J Physiol* 1971;221:470–479.

21. Stone JR, Marletta MA. Soluble guanylate cyclase from bovine lung: Activation with nitric oxide and carbon monoxide and spectral characterization of the ferrous and ferric states. *Biochemistry* 1994;33:5636–5640.

22. Marks GS, Brien JF, Nakatsu K, et al. Does carbon monoxide have a physiological function? *Trends Pharmacol Sci* 1991;12:185–188.

23. Chang S-W, Dutton D, Wang H-L, et al. Intact lung cytochrome P-450 is not required for hypoxic pulmonary vasoconstriction. *Am J Physiol* 1992; 263:L446-L453.

24. Harder DR, Narayanan J, Birks EK, et al. Identification of a putative microvascular oxygen sensor. *Circ Res* 1996;79:54–61.

25. Coceani F, Armstrong C, Kelsey L. Endothelin is a potent constrictor of the lamb ductus arteriosus. *Can J Physiol Pharmacol* 1989;67:902–904.

26. Coceani F, Kelsey L. Endothelin-1 release from lamb ductus arteriosus: Relevance to postnatal closure of the vessel. *Can J Physiol Pharmacol* 1991; 69:218–221.

27. Coceani F, Kelsey L, Seidlitz E. Evidence for an effector role of endothelin in closure of the ductus arteriosus at birth. *Can J Physiol Pharmacol* 1992; 70:1061–1064.

28. Clyman RI, Mauray F, Demers LM, et al. Developmental response to indomethacin: A comparison of isometric tension with PGE_2 formation in the lamb ductus arteriosus. *Prostaglandins* 1979;18:721–730.

29. Coceani F, Huhtanen D, Hamilton NC, et al. Involvement of intramural prostaglandin E_2 in prenatal patency of the lamb ductus arteriosus. *Can J Physiol Pharmacol* 1986;64:737–744.

30. Hirata Y, Yoshimi H, Takaichi S, et al. Binding and receptor down-regulation of a novel vasoconstrictor endothelin in cultured rat vascular smooth muscle cells. *FEBS Lett* 1988;239:13–17.

31. Goligorsky MS, Tsukahara H, Magazine H, et al. Termination of endothelin signaling: Role of nitric oxide. *J Cell Physiol* 1994;158:485–494.

32. Gandhi CR. Vascular smooth muscle cells metabolize endothelin-1 in the absence of a functional receptor. *Biochim Biophys Acta* 1995;1269:290–298.

33. Hahn AWA, Resink TJ, Scott-Burden T, et al. Stimulation of endothelin mRNA and secretion in rat vascular smooth muscle cells: A novel autocrine function. *Cell Regul* 1990;1:649–659.

34. Iwasaki S, Homma T, Matsuda Y, et al. Endothelin receptor subtype B mediates autoinduction of endothelin-1 in rat mesangial cells. *J Biol Chem* 1995;270:6997–7003.

35. Kovalcik V. The response of the isolated ductus arteriosus to oxygen and anoxia. *J Physiol* 1963;169:185–197.

36. Hughes AK, Stricklett PK, Padilla E, et al. Effect of reactive oxygen species on endothelin-1 production by human mesangial cells. *Kidney Int* 1996;49: 181–189.
37. Love GP, Keenan AK. Cytotoxicity-associated effects of reactive oxygen species on endothelin-1 secretion by pulmonary endothelial cells. *Free Radic Biol Med* 1998;24:1437–1445.
38. Yasuda N, Kasuya Y, Yamada G, et al. Loss of contractile activity of endothelin-1 induced by electrical field stimulation-generated free radicals. *Br J Pharmacol* 1994;113:21–28.
39. Macarthur H, Warner TD, Wood EG, et al. Endothelin-1 release from endothelial cells in culture is elevated both acutely and chronically by short periods of mechanical stretch. *Biochem Biophys Res Comm* 1994;200:395–400.
40. McClellan G, Weisberg A, Rose D, et al. Endothelial cell storage and release of endothelin as a cardioregulatory mechanism. *Circ Res* 1994;75:85–96.
41. Haynes WG, Webb DJ. Venoconstriction to endothelin-1 in humans: Role of calcium and potassium channels. *Am J Physiol* 1993;265:H1676-H1681.

Chapter 21

Maturational Changes in the Human Pulmonary Vascular Resistance

James C. Huhta, MD, and Juha Rasanen, MD

Background

Basics of Lung Pathology and Arteriolar Development

Human fetal pulmonary development includes the rapid increase in air-exchange surface area by the arborization and multiplication of small airways and air sacs, the multiplication of pulmonary arterioles, and the increase in the cross-sectional area of the pulmonary vascular bed. In the human fetus, this process is a continuum, but is most active in the time-frame of from 20 to 30 weeks of gestation. The ability of the premature newborn to exchange air is the fundamental step in the establishment of viability outside the uterus. Much of the research into improving air exchange in this patient group has been directed at enhancing the maturity of the air-liquid interface by using compounds that naturally decrease this surface tension, such as surfactant. Each air sac is accompanied by a vascular net, which is the primitive pulmonary vascular bed including the pulmonary arteriole (where the vascular resistance change will occur), the capillary bed, and the pulmonary venule.

Maturation of the pulmonary vascular bed is poorly understood, but is manifested by an increasing number of vessels and the beginning of a control mechanism to adjust the pulmonary vascular resistance (and hence, the flow to the region). Intuitively, it is apparent that the pulmonary vascular units adjust the flow to the portions of lung that are ventilated, and this control is acquired prior to birth. This control

From: Weir EK, Archer SL, Reeves JT (eds). *The Fetal and Neonatal Pulmonary Circulations.* Armonk, NY: Futura Publishing Company, Inc.; ©1999.

mechanism is now known to be partially related to the local environment including the alveolar pH, P_{CO_2}, and P_{O_2}. There are also neurogenic and humoral effects on the arteriolar smooth muscle in the path of blood flow which can raise the resistance to a local area or to the entire lung when the stimulus is generalized. There is little effect, however, of the content of the blood flowing in the vessels on the control of the pulmonary vascular resistance.

The original experiments of Dawes showed that the fetal pulmonary resistance changes around the time of birth are modulated by the ventilation of the lungs and the oxygenation of the air ventilating the lungs, and not significantly influenced by the content of blood which perfuses the arterioles. Others have suggested that fetal pulmonary vascular responses to hyperoxemia and hypoxemia, as well as to vasoactive agents, change with advancing gestational age.[1,2] In the beginning of the third trimester, the fetal lamb pulmonary circulation does not respond to changes in the oxygen tension or to intravenous acetylcholine injection, whereas at term, a rise in the fetal lamb oxygen tension can induce an increase in pulmonary blood flow similar to that seen with the onset of breathing at birth.[2] Similarly, reductions in the fetal oxygen tension cause a decrease in the pulmonary blood flow and an increase in the pulmonary vascular resistance at near-term gestation. Also, the sensitivity of the pulmonary circulation to acetylcholine is increased in older fetuses.[1]

Fetal lamb research has shown that the pulmonary blood flow is a small percentage of the combined cardiac output in lambs. Little information is available concerning the changes in distribution which may occur during gestation.

Fetal Disease Models

Fetal ductal ligation experiments can produce pulmonary vascular disease through changes in pulmonary pressure and flow. Levin et al[3] and Morin[4] have published extensively concerning the fetal pulmonary vascular changes that occur following elevation of pulmonary pressure by occlusion of the ductus arteriosus. By inducing ductal constriction or occlusion, these authors have shown that changes in the vascular bed in the lungs can occur rapidly and normal patterns of arborization and angiogenesis are inhibited.

Models of diaphragmatic hernia have been shown to simulate neonatal pulmonary hypoplasia. Using a fetal lamb model, investigators[5] have created in utero simulations of the effects of a diaphragmatic hernia on the developing fetus. These experiments have shown that the fetus is usually not affected hemodynamically by the creation of a diaphragmatic hernia early in utero, but the postnatal physiology is altered dramatically in terms of the lung and arteriolar hypoplasia on the side of the hernia. Currently, efforts are under way to understand how the pulmonary hypoplasia in this clinical situation could be treated. One example of this research is the palliation of congenital diaphragmatic hernia (CDH) using obstruction of the trachea to reexpand the lungs.[6]

Most human fetuses with CDH diagnosed before 24 weeks of gestation die despite optimal postnatal care. In fetuses with liver herniation into the chest, prenatal repair has not been successful. In the course of exploring the pathophysiology of CDH and its repair in fetal lambs, it has been found that obstruction of the normal egress of fetal lung fluid enlarges developing fetal lungs, reduces the herniated viscera, and accelerates lung growth, resulting in improved pulmonary function after birth. Harrison et al[6] developed and tested experimentally a variety of methods to temporarily occlude the fetal trachea, allow fetal lung growth, and reverse the obstruction at birth. The authors applied this strategy of temporary tracheal occlusion in eight human fetuses with CDH and liver herniation at 25–28 weeks of gestation. With ongoing experimental and clinical experience, the technique of tracheal occlusion evolved from an internal plug (two patients) to an external clip (six patients), and a technique was developed for unplugging the trachea at the time of birth (Ex Utero Intrapartum Tracheoplasty [EXIT]). Two fetuses had a foam plug placed inside the trachea. The first showed dramatic lung growth in utero and survived; the second (who had a smaller plug to avoid tracheomalacia) showed no demonstrable lung growth and died at birth. Two fetuses had external spring-loaded aneurysm clips placed on the trachea; one was aborted due to tocolytic failure, and the other showed no lung growth (presumed leak) and died 3 months following birth. Four fetuses had metal clips placed on the trachea. All showed dramatic lung growth in utero, with reversal of pulmonary hypoplasia documented after birth; however, these four fetuses died of nonpulmonary causes. Temporary occlusion of the fetal trachea accelerates fetal lung growth and ameliorated the often fatal pulmonary hypoplasia associated with severe CDH. Although the strategy was physiologically sound and technically feasible, the authors cited complications encountered during the evolution of these techniques which limited the survival rate. Further evolution of this technique is required before it can be recommended as therapy for fetal pulmonary hypoplasia. Such experience highlights the need for more detailed understanding of the mechanical and biochemical changes associated with fetal lung growth.

Normal Human Fetal Changes

Doppler Blood Velocity Methods for Calculating Fetal Pulmonary Flow/Resistance/Impedance

Rasanen et al[7] first measured pulsatility index (PI) calculations in the human fetal pulmonary circulation and showed that the fetal branch pulmonary arterial vascular impedance decreases significantly during the second half of pregnancy. The linear decrease in vascular impedance during the second trimester and in the beginning of the third trimester may be related to the growth of the lung and the increase in the number of resistance vessels. During the latter part of the third trimester, pulmonary vascular impedance did not decrease. Identical data was obtained from the left and right lungs.

Fetal Pulmonary Flow Measurements

Pulsed Doppler can be used to estimate the flow through a blood vessel using the relation that the flow is equal to the product of the mean velocity integrated over the entire lumen and the cross-sectional area of the vessel. With newer ultrasound equipment, submillimeter resolution is possible, and the diameter of small proximal pulmonary arteries (2–5 mm) can be measured. The best measurement is an orthogonal image which enhances the axial resolution of the lumen and is made using the leading edge to leading edge methodology. The blood velocity is obtained with pulsed Doppler in a plane that is as close as possible to the direction of blood flow.

In the Rasanen et al studies,[7,8] image-directed pulsed and color Doppler equipment with a 5- or 7-MHz probe was used to obtain blood velocity waveforms at the levels of the aortic and pulmonary valves, the proximal right pulmonary artery (RPA), left pulmonary artery (LPA) (after the main pulmonary bifurcation), distal pulmonary artery (DPA), and the ductus arteriosus (DA). The lowest high pass filter level was used (100 Hz) and the spatial peak temporal average power output for color and pulsed Doppler was kept at < 100 mW/cm^2. An angle of $<$ 15° was accepted between the vessel and the Doppler beam as assessed by color Doppler.

Calculations

From Doppler tracings, fetal heart rate and time velocity integral (TVI) could be calculated. The TVI was considered to be a measure of the length of the column of ejected blood and was measured as the integral under the Doppler spectrum in systole and diastole. The aortic and pulmonary valve annuli, ductus, and pulmonary artery diameters were measured from frozen images during systole using the leading edge to leading edge method. Three separate measurements of the diameters were made and the results were averaged. Calculation of the cross section of the vessel in square centimeters was based on the assumption that the cross-sectional area was circular. Volumetric flow, Q, was calculated using the formula:

$$Q = FHR \times CSA \times TVI$$

where FHR is fetal heart rate, and CSA is the cross-sectional area of the vessel. The volume flow through the aortic valve was the left ventricular cardiac output (LVCO), and through the pulmonary valve was the right ventricular cardiac output (RVCO). Total pulmonary blood flow (QP) was the sum of the calculated RPA and LPA flows. All Doppler measurements were performed during fetal apnea and in the absence of fetal body movements. The validity of the volume measurements was tested by comparing the independent results from calculations of the right ventricular flow and the sum of the ductus, and the pulmonary artery flows,

Utilizing these methods, Rasanen et al[7] determined the normal distribution of human fetal combined cardiac output (CCO) from the left and right ventricles. They also established weight-indexed pulmonary and systemic vascular resistances (Rpi and Rsi, respectively) and changes during the second half of pregnancy. Blood flows at the aortic and pulmonary valve annuli (LVCO and RVCO, respectively), right and left pulmonary arteries (QP), and ductus arteriosus (QDA) were calculated in 63 normal fetuses. Foramen ovale blood flow (QFO = LVCO − QP) was estimated.

They found that from 20 to 30 weeks of gestation, the proportion of QP of the CCO increased (from 13% to 25%, p<0.001), while the proportion of QFO decreased (from 34% to 18%, p<0.001). After 30 weeks, the proportions of QP and QFO were unchanged. At 38 weeks, the proportion of RVCO (60%) was higher (p<0.05) than that of LVCO (40%). The proportion of QDA did not change significantly. The correlation between RVCO calculated from blood flow through the pulmonary valve and from QDA and QP was good (r=0.97, p<0.0001). Rpi (p<0.001) decreased from 20 to 30 weeks of gestation. From 30 to 38 weeks, Rpi increased (p<0.0001). Rsi increased (p<0.001) from 20 to 38 weeks. The ratio of Rpi to Rsi decreased (p<0.01) from 20 to 30 weeks, and later remained unchanged. They concluded that the human fetal pulmonary circulation has an important role in the distribution of cardiac output and that there are predictable changes in normal gestation.

The hypothesis that fetal blood in the lungs in utero is small in amount is rejected by this data.

Normal Human Fetal Vascular Reactivity

The effects of oxygen on the fetal circulation have been studied in a variety of ways. Maternal hyperoxygenation at 50% oxygen for 5 minutes increased maternal transcutaneous oxygen partial pressure approximately 3-fold.[9] After 5 minutes of maternal hyperoxygenation with 100% oxygen, intervillous space oxygen tension rose 41% from the baseline values.[10] Transcutaneously measured fetal oxygen partial pressure has been found to increase during maternal hyperoxygenation.[11,12] In addition, maternal administration of 55% humidified oxygen has been shown through umbilical cord sampling in utero to increase human fetal partial pressure of oxygen.[13]

Rasanen and coworkers[8] went on to test the pulmonary vascular response to oxygen early and late in gestation. Twenty fetuses were studied between 20 and 26 weeks of gestation, 20 fetuses were studied between 31 and 36 weeks of gestation, and all were divided into four groups (see below).

Group I   20–26 weeks, oxygen
Group II   20–26 weeks, room air
Group III 31–36 weeks, oxygen
Group IV   31–36 weeks, room air

Each fetus was appropriate for gestational age in size according to fetal biometry. Fetal anatomic survey did not reveal any abnormalities and all newborns were normal on the basis of physicial examination.

After a baseline Doppler study, randomization was performed with sealed envelopes; 10 mothers received medical compressed air (21% oxygen) and 10 received 60% humidified oxygen via face mask in each gestational age group. The examiners were unaware of the randomization. All studies were performed after 5 minutes on the new setting or after the last Doppler measurement, and the randomization was revealed after analysis.

Pulsatility Index Results

The baseline values of the measured parameters did not differ significantly between groups I and II, or groups III and IV. The PI values of the RPA, LPA, DPA, and DA did change significantly in groups I and II. In group III, the PI values of RPA, LPA, and DPA decreased signifi-

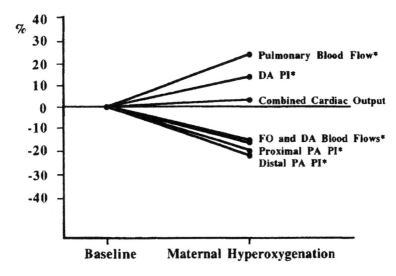

Figure 1. Mean percentage change from baseline during 60% oxygen at 31–36 weeks. DA = ductus arteriosus; FO = foramen ovale; PA = pulmonary artery; PI = pulsatility index. *Baseline and maternal hyperoxygenation values are different (p < 0.05).

cantly (p<0.0001) during maternal hyperoxygenation (Figure 1). The decrease was between 18% and 21% for these values and, at the same time, the value of DA increased significantly (14%). After return to room air, all values returned to baseline. In group IV, the PI values of RPA, LPA, and DPA, and DA remained unchanged.

Blood Flow Results

In groups I and II, LVCO, RVCO, QDA, and QP did not change significantly. In group III, maternal hyperoxygenation increased QP significantly (p<0.001) and decreased QDA (p<0.01). The mean increase in QP was 25% from the baseline value, and the mean decrease in the QDA was 17%. All changes returned to baseline with resumption of room air.

The intraobserver variability was < 4% for the PI values and < 9% for volumetric blood flow calculations. Two independent RVCO calculations (n=40) demonstrated a significant correlation at every study point with an R value of > 0.95 (p<0.0001).

We concluded that maternal hyperoxygenation with 60% oxygen did not affect the human fetal pulmonary vascular impedance as assessed by the PI, nor was there change in QP, between 20 and 26 weeks of gestation. Between 31 and 36 weeks of gestation the pulmonary vascular resistance/impedance decreased and the QP increased significantly. This effect was completely reversible with withdrawal of oxygen. Compensatory changes in foramen ovale flow were measured during increases in QP.

These results showed that the human fetal vascular circulation is under acquired vasoconstriction, at least after 31 to 36 weeks of gestation. In this way, blood flow is directed from the pulmonary circulation to the systemic circulation preferentially. Fetal oxygen tension has a role in the regulation of the pulmonary circulation during the latter part of the third trimester. Exactly how these maturational changes in the reactivity of the vascular bed are mediated is not yet clear.

Human Fetal Disease with Abnormal Resistance

Rizzo et al studied pulmonary vascular findings by Doppler in normally grown and growth-retarded fetuses.[14] Doppler studies were performed in 182 normally grown fetuses (gestational age 18–40 weeks), and in 61 growth-retarded fetuses (gestational age 24–36 weeks) that were free from structural and chromosomal abnormalities, and whose umbilical and middle cerebral artery Doppler findings suggested uteroplacental insufficiency as the most likely etiology of the growth defect. The PI was used to quantify the velocity waveforms. Successful recordings were obtained in 90.1% of the normally grown and 93.4% of the growth-retarded fetuses. In the normally grown fetuses, the PI values significantly decreased with advancing gestation. In growth-retarded fetuses, the PI values were significantly elevated compared to those of normal fetuses. A significant relationship was observed between the severity of hypoxia and PI values from the peripheral pulmonary arteries in 29 fetuses in which Doppler recordings were obtained immediately before cordocentesis. In conclusion, these data show that, in normal fetuses, the Doppler-measured impedance to flow in the peripheral pulmonary circulation decreases with advancing gestation. Rizzo concluded that impedance to flow in the lungs is elevated in the presence of growth retardation and this increase is related to the severity of fetal hypoxia.

Ductal Response to Prostaglandin Inhibitors

Maturational changes in the fetal circulation have been studied with regard to the DA and its response to prostaglandin inhibition. No human fetal ductal constriction has been reported prior to 25 weeks of gestation. Thereafter, the chance of ductal constriction with exposure of the fetus to indomethacin increases with gestational age. After 32 weeks of gestation, constriction is common, and most obstetricians avoid this drug in older fetuses. After extensive studies, it is now known that the ductal constriction is dose-dependent and reversible, with no significant residua. Rarely, occlusion of the ductus may occur after high dose indomethacin. In these fetuses, the resulting pulmonary hypertension can result in changes in the pulmonary vascular bed, which could predispose to pulmonary hypertension after birth. Direct effects of indomethacin on the pulmonary vascular bed have been hypothesized, but no direct evidence is available from human studies.

Oligohydramnios

Premature rupture of membranes with oligohydramnios or decreased amounts of amniotic fluid is known to cause reduction in the lung volumes. It is hypothesized that the fetal lungs need the constant flow of amniotic fluid to develop normally and stimulate air sac development. With the loss of amniotic fluid volume, the lungs are at risk and the resulting hypoplasia of the lung volume is associated with abnormal pulmonary vascular development.

New Techniques to Study the Fetal Lungs

Recent developments may complement the pulsed Doppler methodology that has been summarized in this chapter. For example, fetal lung volumetry by three-dimensional ultrasound has been attempted using new equipment.[15] The aim of this study was to establish a method for determination of fetal lung volume by three-dimensional ultrasound. The thoraces of 113 fetuses (singleton pregnancies, 11–41 weeks of gestation without any signs of malformation or oligohydramnios) were examined by three-dimensional ultrasound. Volumetric evaluation of each lung was performed in each of three perpendicular planes (six measurements in total). There were significant differences in all three measurements between the left and right lungs. Especially in the second and third trimesters, measurement of the frontal and the sagittal planes was sometimes prevented by poor imaging conditions. The scan volume was always too small for fetuses of more than 34 weeks of gestation. With these problems considered, nomograms of fetal lung volume for the left and the right lungs were calculated. Lung volumes in the present study showed good correlation with published autopsy findings. Therefore, fetal lung volume may have a role to play in the detection of pulmonary hypoplasia.

A new method for assessing the perfusion of the fetal lungs noninvasively has been reported. Dubiel et al[16] evaluated fetal lung perfusion with color Doppler energy (CDE) imaging and then tested the effects of betamethasone treatment, a commonly used therapy to prevent prematurity of the lungs. The aim of their study was semiquantitative evaluation of tissue blood flow in the fetal lung before and after administration of betamethasone. This was carried out by means of computer analysis of ultrasound Doppler signals obtained by the CDE technique. CDE signals were recorded in 20 singleton pregnancies with appropriate growth and imminent preterm delivery between 26 and 33 weeks of gestation. The CDE signal recordings were made before and after intramuscular administration of betamethasone 8 mg/day for 3 days. Fixed, preset CDE system control settings for the fetal right lung were used during the examinations. Images from CDE scans were recorded on S-VHS videotape and transmitted for computer analysis of 8-bit images at 256 gray-scale levels. The mean flow signal intensity was recorded for the fetal lung before and after betamethasone administration. Additionally, blood velocity waveforms were measured in the intrapulmonary arteries and veins in the peripheral part of the lung. CDE signals from the fetal lung indicated increased energy values after corticosteroid treatment in 16 cases. In 3 cases, there was no change in CDE signal values, and in 1 case, a fall of the signal value was noted. Blood velocity waveforms from the intrapulmonary arteries showed decreased resistance to flow in 15 cases, increased resistance to flow in 4 cases, and no change in 1 case. No significant differences in venous blood flow velocities were found. In conclusion, the results suggest that there was an increase in fetal lung blood perfusion after maternal corticosteroid administration.

At the present time, there is limited pathological evaluation of fetal lungs to confirm the validity of these newer, noninvasive methods. Recently, Laudy et al[17] used combined color-coded Doppler and pulsed Doppler ultrasonography to allow visualization of the fetal pulmonary circulation and study pulmonary blood flow velocity waveforms. Systolic and diastolic changes were observed in fetal pulmonary artery flow velocity waveforms in a case of fetal pulmonary hypoplasia at 34 weeks of gestation. Their observation supported our hypothesis that Doppler blood velocity data can detect lung hypoplasia based on postmortem examination of decreased total size of the pulmonary vascular bed, decreased number of pulmonary vessels per unit of lung tissue, and increased pulmonary vascular muscularization.

References

1. Lewis AB, Heymann MA, Rudolph AM. Gestational changes in pulmonary vascular responses in fetal lambs in utero. *Circ Res* 1976;39: 536–541.
2. Morin FC III, Egan EA, Ferguson W, et al. Development of pulmonary vascular response to oxygen. *Am J Physiol* 1988;254:H542-H546.

3. Levin DL, Rudolph AM, Heymann MA, et al. Morphological development of the pulmonary vascular bed oxygen in fetal lambs. *Circulation* 1976;53:144–151.
4. Morin FC. Ligating the ductus arteriosus before birth causes persistent pulmonary hypertension in the newborn lamb. *Pediatr Res* 1989;25:245–250.
5. Rasanen J, Huhta JC, Weiner S, et al. Fetal branch pulmonary arterial vascular impedance during the second half of pregnancy. *Am J Obstet Gynecol* 1996;174(5):1441–1449.
6. Harrison MR, Adzick NS, Flake AW, et al. Correction of congenital diaphragmatic hernia in utero VIII: Response of the hypoplastic lung to tracheal occlusion. *J Pediatr Surg* 1996;31(10):1339–1348.
7. Rasanen J, Wood DC, Weiner S, et al. Role of the pulmonary circulation in the distribution of human fetal cardiac output during the second half of pregnancy. *Circulation* 1996;94(5):1068–1073.
8. Rasanen J, Wood DC, Debbs RH, et al. Reactivity of the human fetal pulmonary circulation to maternal hyperoxygenation increases during the second half of pregnancy: A randomized study. *Circulation* 1998;97:257–262.
9. Polvi HJ, Pirhonen JP, Erkkola RU. The hemodymanic effects of maternal hypo- and hyperoxygenation in healthy term pregnancies. *Obstet Gynecol* 1995;86:795–799.
10. Vasicka A, Quilligan EJ, Aznar R, et al. Oxygen tension in maternal and fetal blood, amniotic fluid, and cerebrospinal fluid of the mother and the baby. *Am J Obstet Gynecol* 1960;79:1041–1047.
11. Huch A, Huch R, Schneider H, et al. Continuous transcutaneous monitoring of fetal oxygen tensions during labour. *Br J Obstet Gynaecol* 1977;84: (suppl 1):1–39.
12. Wilcourt RJ, King JC, Queenan JT. Maternal oxygen administration and the fetal transcutaneous pO2. *Am J Obstet Gynecol* 1983;146:714–715.
13. Nicolaides KH, Bradley RJ, Soothill PW, et al. Maternal oxygen therapy for intrauterine growth retardation. *Lancet* 1987;1:942–945.
14. Rizzo G, Capponi A, Chaoui R, et al. Blood flow velocity waveforms from peripheral pulmonary arteries in normally grown and growth-retarded fetuses. *Ultrasound Obstet Gynecol* 1996;8(2):87–92.
15. Pohls UG, Rempen A. Fetal lung volumetry by three-dimensional ultrasound. *Ultrasound Obstet Gynecol* 1998;11(1):6–12.
16. Dubiel M, Gudmundsson S, Pirhonen J, et al. Betamethasone treatment and fetal lung perfusion evaluated with color Doppler energy imaging. *Ultrasound Obstet Gynecol* 1997;10(4):272–276.
17. Laudy JA, Gaillard JL, v.d. Anker JN, et al. Doppler ultrasound imaging: A new technique to detect lung hypoplasia before birth? *Ultrasound Obstet Gynecol* 1996;7(3):189–192.

Chapter 22

The Pulmonary Vasculature in Congenital Diaphragmatic Hernia

Dick Tibboel, MD, PhD, Sherif M.K. Shehata, MD, MCh, and Alexandra H. Guldemeester, MD

Morphological Aspects of Normal Pulmonary Vascular Development

Angiogenesis is first detected in coats of developing trachea, esophagus, and lung buds at stage 14 (gestational age of approximately 32 days). A vascular plexus is formed receiving its blood supply both from branches of the aortic sac and from numerous branches of the dorsal aorta. Primitive pulmonary arteries become incorporated into the sixth aortic arch and intersegmental arteries involute by the end of the 5th week of gestation. Connections with systemic arteries may persist in abnormal situations.

According to Reid's third law, preacinar vessels (both arteries and veins) develop at the same time as airways, so after the 16th week all preacinar artery branches are present.[1] The relationship of the blood vessels to the airways and air spaces permits useful landmarking or timing of critical events in the development and function of the pulmonary circulation.[2]

Structure of pulmonary arteries varies with vessel size and developmental stage of the lung. The muscular coat of an artery develops during the canalicular stage. Axial arteries from hilum to the 7th generation are elastic; more peripheral arteries are muscular, partially muscular or, at the level of intra-acinar artery, predominantly nonmuscular. By definition, an elastic artery has more than five elastic laminae in its media, a muscular artery has between two and five. A partially muscular artery has smooth muscle cell (SMC) tissue in only one part of its·circumference;

From: Weir EK, Archer SL, Reeves JT (eds). *The Fetal and Neonatal Pulmonary Circulations.* Armonk, NY: Futura Publishing Company, Inc.; ©1999.

at this level the continuous muscular coat has been replaced by a spiral of SMCs. A nonmuscular artery is similar in structure to an alveolar capillary, except for its (larger) diameter.[3,4] Smaller muscular, and probably also partially muscular, arteries represent the so-called resistance arteries. This muscularization decreases towards the periphery. A newborn has one artery for every 20 alveoli. Due to formation of new alveoli postnatally, this ratio is reduced to 1:8 in an adult human being.[3–6]

Two types of pulmonary arteries can be distinguished: conventional arteries, which accompany airways branching from the axial airway, and additional or supernumerary arteries which are lateral branches that arise between conventional arteries and run a short course to supply the capillary bed of alveoli immediately adjacent to the pulmonary artery at the peribronchial parenchyma.[2] The latter are considerably more numerous and contribute in a significant way to the cross-section of the totally recruited vascular bed. Branching is more frequent towards the periphery. Supernumerary arteries constitute approximately 25% of the cross-sectional area total at the preacinar level, whereas at the intra-acinar level they comprise approximately 33%. In the normal lung, according to Hislop and Reid, 23 generations of conventional arteries exist along the posterior basal artery and 64 supernumerary branches. It has also been suggested that supernumerary arteries facilitate blood oxygenation by allowing passage of venous blood to the more remote alveoli adjacent to large arteries, veins, and airways.[2,6,7] The intra-acinar arteries represent the resistance arteries in the pulmonary vascular bed. The external diameter of preacinar arteries is usually > 200 μm, while arteries running with respiratory bronchioli represent intra-acinar arteries with a diameter of 50–200 μm.[8,9] These intra-acinar arteries, together with supernumerary arteries, rapidly increase in number and dilate near term, thus accommodating postnatal demands of the pulmonary circulation.[10–12]

Following the description of morphological changes in the developing pulmonary vasculature, the role(s) of growth factors, especially the isoforms of fibroblast growth factor (FGF), transforming growth factor-β (TGF-β) and isoforms of platelet-derived growth factor (PDGF) were investigated. The differences in animal models, as well as the variety of techniques and culture systems used in these experiments, make the definitive role of growth factors in normal and abnormal pulmonary vascular development hard to define.[13–17]

Abnormal Lung Development

Developmental defects of the lung include: (1) agenesis or hypoplasia of one or both lungs, or of single lung lobes; (2) tracheal and bronchial anomalies; (3) vascular anomalies; and (4) congenital cysts.

Pulmonary hypoplasia in newborns is seen in a number of malformation syndromes. It is diagnosed in 7.8–10.9% of neonatal necropsies and in about 50% of the necropsied neonates with congenital anomalies.[18–20] Factors affecting lung growth include: (1) those unfavorably influencing the amount of intrathoracic space (as in congenital diaphragmatic hernia [CDH] and cystic malformations of the lung),[21,22] or the amniotic space (as in oligohydramnios due to rupture of the membranes or Potter's syndrome)[23–25]; and (2) decreased pulmonary arterial flow in cardiovascular malformations (as in tetralogy of Fallot or hypoplastic right heart).[26,27]

Pulmonary weight with reference to total body weight has always been used as a parameter to define pulmonary hypoplasia.[20] Several investigators performed a radial alveolar count of distal airways to further characterize these affected lungs.[28,29] Normal lung weight or lung weight/body weight (LW/BW) ratios in different series are reported to be between 0.018 and 0.022. Emery and Mithal excluded lungs with edema and exudate and found mean LW/BW ratios of 0.013.[30] The radial alveolar count provides a more distinct definition of hypoplastic and normal lungs than the LW/BW ratio alone. Wigglesworth and Desai found that total lung DNA near term in many cases of pulmonary hypoplasia was similar to that in normal fetuses at about 20 weeks of gestation.[31,32] They concluded that lung growth must have been impaired at some time before 20 weeks and defined two groups of patients with pulmonary hypoplasia. The first group consists of fetuses with oligohydramnios due to renal agenesis, urethral obstruction, or amniotic fluid leakage in early pregnancy without other malformations. The lungs of these fetuses have a characteristic histological pattern of narrow airways and impaired maturation of respiratory epithelium, associated with lack of interstitial tissue and failure of normal elastic tissue development around the airways and terminal sacs. The second group (including CDH) has a normal or increased volume of amniotic fluid. In this group, the lungs, although small, are usually of appropriate maturity for gestational age, with normal epithelial maturation, phospholipid content, and elastin development. Thus, lung growth and maturation during the early period may be critically dependent on influences outside the lung, such as fetal breathing movements and lung liquid secretion.[33,34]

Abnormal Pulmonary Vascular Development

In abnormal pulmonary development it is especially important to compare the possible differences in pulmonary artery structures in a standardized way. Four main features need to be assessed in this respect in order to determine postconceptional age: (1) branching pattern; (2) number or density of arteries; (3) wall structure; and (4) arterial size.[2] Hislop and Davies described a way to process lung tissue into histological slides resulting in barium-gelatin filled arteries and dark stained elastin layers easy to distinguish from the surrounding, but empty lung veins.[5,6] In these slides, external diameter, wall thickness, and wall structure regarding the muscle coat (muscular, partially muscular, or nonmuscular) are registered for each artery, as is the type of the accompanying airway. The percentage wall thickness ($2\times$ wall thickness/external diameter) is calculated. In addition, the use of a radiopaque injection medium allows rapid assessment of the pulmonary circulation through arteriograms.[3,35]

Geggel and Reid distinguished between maladaptation, maldevelopment, and underdevelopment.[9] Maladaptation is represented by a structurally normal lung at birth, in which no increase in compliance of small resistance arteries occurs. Therefore, the pulmonary vascular bed is highly reactive and a vicious circle of acidosis, hypoxia, hypercarbia, pulmonary vasoconstriction and pulmonary hypertension may develop. Maldevelopment indicates new and precocious muscularization as seen in idiopathic persistent pulmonary hypertension of the newborn (PPHN). Excessive muscularization is seen in hypoplastic left heart syndrome, chronic intrauterine hypoxia, and also following meconium aspiration syndrome. Underdevelopment represents the reduced size of arteries seen in congenital anomalies associated with pulmonary hypoplasia, such as CDH, renal agenesis, or dysplasia. This relation could, in part, be explained by studies confirming the renal hypoplasia-lung hypoplasia relationship[36] (Table 1).

Vascular Morphology in Human CDH

The main pathological findings in CDH lungs are hypoplasia and vascular abnormalities. The latter consist of: (a) reduced total pulmonary vascular bed and decreased number of vessels per volume unit of lung; and (b) medial hyperplasia of pulmonary arteries together with peripheral extension of muscle layer into small arterioles. Adventitial thickening has also been reported.[37,38]

Intra-acinar arteries in healthy newborns are virtually all nonmuscular; however, in PPHN most of these arteries are completely muscularized. Geggel et al gave a detailed morphometric analysis of the lungs in a series of 7 infants with CDH.[8] They divided these patients into two groups: 4 infants who were never able to be adequately ventilated (the no-honeymoon group), and 3 who did well initially following repair of their diaphragmatic hernia, but then developed increased pulmonary vascular resistance and died (honeymoon group). No-honeymoon patients have smaller lungs, increased muscularization of intra-acinar ar-

Table 1

Arterial and Bronchial Morphometrics in Different Forms of Perinatal Pulmonary Hypertension*

Cause	Airway		Intraacinar Artery			
	Number of Bronchial Generations	Number of Alveoli per Acinus	Muscle Extension by Position	External Diameter	Medial Wall Thickness	Number
Excessive muscularization						
Idiopathic PPHN	N	N	↑	N	↑	N
Meconium aspiration	N	N	↑	N	↑	N
TAPVC-SD	N	↑	↑	↑	N	
TAPVC-ID	N	↑	↑	↑	N	
Coarctaion, VSD, PDA	N	N	N,↑	↑	↑[1],↓[2]	N
Underdevelopment						
CDH	↓	N	N,↑	↓[3]	↑	↓
Renal agenesis/dysplasia	↓	↓	↑,N,↓	↓[4]	↑,N,↓	↓
Rhesus isoimmunization	↓	N,↓	N	↓[3]	N[5]	↓
Idiopathic (primary)	↓		NA	NA	NA	NA
Maladaption						
VSD	N	↑	↓	↑	↑,N	

CDH = congenital diaphragmatic hernia; ID = infradiaphragmatic; PDA = patent ductus arteriosus; PPHN = persistent pulmonary hypertension of the newborn; SD = supradiaphragmatic; TAPVC = total anomalous pulmonary venous connection; VSD = ventricular septal defect; N = normal; NA = not available; ↑ = increase; ↓ = decrease.

Notes: 1, dependent on the severity of coarctation; 2, preacinar arteries; 3, small for age but appropriate for lung volume; 4, small for age but large for lung volume; 5, preacinar medical hypertrophy.

*(Adapted from Reference 9.)

teries, and decreased luminal area of preacinar and intra-acinar arteries. Persistent hypoxemia in the no-honeymoon group is determined by severity of pulmonary hypoplasia and structural remodeling of pulmonary arteries.

While studying lungs of CDH patients, Kitagawa et al first observed abnormalities in both number and muscularization of arterial branches.[21] They reported that the number of conventional branches was reduced to 14 in the right lung and to 12 in the left lung. Furthermore, a reduction of supernumerary branches to 17 in the right lung, but only to 36 in the left lung was seen. Thicker muscular walls in smaller diameter arteries (external diameter < 300 μm) were also described by this group.

Other investigators reported reduction in the cross-sectional area of the pulmonary vascular bed and uniform thickening of the pulmonary artery muscle mass in their study of CDH lungs.[39-41]

Cellular and Molecular Mechanisms of Cell Proliferation in Pulmonary Vasculature

Although many studies have focused on morphological changes that occur in the pulmonary vasculature during normal transition to extrauterine life, signaling mechanisms that may lead to these changes have not yet been sufficiently addressed. Several observations suggest distinct mechanisms that operate to control growth during development. Differences in production of growth factors and/or activation of second messenger pathways may underlie particular growth patterns in various developmental stages.

Adaptation of the pulmonary circulation to postnatal life requires growth and differentiation of blood vessels and a transition in SMCs from a fetal to an adult phenotype.[42-44] Several studies have demonstrated that when the normal transition to postnatal life is interrupted by hypoxia or increased pulmonary blood flow, marked proliferative changes in pulmonary artery SMCs (PA SMCs) are observed.[45] Similarly, SMCs derived from neonatal pulmonary arteries are less differentiated and exhibit enhanced growth responses to mitogenic stimuli when compared with the relatively differentiated and quiescent SMCs derived from the adult pulmonary artery.[46] Thus, the increased growth capacity of neonatal PA SMCs likely contributes both to the normal pulmonary vascular development and the predisposition to develop exorbitant pulmonary vascular remodeling in response to injury in the neonatal period, such as is observed in idiopathic PPHN, congenital heart disease, and lung hypoplasia with or without CDH.[45,47,48]

While it is generally appreciated that "immature" cells possess increased growth capacity, the relevant intracellular signaling mechanism(s) are poorly understood. Compared with adult cells, neonatal PA SMCs exhibit increased basal protein kinase C (PKC) activity and an increased PKC response to phorbol esters. This increase in PKC activity apparently contributes to the enhanced growth responses in these cells, yet the mechanism(s) through which PKC exerts growth promoting effects are unknown. One possible mechanism is PKC stimulation of cellular adenosine 3′,5′-cyclic monophosphate (cAMP).[49]

Cyclic AMP is a second messenger associated with cell growth. However, the role of cAMP on SMC proliferation is controversial; previous reports suggested that cAMP might have either a negative or positive influence on proliferation. Owen showed that, in growth arrested vascular SMCs, cAMP stimulates DNA synthesis, whereas in growing vascular cells cAMP inhibits DNA synthesis.[50] Furthermore, in neural cells it was recently demonstrated that cAMP-induced growth might be developmentally regulated.[51] Thus, the effect of cAMP on proliferation may differ depending on cell type, state of cell differentiation, and stage of cell cycle.[52]

Recent identification of multiple isoforms of adenylyl cyclase, the enzyme responsible for cAMP synthesis, demonstrated that two adenylyl cyclase isoforms are stimulated by PKC providing a putative linkage between PKC and cellular cAMP production.[53,54]

Endothelin-1 (ET-1) and angiotensin II (ANG II) are potent vasoconstrictors, and are generally believed to stimulate growth in adult SMCs derived from the systemic circulation. Indirect evidence for the involvement of ET-1 and ANG II in medial thickening of pulmonary arteries has been shown in adult rats, but direct effects of the polypeptides on PA SMC proliferation are less clear. For example, ET-1 was previously reported to increase growth in adult swine PA SMCs in the presence of 0.5% serum, whereas ET-1 and ANG II were not pro-proliferative in adult bovine PA SMCs in the presence of 0.1% serum. The reason for this discrepancy is unclear, although it is possible that these agents act as co-mitogenic stimuli requiring other growth factors to stimulate proliferation.[55–58] Independent support for this idea comes from the work of Morrell et al, who observed that ANG II stimulated proliferation of adult rat PA SMCs only when cells were primed by preincubation with 10% serum, but not under serum-deprived conditions (0.1%).[59,60] It is unclear whether the pulmonary vasculature possesses a developmentally regulated susceptibility to ANG II, although a previous report suggests that pulmonary vasoconstrictor responses to ET-1 may be developmentally regulated.[61–63]

Intracellular signaling mechanisms linking ET-1 and ANG II to increased proliferation in neonatal PA SMCs are poorly understood. Previous studies have demonstrated that PKC activity is increased in neonatal versus adult PA SMCs and that ET-1 and ANG II can activate PKC. Following receptor binding of ET-1 and/or ANG II to their respective receptors, the signal transduction involves activation of G-proteins, including diacylglycerol, resulting in elevation of intracellular PKC. Furthermore, activation of PKC is generally found to increase proliferation. Activation of PKC in some cells may increase cAMP content, which supports the idea that second messenger pathways may be developmentally controlled.[64,65]

PDGF is well recognized as an inducer of DNA synthesis and mitogenesis, especially in its role in the regulation of vascular endothelial growth factor (VEGF), which leads to angiogenesis (Figure 1). Previous work has demonstrated that PDGF activates mitogen-activated protein (MAP) kinase, which in turn plays a crucial role in regulating the entry of cells into the growth cycle.[66] In a number of cells it has been proposed that the kinetics of MAP kinase activation may dictate the relative efficacies of both growth factor and G-protein-coupled receptor agonists as mitogens.

The effect of prostaglandins on cell growth has been under study for many years and notwithstanding differences in animal species and methodology, it is clear that many prostaglandins have inhibitory ef-

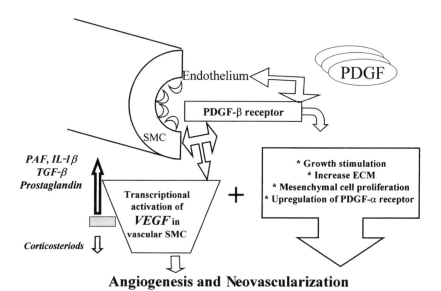

Angiogenesis and Neovascularization

Figure 1. Diagram showing the interregulation of both platelet-derived growth factor (PDGF) and vascular endothelial growth factor (VEGF) in angiogenesis. SMC = smooth muscle cell; PAF = platelet activating factor; IL = interleukin; TGF = transforming growth factor; ECM = extracellular matrix; α and β = types of PDGF receptors.

fects on cell growth. However, Pasricha et al[68] and Palmberg et al[69] demonstrated stimulation of PA SMC growth by PGI_2 and PGE_2. These various results may involve different receptors at the cell membrane, different signaling pathways, or hypothetically, direct effects of prostaglandins on the nucleus.[67–69]

In view of pro-proliferative effects, another growth factor of considerable interest that may be regulated by prostaglandins is VEGF. Its effects are mitogenic in nature and appear to be regulated at the receptor level. VEGF, a potent angiogenic growth factor, has been reported to have a narrow target cell specificity to endothelial cells. Moreover, VEGF regulates vasculogenesis and postnatal vascular remodeling.[70,71] Fms-like tyrosine kinase (FLT-1) and FLK-1 are receptors for VEGF and are known to be expressed during early vascular development in the mouse embryo.[72] The expression of FLT-1 is restricted to vascular endothelial cells. ET-1 has been demonstrated to stimulate the synthesis of VEGF protein in human adult vascular SMCs. However, little is known about the molecular regulation of endothelial-specific gene expression during development.

Generalizations about signal transduction pathways in cultured cells must be made with much care since species variations and different experimental protocols, specifically the presence or absence of defined growth factors to stimulate DNA synthesis, will markedly influence responses.

The earliest and most striking proliferative changes in the neonatal pulmonary arterial wall occur in the adventitia where the fibroblast resides.[73–75] Thus, the specific signaling mechanisms in the fibroblast need to be elucidated, since it is known that growth factors and receptor expression are not alike in these cells and are probably of great importance in our understanding of the normal and abnormal development of the pulmonary vasculature.

Studies in Rats

We used the nitrofen rat model in order to unravel the pathogenesis of CDH.[76] In this model, CDH rats show respiratory insufficiency directly after birth. Newborn rats were killed by an intraperitoneal injection of sodium pentothal (200 mg/kg of body weight). We studied the pulmonary arterial bed in a control and a nitrofen-treated group. The latter was subdivided on the basis of the presence or absence of CDH. The chest wall was removed and the pulmonary arterial bed was injected and perfused through a cannula in the right ventricle, with a barium-gelatin mixture at 60°C and constant pressure. Perfusion was stopped when this solution reached the visceral pleura in all segments resulting in so-called "snow flocks." Subsequently tracheal cannulation and lung fixation with Davidson solution (40 vol % ethanol 100%; 5 vol % acetic acid 96%; 10 vol % formaldehyde 37%; 45 vol % saline; pH 7.3) was performed; fixation was maintained under constant pressure of 20-cm water. After fixation, the lungs were dissected out of the thoracic cavity. Then, the number of animals with a diaphragmatic defect, the position (right- or left-sided) and size of the defect, as well as the contents of the thorax (liver, bowel, stomach) were observed. An arteriogram was taken of each pair of lungs. Dissected lungs were processed for routine histology resulting in paraffin embedding of total lungs. Six μm frontal sections showing both lungs were made and stained with hematoxylin-eosin and Lawson, combined with van Gieson staining. Analysis of each section was carried out in a blind fashion by means of an ocular micrometer (1 unit is 1.48 μm, Zeiss Optical Industry) and standard magnification (10 × 63). A total of at least 35 arteries of each animal (15 from each section) were examined. For each artery, external diameter, wall thickness, wall structure (muscular, partially muscular, or nonmuscular), and the accompanying airway was noted. Wall thickness was defined as the distance between luminal surface and adventitia. External diameter was defined as the distance between the outer edges of the adventitia. The percentage wall thickness (2× wall thickness/external diameter) × 100% was calculated. The mean value for each group was calculated with respect to the accompanying structure. No correction was made for processing and shrinkage factors. A frequency tabulation of the artery structure was made with respect to the accompanying airway structure.

At the level of the respiratory bronchioles, significant differences in the vessels were found. Decreased external diameter and increased wall thickness were seen in CDH, but not in control lungs. Abnormal muscularization of the peripheral branches of the CDH pulmonary arteries was also found (Table 2).

Functional Studies

Morphological abnormalities in the pulmonary vasculature in CDH are well documented. However, the question remains whether these morphological features are directly correlated to responses of the pulmonary vasculature during the perinatal period.[76] It has been observed clinically that reactions to various vasoactive agents including inhaled nitric oxide (NO) are highly unpredictable.[77,78]

The exact mechanisms that control normal and abnormal tone in the neonatal pulmonary circulation are unknown. Presence of SMC and connective tissue in the vessel wall may be highly important and influenced by various mediators (eg, bradykinin, ANG II, ET-1, epinephrine,

Table 2

Number, Size, and Structure of Arteries in Three Groups of Newborn Rats in Relation To Airways

Accompanying Airway Landmark	No. Of Examined Arteries per Animal	External Diameter (μm)	Wall Thickness (% external diameter)	Wall Structure		
				Muscular (%)	Partial Muscular (%)	Nonmuscular (%)
Conducting airways						
Control	20	115 (59)	8.1 (2.1)	76	14	10
Nitrofen	21	98 (45)*	9.4 (3.6)	75	18	7
CDH	19	65 (29)*†	18.9 (7.3)*†	90	6	4
Respiratory bronchioli						
Control	22	46 (14)	11.7 (6.4)	13	23	64
Nitrofen	24	46 (19)	11.1 (3.7)	20	47	33
CDH	20	39 (14)*†	18.3 (7.6)*†	45	24	31

All values are mean (SD). Wall structure is expressed in relative frequency.

N = number; CDH = congenital diaphragmatic hernia.

*Indicates significance of CDH vs control; †indicates significance of CDH vs nitrofen; both at p < 0.05. (Adapted from Reference 76.)

thromboxane B_2, and metabolites of arachidonic acid) in a complex and yet not completely understood mechanism.

Although high levels of circulating immunoreactive ET-1 have been reported in human neonates with PPHN and CDH,[79] pulmonary expression of ET-1 and the exact mechanisms through which ET-1 and its receptors interact to regulate pulmonary vascular tone are not fully known.[77]

We hypothesized that in CDH, altered pulmonary vascular reactivity might be related to differential expression of ET-1 and its receptors. Therefore, we examined the pulmonary expression of ET-1, ET_A, and ET_B receptor mRNAs in a rat model of CDH and compared the expression pattern with age-matched controls.[80] Significantly ($p<0.05$) enhanced levels of ET-1 mRNA were observed in CDH rat lungs as compared to controls. No significant difference in expression of ET-1 mRNA between right and left lung (the most hypoplastic) in CDH rats was observed. A 3.0 ± 0.9-fold increase in ET_A mRNA was observed in CDH as compared to controls, whereas ET_B mRNA levels remained unchanged in both CDH and control rats.

Gosche revealed that in the nitrofen model, responses to potassium-induced depolarization, phenylephrine, ANG II, serotonin, and U46619 were not different in pulmonary arterioles derived from control and CDH rats (personal communication). These data suggest that structural alterations of the pulmonary vasculature observed in infants with CDH may not necessarily be responsible for exaggerated vasoconstrictive responses to normal stimuli. Using the same model, Karamanoukian et al detected both decreased NOS expression and activity in CDH rat lungs using a [14C]-L-arginine to [14C]-L-citrulline conversion assay and Western blots, suggestive of an absence of primary NO deficiency in CDH.[77]

In other studies, levels of several eicosanoids in lung homogenates and in bronchoalveolar lavage fluid of controls and rats with CDH were measured.[81,82] In controls, concentrations of a stable metabolite of prostacyclin (6-keto-$PGF_{1\alpha}$), thromboxane A_2 (TXB_2), PGE_2, and leukotriene B_4 (LTB_4) decreased after birth. CDH lungs demonstrated higher levels of 6-keto-$PGF_{1\alpha}$ compared to controls. We concluded that in CDH, abnormal lung eicosanoid levels are present perinatally.[83,84] Elevated levels of 6-keto-$PGF_{1\alpha}$ in CDH may reflect a compensatory mechanism for increased resistance in the pulmonary vascular bed.[85,86]

Studies in Lambs

This model has mainly been used to study the effect of prenatal repair of the diaphragmatic defect and consequent catching up of lung growth. Glick and his colleagues have studied pulmonary vascular re-activity in newborn lambs with CDH and suggested that an abnormal-ity of the NO pathway in CDH may be present.[77] They investigated the influence of NO on pulmonary vasodilatation in CDH lambs in utero. Both the endothelium-dependent and endothelium-independent path-ways appeared to be intact in this model. Production of NO using an arginine-citrulline conversion assay was also examined. No difference could be demonstrated between control and CDH lungs.[87,88]

Wilson and coworkers evaluated the pulmonary vasculature in newborn CDH lungs by combining surgical induction of CDH with tra-cheal ligation (TL).[89] After establishing that alveolar growth had oc-curred, they reviewed the pulmonary vasculature. Analysis of larger vessels was carried out by computer digital evaluation of angiogram lung slices, and showed that the total area of large vessels was in-creased in the CDH/TL group, compared with normal control animals, or the CDH group. The ratio of large vessel to lung area was however similar in all groups. While the number of capillaries per alveolus was also similar in all groups, microscopic morphometric analysis revealed that total number of capillaries was increased in CDH/TL lungs com-pared with both CDH and control. In addition, the percentage of ves-sels that were < 100 μm in diameter and muscularized in the capillary wall and capillary-alveolar interface appeared normal in the CDH/TL group, in contrast to the CDH group.[89]

Studies in Humans

We carried out a number of studies in human specimens of CDH in order to investigate the structural remodeling of pulmonary arterial morphology in CDH and control neonates during different periods of gestational and postnatal age. DeMello and Reid posed the following: ".. An intriguing question is how ECMO [extracorporeal membrane oxygenation] in some cases allows resolution of pulmonary hyperten-sion of the newborn and whether this occurs by allowing growth or by (resting) the microcirculation and the small resistance arteries to avoid exposure to blood pressure is not clear."[2] We therefore also studied possible arterial structural changes imposed on pulmonary arteries in CDH by ECMO treatment.

Twenty-nine neonatal lung autopsy specimens of CDH neonates with lung hypoplasia confirmed by a LW/BW index ≤ 0.012, were re-trieved from the archives of the Department of Pathology, Erasmus University Medical School, Rotterdam, The Netherlands. These neo-nates represented the CDH cases collected over a period of 25 years. Specimens were divided into three groups: (1) group A, tissue from 5

CDH neonates of gestational age < 34 weeks (mean 31.6 ± 0.87 weeks); (2) group B, 20 CDH neonates of gestational age ≥ 34 weeks (mean 38.6 ± 0.41 weeks), including 5 newborns who died ≤ 1 hour after birth. None of these received ECMO treatment; and (3) group C, 4 CDH term neonates (mean gestational age 39 ± 2.04 weeks) who received ECMO treatment for an average bypass time of 270 hours.

Ten neonates without lung hypoplasia (which was proved histologically), who died either from acute placental insufficiency or infection within the first 24 hours after birth, served as controls. Controls were divided into two groups of 5 cases each: (1) group A, neonates with gestational age < 34 weeks (mean 25.9 ± 0.85 weeks); and (2) group B, neonates with gestational age ≥ 34 weeks (mean 38.8 ± 0.61 weeks). All autopsy lung specimens were fixed by immersion in formalin, and embedded in paraffin. Serial sections of 6 μm in diameter were mounted for histopathological examination and counterstained by hematoxylin-eosin. Examination revealed thickened media and adventitia in the CDH cases. We found thickening in intra-acinar pulmonary arteries of the preterm controls, in contrast to thin adventitia in the term neonates. The lungs of the CDH term neonates showed the thickest adventitia (Figures 2A and 2B). This adventitial thickening decreased during

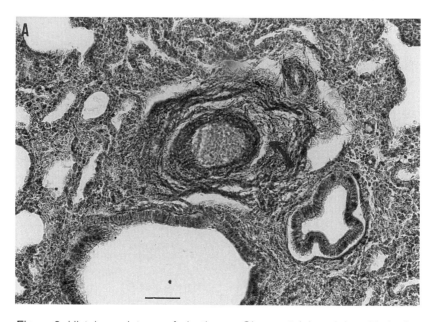

Figure 2. Histology pictures of elastic van Gieson staining. Adventitia is denoted by an arrow. A: Term CDH lung specimen without ECMO treatment with thick adventitia of intra-acinar pulmonary artery. (*continued*)

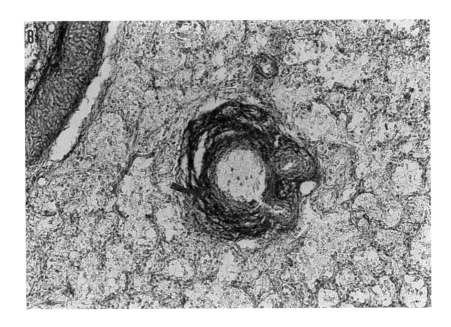

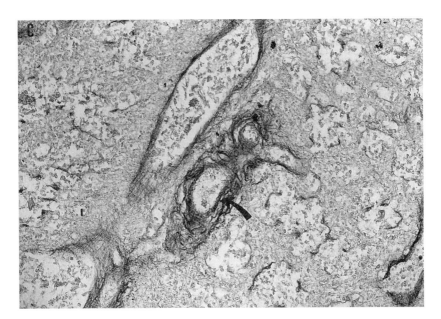

Figure 2 (continued). B: Term control lung showing the thin adventitia in a comparable size artery. **C:** Term CDH lung specimen with ECMO treatment denoting the reduction in the adventitial thickness of the same diameter artery. Bar = 50 μm.

ECMO treatment (Figure 2C). Adventitial thickening was also observed in pulmonary supernumerary arteries in the CDH cases. In the CDH group, we found, at the level of the intra-acinar pulmonary arteries, significant persistence of the abnormal high measurements of adventitial, medial, and total arterial wall thickness until term, as compared to the age-matched control group. Intra-acinar arteries together with supernumerary arteries are known to have a major role in regulating the pulmonary resistance and pressure.[10–12] Adventitial thickening as seen in supernumerary arteries in CDH could explain the reduction in the arterial ability to open and/or dilate the vascular bed, resulting in increased pulmonary pressure. This could, in part, be explained by the physical property of lower resilience of the adventitial collagen fibers.[75]

Yamataka and Puri recently reported that newly synthesized procollagen (M-57) was detected in media and adventitia of pulmonary arteries of 21 newborns with CDH and in neointima in 2 patients with PPHN.[90] M-57 staining was not observed in media of pulmonary arteries of the lungs of 8 sudden infant death syndrome patients. These observations suggest a potential role for TGF-β3, but not TGF-β1 or TGF-β2, in pulmonary vascular remodeling, and furthermore indicate that SMCs in muscular pulmonary arteries may actively synthesize collagen in patients with CDH and PPHN.[90]

The role of VEGF in fetal vasculogenesis and angiogenesis has been described extensively.[70–72] Previous reports revealed that VEGF is expressed in mid-gestation to initiate new vessel formation.[91,92] We investigated the expression of VEGF in human specimens of CDH and age-matched controls. Distinct VEGF immunostaining was identified in bronchial epithelium and media of pulmonary arteries in CDH (Figure 3A). Staining for VEGF was most intense in smaller arterial branches of pulmonary arteries (Figure 3A). Immunoreactivity for VEGF was significantly more intense in CDH cases compared to controls (Figures 3A and 3B). Furthermore, VEGF expression in endothelium of pulmonary vessels was only detected in CDH cases. Weak VEGF expression was observed in the media of large pulmonary veins in CDH cases. No differences in VEGF expression pattern between CDH cases who were artificially ventilated up to 48 hours and the 4 who received such treatment for < 1 hour were observed.[93]

A previous study reported that VEGF is not expressed in the normal endothelium of the developing fetus.[91] However, it was demonstrated in endothelial cells derived from microvessels that VEGF expression was upregulated by hypoxia and adenosine.[91,92,94–96] Nauck et al indicated an inhibitory effect on VEGF expression by corticosteroids.[97] We demonstrated positive VEGF staining in endothelium of pulmonary vessels of human hypoplastic lungs in CDH, but not controls (Figure 3B). Increased expression of VEGF in CDH could not be attrib-

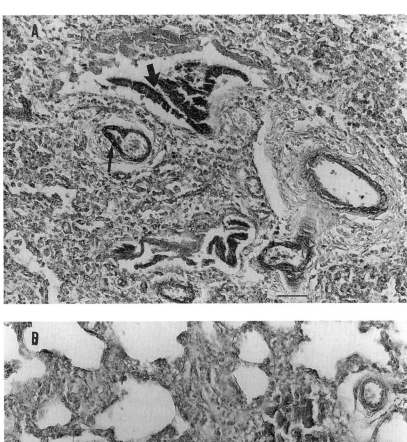

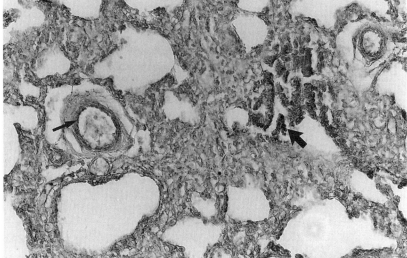

Figure 3. Immunohistochemical staining using VEGF. **A:** CDH lung specimen with increased expression of VEGF in medial SMC of intra-acinar artery (thin arrow) and bronchial epithelium (thick arrow). **B:** Control specimen with the faint expression of VEGF in both medial SMC of intra-acinar artery (thin arrow) and bronchial epithelium (thick arrow). Bar = 50 μm.

uted to hypoxia or barotrauma, since controls were also subject to ventilation for varying periods up to 16 hours. We speculate that VEGF expression may reflect an unsuccessful attempt of the developing fetus to compensate for decreased lung vessel growth. In contrast, we, and other investigators, reported that in normal fetal rat lung, VEGF was expressed in vitro and in vivo and was mainly localized in bronchial epithelium and SMCs.[98] Paradoxically, expression of VEGF could not be detected within media or endothelium in a CDH rat model.[98]

Functional Studies in Humans

In a recent comparative study of human cases of CDH, we observed high levels of 6-keto-$PGF_{1\alpha}$, a vasodilatory eicosanoid, in bronchoalveolar lavage fluid in a CDH patient with PPHN,[84] suggestive of an attempt of the body to overcome the vasoconstrictive status of the pulmonary vasculature. We hypothesized that an imbalance in vasoconstrictor and vasodilator eicosanoids may be involved in PPHN in CDH patients.

Conclusion

Although morphological changes in CDH are well documented, there is little conceptual understanding of the development of abnormal vessels during gestation in humans. The question then remains whether the vascular abnormalities result from maturational arrest or coincide with abnormal development of lung parenchyma. Normal remodeling of the pulmonary vasculature towards the end of fetal development does not take place, possibly because genes responsible for the first process are not switched off. Thus, the genes responsible for these abnormalities need to be found in order to clarify when the system can be expected to go awry.

Even when more detailed information on morphology becomes available, clinicians still have to deal with unpredictable pulmonary reactivity in CDH and variable responses to NO and ECMO treatment. Clinical experience in many centers worldwide has provided well-documented cases of patients who were responders, and others who continued to be nonresponders, to known therapies. Our studies demonstrated that, after ECMO treatment, decreased adventitial thickening of pulmonary arteries could be seen. This may result from ECMO and/or reflect delayed remodeling after birth. Whether this phenomenon can be correlated to distinct morphological changes or differences in expression of a variety of growth factors still needs to be elucidated.

References

1. Reid L. The lung: Its growth and remodeling in health and disease. *Am J Roentgenol* 1977;129:777–788.
2. deMello D, Reid L. Arteries and veins. In: Crystal RG, West JB, eds: *The Lung: Scientific Foundation*. New York: Raven Press; 1991:767–777.
3. Reid L. The pulmonary circulation: Remodeling in growth and disease. *Am Rev Respir Dis* 1979;119:531–553.
4. Reid L. Lung growth in health and disease. *Br J Dis Chest* 1984;78:113–134.
5. Davies G, Reid LM. Growth of the alveoli and pulmonary arteries in childhood. *Thorax* 1970;25:669–681.
6. Hislop A, Reid LM. Pulmonary arterial development during childhood: Branching pattern and structure. *Thorax* 1973;28:129–135.
7. Hislop A, Reid L. Persistent hypoplasia of the lung after repair of congenital diaphragmatic hernia. *Thorax* 1976;31:450–455.
8. Geggel RL, Murphy JD, Reid L. Congenital diaphragmatic hernia: Arterial structural changes and persistent pulmonary hypertension after surgical repair. *J Pediatr* 1985;107:457–464.
9. Geggel RL, Reid LM. The structural basis of PPHN. *Clin Perinatol* 1984;3:525–549.
10. Wagenvoort CA, Neufeld HN, Edwards JE. The structure of the pulmonary arterial tree in fetal and early postnatal life. *Lab Inves t* 1961;10:751–762.
11. Wagenvoort CA, Mooi WJ. The normal lung vessels. In: Wagenvoort CA, Mooi WJ, eds: *Biopsy Pathology of Pulmonary Vasculature. 1st ed.* London, New York: Chapman and Hall Medical; 1989:24–50.
12. Wagenvoort CA, Wagenvoort N. Arterial anastomoses, bronchopulmonary arteries and pulmobronchial arteries in perinatal lungs. *Lab Invest* 1967;16:13–24.
13. Klagsbrun M. The fibroblast growth factor family: Structural and biological properties. *Prog Growth Factor Res* 1989;1:207–235.
14. Heine UI, Munoz EF, Flanders KC, et al. Role of transforming growth factor-β in the development of the mouse embryo. *J Cell Biol* 1987;105:2861–2876.
15. Buch S, Jones C, Sweezey N, et al. Platelet-derived growth factor and growth-related in rat lung. I. Developmental expression. *Am J Respir Cell Mol Biol* 1991;5:371–376.
16. Han RN, Mawdsley C, Souza P, et al. Platelet-derived growth factors and growth-related genes in rat lung: III. Immunolocalization during fetal development. *Pediatr Res* 1992;31:323–329.
17. Ross R, Raines EW, Bowen-Pope DF. The biology of platelet-derived growth factor. *Cell* 1986;46:155–169.
18. Driscoll SG, Smith CAA. Neonatal pulmonary disorders. *Pediatr Clin North Am* 1963;9:325–352.
19. Pryse-Davies J. Pathology of the perinatal lung. *Proc R Soc Med* 1972;65:823–824.
20. Wigglesworth JS, Desai R, Guerrine P. Fetal lung hypoplasia: Biochemical and structural variations and their possible significance. *Arch Dis Child* 1981;56:606–615.
21. Kitagawa M, Hislop A, Boyden EA, et al. Lung hypoplasia in congenital diaphragmatic hernia: A quantitative study of airway, artery, and alveolar development. *Br J Surg* 1971;58:342–346.
22. Reale FR, Esterly JR. Pulmonary hypoplasia: A morphometric study of the

lungs of infants with diaphragmatic hernia, anencephaly, and renal mal-formations. *Pediatrics* 1973;51:91–96.
23. Potter EL. Bilateral renal agenesis. *J Pediatr* 1946;29:68–72.
24. Fantel AG, Shepard TH. Potter syndrome: Non renal features induced by oligoamnios. *Am J Dis Child* 1975;129:1346–1347.
25. Tibboel D, Gaillard JLJ, Spritzer R, et al. Pulmonary hypolasia secondary to oligohydramnios with very premature rupture of fetal membranes. *Eur J Pediatr* 1990;149:496–499.
26. Hislop A, Sanderson M, Reid LM. Unilateral congenital dysplasia of lung associated with vascular anomalies. *Thorax* 1973;28:435–441.
27. Haworth SG, Reid LM. Quantitative structural study of pulmonary circulation in newborn with pulmonary atresia. *Thorax* 1977;32:129–133.
28. Areechon W, Reid LM. Hypoplasia of lung with congenital diaphragmatic hernia. *Br Med J* 1963;1:230–233.
29. Askenazi SS, Perlman M. Pulmonary hypoplasia: Lung weight and radial alveolar count as criteria of diagnosis. *Arch Dis Child* 1979;54:614–618.
30. Emery JL, Mithal A. The number of alveoli in the terminal respiratory unit of man during late intra uterine life and childhood. *Arch Dis Child* 1960;35:544–547.
31. Wigglesworth JS, Desai R. Use of DNA estimation for growth assessment in normal and hypoplastic fetal lungs. *Arch Dis Child* 1981;56:601–605.
32. Enesco M, Leblond CP. Increase in cell number as a factor in the growth of the organs and tissues of the young male rat. *J Embryol Exp Morphol* 1962;10:530–562.
33. Potter EL, Bohlender GP. Intrauterine respiration in relation to development of the lung. *Am J Obstet Gynecol* 1941;42:14–22.
34. Wigglesworth JS, Desai R. Is fetal respiratory function a major determinant of perinatal survival? *Lancet* 1982;1:264–267.
35. Thibeault DW, Haney B. Lung volume, pulmonary vasculature and factors affecting survival in congenital diaphragmatic hernia. *Pediatrics* 1998;101–2:289–295.
36. Hosoda Y, Rossman JE, Glick PL. Pathophysiology of congenital diaphragmatic hernia IV: Renal hypoplasia is associated with pulmonary hypoplasia. *J Pediatr Surg* 1993;28(3):464–470.
37. Yamataka T, Puri P. Pulmonary artery structural changes in pulmonary hypertension complicating congenital diaphragmatic hernia. *J Pediatr Surg* 1997;32:387–390.
38. Taira Y, Yamataka T, Miyazaki E, et al. Adventitial changes in pulmonary vasculature in congenital diaphragmatic hernia complicated by pulmonary hypertension. *J Pediatr Surg* 1998;33:382–387.
39. Naeye RL, Sochat SJ, Whitman V. Unsuspected pulmonary vascular abnormalities associated with diaphragmatic hernia. *Pediatrics* 1976;58:902–904.
40. Levin DL. Morphologic analysis of the pulmonary vascular bed in congenital left-sided diaphragmatic hernia. *J Pediatr* 1978;92:805–809.
41. Nakamura Y, Yamamoto I, Fukuda S, et al. Pulmonary acinar development in diaphragmatic hernia. *Arch Pathol Lab Med* 1991;115:372–376.
42. Allen K, Haworth SG. Human postnatal pulmonary arterial remodeling: Ultrastructural studies of smooth muscle cell and connective tissue maturation. *Lab Invest* 1988;59(5):702–709.
43. deMello D, Reid L. Pre- and postnatal development of the pulmonary circulation. In: Chernick V, Mellins R, eds: *Basic Mechanisms of Pediatric Respiratory Disease*. Vols. II, V. Philadelphia: BC Decker, Inc; 1991:36–54.

44. Haworth S. Development of the pulmonary circulation: Morphologic aspects. In: Polin R, Fow W, eds: *Fetal and Neonatal Physiology*. Philadelphia: WB Saunders; 1991:671–682.
45. Stenmark KR, Mecham RP. Cellular and molecular mechanisms of pulmonary vascular remodeling. *Annu Rev Physiol* 1997;59:89–144.
46. Dempsey EC, Badesch DB, Dobyns EL, et al. Enhanced growth capacity of neonatal pulmonary artery smooth muscle cells in vitro: Dependence on cell size, time from birth, insulin-like growth factor I, and auto-activation of protein kinase C. *J Cell Physiol* 1994;160(3):469–481.
47. Haworth S. Pulmonary remodeling in the developing lung. *Eur Respir Rev* 1993;3(16):550–554.
48. Reid LM. The pulmonary circulation: Remodeling in growth and disease. The 1978 J. Burns Amberson lecture. *Am Rev Respir Dis* 1979;119(4):531–546.
49. Morimoto BH, Koshland DE. Conditional activation of cAMP signal transduction by protein kinase C. *J Biol Chem* 1993;269(6):4065–4069.
50. Owen NE. Effect of prostaglandin E1 on DNA synthesis in vascular smooth muscle cells. *Am J Physiol* 1986;250(4 Pt 1):C584-C588.
51. Yamada H, Suzuki K. Age-related differences in mouse Schwann cell response to cyclic AMP. *Brain Res* 1996;719(1–2):187–193.
52. Pyne NJ, Moughal N, Stevens PA, et al. Protein kinase C-dependent cyclic AMP formation in airway smooth muscle: The role of type II adenylate cyclase and the blockade of extracellular-signal-regulated kinase-2 (ERK-2) activation. *Biochem J* 1994;304(Pt 2):611–616.
53. Roger PP, Reuse S, Maenhaut C, et al. Multiple facets of the modulation of growth by cAMP. *Vitam Horm* 1995;51:59–191.
54. Yoshimura M, Cooper DMF. Type-specific stimulation of adenylyl cyclase by protein kinase C. *J Biol Chem* 1993;268(8):4604–4607.
55. Dubey RK, Roy A, Overbeck HW. Culture of renal arteriolar smooth muscle cells: Mitogenic responses to angiotensin II. *Circ Res* 1992;71(5):1143–1152.
56. Zamora MR, Stelzner TJ, Webb S, et al. Overexpression of endothelin-1 and enhanced growth of pulmonary artery smooth muscle cells from fawn-hooded rats. *Am J Physiol* 1996;270(1 Pt 1):L101-L109.
57. Assender JW, Irenius E, Fredholm BB. Endothelin-1 causes a prolonged protein kinase C activation and acts as a co-mitogen in vascular smooth muscle cells. *Acta Physiol Scand* 1996;157(4):451–460.
58. Toga H, Ibe BO, Raj JU. In vitro responses of ovine intrapulmonary arteries and veins to endothelin-1. *Am J Physiol* 1992;263(1 pt 1):L15-L21.
59. Morrell NW, Morris KG, Stenmark KR. Role of angiotensin-converting enzyme and angiotensin II in development of hypoxic pulmonary hypertension. *Am J Physiol* 1995;269(4 Pt 2):H1186-H1194.
60. Morrell NW, Stenmark KR. Angiotensin II stimulates proliferation of rat pulmonary microvascular smooth muscle cells. *Am J Respir Crit Care Med* 1997;155(4):A636.
61. Griendling KK, Tsuda T, Alexander RW. Endothelin stimulates diacylglycerol accumulation and activates protein kinase C in cultured vascular smooth muscle cells. *J Biol Chem* 1989;264 (14):8237–8240.
62. Griendling KK, Tsuda T, Berk BC, et al. Angiotensin II stimulation of vascular smooth muscle cells: Secondary signaling mechanisms. *Am J Hypertens* 1989;2(8):659–665.
63. Janakidevi K, Fisher MA, Del Vecchio PJ, et al. Endothelin-1 stimulates

DNA synthesis and proliferation of pulmonary artery smooth muscle cells. *Am J Physiol* 1992;263(6 Pt 1):C1295-C1301.

64. Simonson MS, Herman WH. Protein kinase C and protein tyrosine kinase activity contribute to mitogenic signaling by endothelin-1: Cross-talk between G protein-coupled receptors and pp60c-src. *J Biol Chem* 1993;268 (13):9347–9357.

65. Delafontaine P, Lou H. Angiotensin II regulates insulin-like growth factor I gene expression in vascular smooth muscle cells. *J Biol Chem* 1993;268 (22):16866–16870.

66. Han RNN, Mawdsley C, Souza P, et al. Platelet derived growth factors and growth related genes in rat lungs. III. Immunolocalization during fetal development. *Pediatr Res* 1992;31(4):323–329.

67. Höper MM, Voelkel NF, Bates TO, et al. Prostaglandins induce vascular endothelial growth factor in a human monocytic cell line and rat lungs via cAMP. *Am J Respir Cell Mol Biol* 1997;17:748–756.

68. Pasricha PJ, Hassoun PM, Teufel E, et al. Prostaglandin E1 and E2 stimulate the proliferation of pulmonary artery smooth muscle cells. *Prostaglandins* 1992;43:5–19.

69. Palmberg L, Lindgren JA, Thyberg J, et al. On the mechanism of induction of DNA synthesis in cultured arterial smooth muscle cells by leukotrines: Possible role of prostaglandin endoperoxide synthase products and platelet derived growth factor. *J Cell Sci* 1991;98:141–149.

70. Klagsbrun M, D_Amore P. Regulators of angiogenesis. *Annu Rev Physiol* 1991;53:217–239.

71. Shweiki D, Itin A, Sofer D, et al. Vascular endothelial growth factor induced by hypoxia may indicate hypoxia-initiated angiogenesis. *Nature* 1992;359:843–845.

72. Quinn TP, Peters KG, De Vries C, et al. Fetal liver kinase 1 is a receptor for vascular endothelial growth factor and is selectively expressed in vascular endothelium. *Proc Natl Acad Sci USA* 1993;90:7533–7537.

73. Stenmark KR, Fasules J, Hyde DM, et al. Severe pulmonary hypertension and arterial adventitial changes in newborn calves at 4,300 m. *J Appl Physiol* 1987;62(2):821–830.

74. Rabinovitch M. Morphology of the developing pulmonary bed: Pharmacologic implications. *Pediatr Pharmacol* 1985;5(1):31–48.

75. Greenwald SE, Berry CL, Haworth SG. Changes in the distensibilty of the intra pulmonary arteries in the normal newborn and growing pig. *Cardiovasc Res* 1982;16:716–725.

76. Tenbrinck R, Gaillard JLJ, Tibboel D, et al. Pulmonary vascular abnormalities in experimentally induced congenital diaphragmatic hernia in rats. *J Pediatr Surg* 1992;27:862–865.

77. Karamanoukian HL, Peay T, Love JE, et al. Decreased pulmonary nitric oxide synthase activity in the rat model of congenital diaphragmatic hernia. *J Pediatr Surg* 1996;31:1016–1019.

78. North AJ, Moya FR, Mysore MR, et al. Pulmonary endothelial nitric oxide synthase gene expression is decreased in a rat model of congenital diaphragmatic hernia. *Am J Respir Cell Mol Biol* 1995;13:676–682.

79. Kobayashi H, Puri P. Plasma endothelin levels in congenital diaphragmatic hernia. *J Pediatr Surg* 1994;29:1258–1261.

80. McCune SK, Servoss SJ, Guldemeester A, et al. Endothelin-1 and endothelin receptors in congenital diaphragmatic hernia. *Am J Respir Crit Care Med* 1997;155:A842. Abstract.

81. IJsselstijn H, Zijlstra FJ, van Dijk JPM, et al. Lung eicosanoids in perinatal rats with congenital diaphragmatic hernia. *Mediators of Inflammation* 1997; 6:39–45.
82. Nakayama DK, Motoyama EK, Evans R, et al. Relation between arterial hypoxemia and plasma eicosanoids in neonates with congenital diaphragmatic hernia. *J Surg Res* 1992;53:615–620.
83. Ford WDA, James MJ, Walsh JA. Congenital diaphragmatic hernia: Association between pulmonary vascular resistance and plasma thromboxane concentrations. *Arch Dis Child* 1984;59:143–146.
84. Bos AP, Tibboel D, Hazebroek FWJ, et al. Congenital diaphragmatic hernia: Impact of prostanoids in the perioperative period. *Arch Dis Child* 1990;65:994–995.
85. IJsselstijn H, Zijlstra FJ, de Jongste JC, et al. Prostanoids in bronchoalveolar lavage fluid do not predict outcome in congenital diaphragmatic hernia patients. *Mediators of Inflammation* 1997;6:217–224.
86. Harrison MR, Adzick NS, Nakayama DK, et al. Fetal diaphragmatic hernia: Pathophysiology, natural history, and outcome. *Clin Obstet Gynecol* 1986;29:490–501.
87. Hedrick MH, Estes JM, Sullivan KM, et al. Plug the Lung Until it Grows (PLUG): A new method to treat congenital diaphragmatic hernia in utero. *J Pediatr Surg* 1994;29:612–617.
88. Karamanoukian HL, Glick PL, Wilcox DT, et al. Pathophysiology of congenital diaphragmatic hernia X: Localization of nitric oxide synthase in the intima of pulmonary artery trunks of lambs with surgically created congenital diaphragmatic hernia. *J Pediatr Surg* 1995;30:5–9.
89. DiFiore JW, Fauza DO, Slavin R, et al. Experimental fetal tracheal ligation reverses the structural and physiological effects of pulmonary hypoplasia in congenital diaphragmatic hernia. *J Pediatr Surg* 1994;29:248–257.
90. Yamataka T, Puri P. Active collagen synthesis by pulmonary arteries in pulmonary hypertension complicated by congenital diaphragmatic hernia. *J Pediatr Surg* 1997;32(5):682–687.
91. Shifren JL, Doldi N, Ferrara N, et al. In the human fetus, vascular endothelial growth factor is expressed in epithelial cells and myocytes, but not vascular endothelium: Implication for mode of action. *J Clin Endocrinol Metab* 1994;79:316–322.
92. Tischer E, Mitchell R, Hartman T, et al. The human gene for vascular endothelial growth factor: Multiple protein forms are encoded through alternative exon splicing. *J Biol Chem* 1991;266:11947–11954.
93. Shehata SMK, Mooi W, Sharma HS, et al. Pulmonary expression of vascular endothelial growth factor in human newborns with congenital diaphragmatic hernia. *Am J Respir Crit Care Med* 1998;157:A591. Abstract.
94. Pedra A, Razandi M, Hu RM, et al. Vasoactive peptides modulate vascular endothelial cell growth factor production and endothelial cell proliferation and invasion. *J Biol Chem* 1997;272:17097–17103.
95. Liu Y, Cox SR, Morita T, et al. Hypoxia regulates vascular endothelial growth factor gene expression in endothelial cells: Identification of a 5′, enhancer. *Circ Res* 1995;77(3):638–643.
96. Fischer F, Sharma HS, Karliczek GK, et al. Expression of vascular endothelial permeability factor/vascular endothelial growth factor in microvasclar endothelial cells and its upregulation by adenosine. *Mol Brain Res* 1995;28:141–148.
97. Nauck M, Roth M, Tamm M, et al. Induction of vascular endothelial

growth factor by platelet activating factor and platelet derived growth factor is downregulated by corticosteriods. *Am J Respir Cell Mol Biol* 1997;16:398–406.

98. Okazaki T, Sharma HS, Aikawa M, et al. Pulmonary expression of vascular endothelial growth factor and myosin isoforms in rats with congenital diaphragmatic hernia. *J Pediatr Surg* 1997;32:391–394.

Index